THIRD EDITION

THERAPEUTIC RECREATION

A Helping Profession

Gerald S. O'Morrow
Radford University

Ronald P. Reynolds
Virginia Commonwealth University

PRENTICE HALL, Englewood Cliffs, New Jersey 07632

Library of Congress Cataloging-in-Publication Data

O'Morrow, Gerald S.
  Therapeutic recreation.

  Includes bibliographies and index.
  1. Recreational therapy.   I. Reynolds, Ronald P.
  II. Title.
RM736.7.046   1989   615.8'5153   88-9975
ISBN 0-13-914896-5

Editorial/production supervision and
  interior design: Serena Hoffman
Cover design: Wanda Lubelska
Manufacturing buyer: Peter Havens

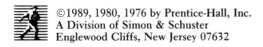

©1989, 1980, 1976 by Prentice-Hall, Inc.
A Division of Simon & Schuster
Englewood Cliffs, New Jersey 07632

Printed in the United States of America

10 9 8 7 6 5 4 3 2 1

ISBN 0-13-914896-5

PRENTICE-HALL INTERNATIONAL (UK) LIMITED, *London*
PRENTICE-HALL OF AUSTRALIA PTY. LIMITED, *Sydney*
PRENTICE-HALL CANADA INC., *Toronto*
PRENTICE-HALL HISPANOAMERICANA, S.A., *Mexico*
PRENTICE-HALL OF INDIA PRIVATE LIMITED, *New Delhi*
PRENTICE-HALL OF JAPAN, INC., *Tokyo*
SIMON & SCHUSTER ASIA PTE. LTD., *Singapore*
EDITORA PRENTICE-HALL DO BRASIL, LTDA., *Rio de Janeiro*

Contents

Preface

Since the two previous editions of this book, the profession of therapeutic recreation has grown and matured dramatically as an area of service within the park and recreation field and the allied health care professions. This development has been the result of continued efforts toward professionalization on the part of therapeutic recreation personnel, as well as a growing recognition by the general public that disabled persons have the right to participate in leisure experiences while contributing to society.

As in earlier editions, *Therapeutic Recreation: A Helping Profession* is written primarily for the student who is considering and preparing for a professional career in therapeutic recreation. It is a comprehensive text for use in colleges and universities offering an introductory course in therapeutic recreation. Its purpose is to inform all who are interested in knowing about therapeutic recreation; for example, parts could be adopted for in-service training programs within health-care and correctional agencies.

Throughout the book, students are exposed to the knowledge that constitutes the field of therapeutic recreation and the abilities they must possess upon entering the profession. However, some of the material may not be provocative or specifically related to therapeutic recreation. Such material is justified, in the opinion of the authors, because therapeutic recreation specialists, like other health-care and correctional specialists, are expected to know matters not always limited to therapeutic recreation. If therapeutic recreation specialists want to be accepted as equals with other health-care and correctional specialists, they should have knowledge and information beyond that of just therapeutic recreation. When exposed to such a diversity of material, stu-dents will realize that a career in therapeutic recreation can be exciting, challenging, stimulating, and satisfying.

Before revising this text, the authors obtained considerable input from faculty and students who used previous editions in classroom settings. Although there was a strong consensus concerning the relevance of the material presented, it became apparent that the rapid development of the field over the past several years necessitated a substantial revision and reorganization of information. Consequently, this third edition varies significantly in content and format from the previous two. In general, the book considers the historical, professional and service-delivery aspects of therapeutic recreation. It is not intended as a program development, leadership, or administrative text, since other books deal exclusively with these subjects. However, some aspects of these subjects are considered to varying degrees so as to familiarize students with them as they relate to professional development and therapeutic recreation as a service.

As noted above, this text represents a major revision. The chapters dealing with historical and professional development have been substantially updated and revised. Much of the material in the previous editions concerning the process and implementation of therapeutic recreation service has been condensed into what the authors feel is a more comprehensive, yet easier to understand chapter. Five new chapters have been added, each dealing with the provision of therapeutic recreation service and the therapeutic recreation process within a particular service delivery model. Finally an entirely new chapter devoted to trends in therapeutic recreation has been added.

In view of these major changes, the authors recommend that the text be divided into four units, each designed to assist the student in understanding the profession of therapeutic recreation from various perspectives. The first unit is comprised of Chapters 1–3. Chapter 1 offers a brief overview of the importance of recreation opportunities in meeting leisure needs and satisfying other requirements for basic growth and development. Chapter 2 addresses such vitally important subjects as the prevalence and characteristics of special populations, the attitude of society toward people with disabilities, and the concept of health/illness and rehabilitation/punishment. Chapter 3 concludes the first unit with a thorough overview of the agencies and institutions that offer rehabilitation and special services to special populations.

Chapters 4 and 5, which comprise the second unit, examine the historical development and the evolution of the field in relation to the criteria of a profession.

Chapters 6 through 11, which form the third unit, describe how therapeutic recreation service is delivered to clients. Chapter 6 describes the basic elements of assessment, goal development, implementation, and evaluation, and overviews the various models of service delivery where this process may be applied. Chapters 7 through 11 then give concrete examples of the application of the process to a variety of clients within the specific models.

Chapter 12, Trends in Therapeutic Recreation, may be considered a fourth and final unit. This chapter examines current developments in credentialling, educational preparation, the development of professional standards, and client service delivery. Students are encouraged to formulate their own opinions on these and other contemporary issues.

Suggested Readings appear at the end of each chapter to help students increase their understanding of the topics discussed and to assist in the preparation of course assignments. These references are not intended to be complete; therefore, outside reading should not be limited to the books and articles listed.

In addition to revisions in the text, changes have also been made in the appendices. The Medical Terminology Appendix has been removed, since students should obtain this information in the social and behavioral courses required for certification. Appendix A introduces students to charting, including abbreviations, terminology, numbers, and symbols. Popular drugs of choice in treating a variety of diseases and disorders, as opposed to only psychotherapeutic drugs, are considered in Appendix B. Appendix C acquaints students with the organizational leaders, past and present, in therapeutic recreation, as well as individuals and agencies that have been recognized by the National Therapeutic Recreation Society (NTRS) throughout the years. The remaining two appendices present the new National Council for Therapeutic Recreation Certification Standards and various therapeutic recreation resources, respectively.

This book can be used as a springboard to other courses and experiences in professional preparation. The authors advocate using outside speakers in the discussion of particular topics, structuring panel discussions around certain issues, scheduling visits to health-care and correctional facilities, and utilizing various kinds of instructional media.

This edition contains the latest facts and reflects present-day concepts in therapeutic recreation, although readers will note differences and divergent thinking among quoted authors. This situation is healthy in such a vibrant and rapidly developing human-service field. It should also be noted that, in some instances, the authors have deliberately avoided discussing the potential implications of specific events and statements; this was done to encourage discussion and debate on the part of those using the text.

As the body of knowledge in this field grows, agreement concerning the nature and process of therapeutic recreation increases. Accordingly, it was sometimes impossible for the authors to offer original ideas, for such ideas are developed and molded by the thoughts of many, and therapeutic recreation educators and practitioners can read their own ideas and convictions into those presented. The authors feel that this is a positive outcome that reflects increasing evidence that we therapeutic recreation specialists are beginning to reach a consensus regarding our mission.

ACKNOWLEDGEMENTS

Revising a book is in some ways a tedious job, especially when revising extensively. We are not sure that it could have occurred without the very competent and enthusiastic assistance of Bonnie Akers and Linda Rothweiler, to whom we are indebted. In addition, because a book is dependent on authors,' editors,' and publishers' permission to reprint materials, we wish to express our gratitude to all who have given permission to quote materials, especially the National Recreation and Park Association/ National Therapeutic Recreation Society, National Council for Therapeutic Recreation Certification, and Leisurability Publications, Inc. Lastly we are indebted to the reviewers of the manuscript: Stephen C. Anderson, Ph.D., C.T.R.S., Indiana University; Vicki Annand, M.S., C.T.R.S., and Fred Humphrey, Ph.D., C.T.R.S., University of Maryland; Lee Lanz-Stewart, Ph.D., Jean R. Tague, Ph.D., C.T.R.S., Ray West, M.S., C.T.R.S., Diane M. Reynolds, B.S., C.T.R.S., Carol A. Taylor, Ph.D., R.N., Dianne M. O'Morrow, M.S.N., R.N., John E. Joyner, M.D.F.A.C.S., and our students.

Gerald S. O'Morrow
Ronald P. Reynolds

1

Introduction

This book is designed to introduce you to the rapidly developing field of therapeutic recreation and to assist you in evaluating this profession as a possible career for yourself. The authors feel that it is a great area of human service and one in which you will find deep satisfaction and personal challenge.

As a beginning student, you may be unclear as to the fundamental nature of therapeutic recreation service and its basic purposes. Therefore, we have provided considerable detail concerning the various disabling conditions our clients may exhibit, the service delivery settings in which we function, and the process through which we provide direct service. In addition to this factual information, the authors hope that you will encounter the spirit of excitement that permeates the field and discover the sources of enthusiasm that members of the profession enjoy. As your course of study progresses, you will learn that the profession offers unlimited opportunities for growth to individuals with an adventurous spirit. In fact, its future development is dependent upon the energies, abilities, and visions of young, imaginative, and dynamic people.

Before we explore the nature and scope of therapeutic recreation, let us briefly consider the contribution that leisure makes to the daily living experience of all individuals.

Although recreation cannot serve as a substitute for useful employment, housing, or medical services, it does have a potential therapeutic benefit for everyone. Specifically, individuals who have acquired adequate recreational interests, knowledge, appreciation, and skills will participate in creative, stimulating, and enjoyable daily living activities. In this fashion, recreation can be viewed as contributing to the physical, mental, and emotional fitness of all human beings.

SATISFACTION OF PERSONAL NEEDS

It is important to recognize that all humans possess needs, interests, and desires that are biologically, physically, and socially determined. These needs, interests, and desires are further conditioned by the individual's environment, scientific and technological advances, and degree of physical, emotional, social, intellectual, and economic development. Although writers in the recreation field have described leisure in different ways, there is strong agreement that individuals can achieve satisfaction of their needs, interests, and desires through participation in recreational experiences. Regardless of the objectives of recreational participation, there is a fundamental notion that leisure enhances life. The ancient Greeks, in fact, believed that the purpose of all education was to teach people how to live well. To philosophers such as Socrates, the only worthwhile objective of living was to live "the Good Life." Thus, choosing and participating in leisure activities can help people to live better lives.

PERSONALITY DEVELOPMENT

Recreation is integrally related to other life activities, and as such, it is a part of living in which certain needs and interests are satisfied. Indeed, upon reading other works in this field, you will discover that recreation may be viewed as a means for providing experiences that benefit the whole person. Thus, recreation has elements that contribute to the total personality of those who participate in it.

Although there is considerable debate and controversy concerning the nature of the human personality and the factors that influence behavior, for our purposes *total personality* or *whole person* may be defined simply as the sum total of all physical, mental, emotional, and social aspects of the individual. These aspects are of equal importance to the overall health of the personality. They are interrelated, and the condition of any one element affects the health of the other elements as well as the personality as a whole. To draw an analogy—a fine automobile runs smoothly because of the quality of its individual parts and because of the precise fashion in which the parts fit and work together.

PHYSICAL WELL-BEING

Active recreational pursuits can have a positive effect upon the personality. Physiologists and cardiac specialists agree that participation in activities and exercise is essential if the individual is to develop and maintain maximum physical efficiency and total fitness for living. Fitness in this sense involves endurance, strength, agility, and coordination. If the body is maintained at a reasonable level of efficiency, it is more likely to meet demands without undue stress or fatigue. Individuals who use all of their energy in performing daily physical tasks operate at a low level of efficiency and therefore have no energy left for recreational and leisure pursuits. In the words of one expert:

> A healthy person with optimal (not necessarily maximum) physical fitness can carry out his usual everyday tasks without undue fatigue and have enough reserve energy left over to enjoy his leisure; and to engage in activities requiring reasonably prolonged, vigorous physical effort when necessary or desired.[1]

Children also require physical activity; for them play is an absolute physiological need. Pediatricians and other experts in child development have repeatedly pointed out that vigorous play is necessary for the satisfactory growth of all the bodily systems. An adequate amount of exercise can normally be obtained through the free play activities of childhood. As children grow, they require a certain degree of muscular strength and cardiovascular endurance to participate in strenuous physical activities, perform work at school and home, and take part in social activities.

EMOTIONAL WELL-BEING

In our culture people must cooperate with each other, work in groups, and maintain their poise under the pressure of modern living. This is particularly difficult in view of the widespread political and economic unrest in the world today. Confusion, fear, and distrust cause tremendous physical and mental strain. According to some physicians, at least 50 percent of all office visits are the result of various kinds of stress. There is reason to believe that many of the restraints necessary for social living—submitting to authority figures, repressing impulses to fight and/or cry out—build up to intolerable levels in individuals. Involvement in leisure pursuits is one opportunity for the release of these emotions under controlled conditions. As the late Dr. William C. Menninger, a world-famous authority on mental health, stated:

> Mentally healthy people participate in some form of volitional activity to supplement their required daily work.... Their satisfaction from these activities meets deep-seated psychological demands, quite beyond the superficial rationalism of enjoyment.[2]

Activities of a recreational nature serve an identical purpose for children who have been exposed to school routines and confined in the classroom. Additionally, participation in activities serves as a learning opportunity to experience the joy of winning, disappointment of defeat, pride of accomplishment, and frustration of failure. Participation in group activities provides the finest training for the development of emotional stability. Participants acquire a feeling of belonging, have an opportunity to develop an independent personality, and realize satisfaction and happiness. In short, leisure activities offer individuals the opportunity to express positive emotions and learn to control negative feelings.

SOCIAL INTERACTION

All aspects of an individual's personality are profoundly influenced by others. Therefore, if you are to have a healthy personality and be happy, your relationships with others must be positive and satisfying. Many social skills are needed to form these high-quality relationships. Recreational activities offer some of the best means for individuals to learn and develop vital social skills. As individuals interact in a leisure activity, they may develop a profound sense of social awareness. Every recreative experience has a potential contribution to make to the social development and adjustment of adults and children. Getting along with others is an essential part of play. The social interaction that is inherent in play is, in fact, one of the reasons for playing.

Social behavior is learned through practice. Leisure pursuits offer opportunities for experiencing both objectionable and desirable forms of behavior. Consequently, these experiences will enable the individual to learn positive means of responding to others. Simply stated, group recreational experiences provide "laboratories" for individuals to exhibit various types of behaviors. Behaviors that are rewarded are apt to be repeated and learned. In social learning, practice is essential. As correct responses are made, the rewards of participation, the making of new friends, and the attainment of respect and prestige serve as positive reinforcement. Ultimately, this learning leads to social adjustment, which is a prerequisite for success in a vocation, in family living, and in community activities.

THE CHALLENGE OF THERAPEUTIC RECREATION

At the outset of this chapter we stated that all human beings possess fundamental needs, interests, and desires that are biologically, physically, and socially determined.

We further stated that these needs, interests, and desires may be affected by other factors. Individuals with a disability may experience factors that prevent them from satisfying their personal needs. The task of the therapeutic recreation specialist then is to assist such individuals to utilize their residual abilities to overcome obstacles that could prevent the achievement of optimal physical, social, and emotional well-being.

People with disabilities should have the same opportunities as the nondisabled to participate in the recreational life of our nation. This point was made strongly by delegates participating in the National Forum on Meeting the Recreation and Park Needs of Handicapped People.[3] Joseph H. Margalis, a member of the National Recreation and Park Association Board of Trustees, commented as follows in testimony before the House Subcommittee on Labor, Health, Education and Welfare on supporting an appropriation of $10 million to expand recreation services for the handicapped, as authorized by the Rehabilitation Act Amendments of 1978:

> Recreation experiences provide an excellent opportunity for the handicapped to associate informally with society as a whole. . . . Those experiences can contribute to the rehabilitation of handicapped individuals and their inclusion in education, employment, and other individual social functions.[4]

Because public health services are concerned with the promotion of wellness as well as the treatment of illness, recreation has implications for everyone. In its broadest sense, the purpose of recreation and leisure service is to help all people achieve fuller, happier, and more harmonious lives. A positive attitude toward life is a prerequisite for physical and mental health. Recreative experiences contribute directly to the achievement of such an attitude.

Students, therefore, should realize that they are in a position to help people with special needs progress toward better physical, emotional, social, and intellectual adjustment through recreation. If we accept the concept stated above—that recreative experiences have values that promote the growth of the whole person—then it follows that the value and significance of leisure and recreation service increase when related to persons with disabilities. Our mission is to facilitate the growth and development of disabled individuals through recreational experiences. Herein lies the challenge of therapeutic recreation as a helping profession.

NOTES

1. Charles B. Wilkinson, "The Quality of Fitness," *Parks and Recreation* 1, no. 2 (1966), 149.

2. William C. Menninger, "Recreation and Mental Health," *Recreation* 41, no. 9 (November 1948), 17.

3. President's Committee on the Employment of the Handicapped and National Recreation and Park Association, *Recreation and Handicapped People*, Proceedings of National Forum on Meeting the Recreation and Park Needs of Handicapped People, Aug. 15–16, 1974 (Washington, D.C.: U.S. Government Printing Office, n.d.).

4. "Trustee Margalis Urges Expansion of Leisure Services for Disabled," *Dateline: NRPA* 2, no. 4 (June–July 1979), 10.

SUGGESTED READINGS

"As Americans Cope with a Changing Population," *U.S. News and World Report* (Jan. 16, 1984), 44.

BAMMEL, GENE, and LEI LANE BURRUS-BAMMEL. *Leisure and Human Behavior*. Dubuque, Iowa: William C. Brown Co., Publishers, 1982.

BARNETT, LYNN A. "Current Thinking about Children's Play: Learning to Play or Playing to Learn?" *Quest* 26 (Summer 1976), 5–16.

CLARK, MARK W., ed. "Coping with Stress Through Leisure," in *Leisure Today: Selected Readings, Vol. 3*, pp. 27–49, Ron Mendell, ed. Reston, Va.: American Association for Health, Physical Education, Recreation and Dance, 1984.

CSIKSZENTMIHALYI, M. *Beyond Boredom and Anxiety.* San Francisco: Jossey-Bass Co., 1982.

DENZIN, N. K. "Play Games and Interaction: The Contexts of Childhood Socialization," *Sociological Quarterly* 16, no. 4 (1975), 458–78.

FIGLER, STEPHEN K. *Sport and Play in American Life.* Philadelphia: Saunders College Publishing Co., 1981.

HEYWOOD, L. A. "Perceived Recreative Experience and the Relief of Tension," *Journal of Leisure Research,* 10, no. 2 (Spring 1978), 86–87.

ISO-AHOLA, S. E. *The Social Psychology of Leisure and Recreation.* Dubuque, Iowa: William C. Brown Co., Publishers, 1980.

KELLY, JOHN R. *Leisure.* Englewood Cliffs, N.J.: Prentice-Hall, 1982.

KRAUS, RICHARD G. *Recreation and Leisure in Modern Society.* Glenview, Ill.: Scott, Foresman & Co., 1984.

MACLEAN, JANET R., JAMES A. PETERSON, and W. DONALD MARTIN, *Recreation and Leisure: The Changing Scene.* New York: John Wiley & Sons, 1985.

MURPHY, JAMES F. *Concepts of Leisure.* Englewood Cliffs, N.J.: Prentice-Hall, 1981.

SHIVERS, JAY S. *Leisure and Recreation Concepts: A Critical Analysis.* Boston: Allyn & Bacon, 1981.

2

Special Populations

All individuals are special in a philosophical and humanitarian sense. However, in this chapter and throughout the text, we will be concerned with special kinds of individuals who are to a greater or lesser degree different from other individuals in one or more important dimensions of human functioning. Frequently these individuals are termed *special populations*. The term *special populations* is used hereafter to describe those individuals who, because of a variety of circumstances, differ from the average in their physical, emotional, social, and intellectual behavior. This definition of special populations encompasses the physically disabled, the emotionally disturbed, the mentally retarded, and the visually impaired, to mention but a few.

No therapeutic recreation specialist can be fully successful in the many roles he or she assumes without accurate information regarding members of special populations. Therefore, this chapter focuses initially on the prevalence of special populations, attitudes of society toward the disabled, attitudes of the disabled toward themselves, and the concepts of health/disease and rehabilitation/punishment. To enable special population persons to achieve and participate in recreative experiences at a level commensurate with their respective abilities, it is important for the specialist to have a general knowledge and understanding about health disorders and the social problems that prevent and limit participation. Thus, the latter part of this chapter considers both health conditions and disorders and social problems.

The student needs to keep in mind that the presentation and discussion of this material is brief and is not a substitute for courses in the biological and behavioral sciences: Human Anatomy and Physiology, Abnormal Psychology, Characteristics of Mental Retardation, Criminology, and the like. This chapter may be considered a review or an introduction to conditions and disorders. Some of the conditions presented here will be considered in later chapters in association with case studies.

PREVALENCE, ATTITUDES, AND CONCEPTS

PREVALENCE OF SPECIAL POPULATIONS

Whether or not individuals or groups want to admit it, every community, large or small, has its special populations. However, research on the extent of such groups suggests that the numbers vary from community to community.

Various attempts to determine the incidence and prevalence of physical, emotional, social, and intellectual disorders in the population have yielded such diverse results that a word of caution is needed concerning the figures presented herein. For purposes of clarification: *incidence* refers to the number of new cases of a disorder or problem reported during a specific time period; *prevalence* is the frequency of a disorder or problem in a particular population.

Much of the difficulty in determining the prevalence of special populations stems from the fact that the line of demarcation between "normal" or "average" individuals and individuals most often considered to be special population members cannot always be agreed upon.

A second difficulty is due to the fact that the law and the definition change. For example, what is defined as mental retardation changes from time to time and from place to place, as we will note in our discussion of the definition of mental retardation later in this chapter. Consequently, increases in the figures shown in some reports may reflect a change in definition, legislative addition or modification, or even the elimination of the disorder. For example, not too many years ago homosexuality was included in the American Psychiatry Association's *Diagnostic and Statistical Manual for Mental Disorders*. Today it is not.

A third difficulty arises because there appears to be no uniform reporting procedure used by all agencies, nor is there a single governmental agency responsible for collecting information. The 1970 and 1980 censuses did attempt to make possible the accumulation of more nearly accurate census data concerning special populations. Voluntary organizations report those illnesses or disabilities in which they are directly involved. Secondary problems associated with the primary problem may be unreported.

Another difficulty is the labeling of figures as national estimates. While such figures may well apply to a state or a geographical district, they will be found lacking in specific instances, especially when applied to certain local communities. For example, the number of mentally retarded children will be much greater in slum areas than in wealthy suburbs of a city. Certain states and parts of states, such as Florida and southern California, attract individuals who are chronically ill.

A fifth difficulty exists because many times additional information is needed if a clear picture of the problem is to be obtained. For years it has been reported that 3 percent of the population of the United States are mentally retarded. This figure is now being questioned in relation to customs, traditions, and environments.

All of these factors, therefore, caution against overdependency on prevalent figures. Those figures should be used only as an index.

Despite the difficulties in determining the prevalence of special populations, investigators have been able to hazard guesses based on different studies. These guesses have provided us with valuable information that can be used as baseline data for the planning, administration, and evaluation of programs as well as for action by legislative bodies.

Disabled Persons

Although dependable statistics on the total number of individuals who fall within the special population category are still lacking, it has been estimated by some investigators that as much as 35 percent of the population may have some form of physical, emotional, social, or intellectual problem. This estimate does not include social offenders.

Not until the 1970 census of the population was there any attempt to identify the numbers of disabled persons in the United States. Studies conducted by the U.S. Public Health Service (PHS) and the Social Security Administration (SSA) between 1963 and 1966 estimated that there were at least 22.6 million and probably over 30 million individuals unable to participate in activities normal for their age group. The 1970 census showed a total adult population in America of 121 million (excluding those in institutions and in military service) between sixteen and sixty-four years of age, the generally accepted employable age range. Of this total, there were nearly 11.3 million persons with disabilities that had existed for six months or longer and affected their ability to work. The census, therefore, concluded that one in every eleven people in the United States—over 9 percent of the population—has a disability. The census also showed, as might be expected, that the disability rate between sixteen and sixty-four

years of age increases by age for both men and women.[1]

It was reported in 1986 that one in five adults suffers some type of disability and that the rate of disabilities continues to increase with age, affecting more than half the people age sixty-five and over. Difficulty in walking is the most common disability encountered, with 19.2 million people having a problem walking a quarter mile and 7.9 million being unable to make such a walk. A close second in disabilities is difficulty in lifting or carrying a weight equivalent to a full bag of groceries. Inability to climb a flight of stairs without stopping to rest was next, followed by visual impairments and hearing problems. Nearly 12.8 million stated they had trouble reading a newspaper with glasses or contact lenses; 7.7 million reported they had hearing problems; and nearly 500,000 said they were unable to hear an ordinary conversation at all.[2]

Table 2.1 provides information regarding the incidence of disabilities in persons with selected chronic conditions, and Table 2.2 considers disability conditions associated with students enrolled in public elementary and secondary special education programs in the United States.

TABLE 2.1.   Persons with Selected Chronic Conditions, by Sex and Age, 1981

	RATE PER 1000 PERSONS						
CHRONIC CONDITIONS	Total	Male	Female	Under 17 years	17–44 years	45–64 years	65 years and over
Heart conditions	76.4	70.7	81.6	20.4	37.9	122.7	277.0
Hypertension	113.4	100.4	125.5	1.4	54.2	243.7	378.6
Chronic bronchitis	35.3	31.7	38.7	38.4	28.1	40.9	46.1
Asthma	32.2	33.9	30.6	37.9	29.0	33.6	28.6
Arthritis	121.0	87.5	152.3	2.8	47.7	246.5	464.7
Diabetes	24.4	21.7	27.0	1.4	8.6	56.9	83.4
Visual impairments	40.4	47.8	33.4	9.9	27.4	55.2	136.6
Hearing impairments	82.9	91.1	75.3	17.7	43.8	142.9	283.8
Deformities or orthopedic impairments	81.8	86.4	77.6	21.1	90.5	117.5	128.2

SOURCE: Bureau of the Census, *Statistical Abstract of the United States, 1985,* (Washington, D.C.: U.S. Government Printing Office, December 1984), p. 115.

TABLE 2.2. **Public Elementary and Secondary Students in Special Education Programs for the Handicapped, by Types of Handicapped, 1983**

Type of Handicap	ALL CONDITIONS (HANDICAPS) 4255 Percent Distribution
Learning disabled	40.9
Speech impaired	26.6
Mentally retarded	17.8
Emotionally disturbed	8.3
Hard of hearing and deaf	1.7
Orthopedically handi- capped	1.3
Other health impaired	1.2
Visually handicapped	.7
Multihandicapped	1.5
Deaf-blind	.1

SOURCE: Bureau of the Census, *Statistical Abstract of the United States,* 1985. (Washington, D.C.: U.S. Government Printing Office, December 1984), p. 129.

Social Offenders

To ascertain the exact dimensions of socially deviant behavior is extremely difficult because of the distinctions drawn between adult and juvenile offenders and between crime and delinquency, and also because of the disparities in criminal codes and in sentencing and release policies from jurisdiction to jurisdiction.

As of 1985 approximately 2.9 million adults were in the correctional system (64.4 percent on probation, 9.6 percent on parole, 8.7 percent in jail, and 17.3 percent in prison). The Department of Justice also reported that 87 percent of the 2.9 million adults were male, and this represented approximately 3 percent of all adult men in the United States.[3]

In 1983, 10,200,000 juveniles and adults were arrested (but not necessarily charged). Of the 8,500,000 males arrested, nearly 16 percent were under eighteen years of age. On the other hand, a greater percentage of females under eighteen years of age were arrested in 1983 than adult females (21.5 percent to 16.6 percent).[4] A side note here is that as a result of the women's movement that began in the late 1960s, the general public and criminal justice personnel have altered their attitude toward women and crime. Thus, there has been a decline in preferential treatment of women in the criminal justice system.[5]

Adult males in federal and state prisons constituted approximately 96 percent (528,945 inmates) of the adult prison population in 1986. Of the total male population, 44,330 were in federal prisons and 484,615 in state institutions. The adult female population was 4.72 percent (25,192 inmates) of the total prison population as of June 30, 1986. The Justice Department report also noted that the racial breakdown of inmates (1984) showed 52 percent white, 45 percent black, 1 percent American Indian, and the rest Asians and other groups.[6]

A profile of the prison population indicated that two-thirds of the male population are between twenty and thirty-four years of age, most have not completed high school, a majority of them earned less than $6000 during the year prior to their arrest, and their jobs were primarily of an unskilled nature.[7]

The number of juveniles incarcerated as of 1982 was over 80,000, with the average age approximately fifteen in both state and private institutions.[8] Further, a study of the juvenile justice system completed in 1978 and concerned with the profile of male delinquents revealed a profile similar to that of delinquents in 1988. The study indicated that most violent delinquents were minority-group males who lived in lower-class or slum neighborhoods of large urban centers and came from broken homes where there was a poor relationship with the only parent. In addition, they were most likely to be school failures with learning disabilities and to have psychological problems. Rage, low self-esteem, lack of empathy, and limited frustration tolerance are typical characteristics of violent youths, the study said.[9]

Because the concept of delinquency is basically a legal notion implying deviance from cultural norms and/or legal restrictions, a term more useful from the standpoint of understanding the individual child/juvenile has emerged. That term, *conduct disorder,* refers to any behavior of a youngster that causes difficulty or disruption in the individual's relationships with parents, family, teachers, or the larger community including law enforcement agencies. Whether the youngster is also delinquent depends on the moral standards of the community and on whether the youngster is apprehended by legal authorities.[10]

The national recidivism rate of those who have been incarcerated is estimated at 65 percent for adults and 75 percent for youth. Further, nearly 80 percent of the crimes are committed by those adults and youth who have previously been through the criminal justice system. Lastly, nearly 75 percent of the prison population is made up of individuals who are economically deprived and who belong to a minority group.[11]

Disadvantaged Persons

Turning our attention to those who are unable to participate fully in American society because of educational, economic, or social barriers, we note that by the federal government's income criteria, in 1973 there were about 23 million people, or one of every seven Americans, living at the poverty level.[12] A decade later, Census Bureau figures show that 15.2 percent of the population, or 35.3 million people, lived below the government's poverty level.[13] According to some investigators, this figure is considerably higher today.

Who are these people? They include the families of black Southern sharecroppers who moved North expecting to find work. They also include members of other ethnic minority groups: Puerto Ricans and other Spanish-speaking Americans, citizens of Oriental extraction, and almost all American Indians. They also include the residents of Appalachia and other economic-disaster areas and the unskilled workers everywhere. Perhaps the most disadvantaged of this latter group are the migrant farm workers.

Since good care early in life is the best protection against subsequent disability and illness, adequate health care for children is basic to the improvement of the nation's health. However, the health needs of poor children are less well met than those of other children for a variety of reasons: lack of facilities and manpower, especially in impoverished rural areas; limited available funds for both tax-supported and voluntary programs; and restrictive eligibility requirements for free or low-cost care. The result is that few poor children receive regular medical supervision, preventive services, and early diagnosis and treatment. They tend to receive medical attention only when their health problems are very serious.[14]

A similar problem of a lack of medical attention also applies to the diet of the poor. Income is a very important determinant of nutritional status. Most indications are that food prices have been rising faster than income for the poor segments of society. The poor are hit especially hard during times of inflation. Finally, the poor often pay more for food than other segments of the population do because they frequently do not have the choice of shopping at large retail supermarkets. Because of transportation difficulties, they are forced to shop at smaller and less efficient local stores that charge higher prices. Further, because of limited education they are less able to analyze false and misleading advertisement claims or to use food discount coupons or even to read the food sections in newspapers. In fact, they probably don't buy newspapers.[15]

ATTITUDES

As we begin our consideration of attitudes, it is well to distinguish between the terms *disability* and *handicap*. This distinction is an important key to understanding all special population persons. A *disability, impair-*

ment, or *disorder* is a defect in makeup or functioning that can be specified and described objectively. A *handicap,* by contrast, is a potential limitation in functioning that may arise when obstacles imposed by the disability or impairment interfere with optimal development. A disability produces complications in growth and development of special population members, but it is only when these complications limit the special population member's development that we can view the individual as handicapped. Many individuals with physical disabilities, for example, dislike the term *handicap* because they feel it is discriminatory or because they do not consider themselves any more handicapped than individuals without significant disabilities. For many the term *impairment* is preferred since it is less value laden.

Attitude of Society

While significant changes have taken place in society's attitudes toward special populations during the past century, the myths, superstitions, and guilt feelings still exist today. These stigmas are reflected in the day-to-day contact with the disabled, the disadvantaged, and the social offender. Many challenges lie ahead in helping society to accept the value of the individual and the philosophy that each individual has the right to the pursuit of his or her best self-realization.

Generally speaking, nobody is against special population members. Yet our attitudes, actions, and institutions show a clear pattern of considering special population members as surplus members of our society who are to be hidden out of sight or isolated. Prejudice toward these persons, with open or hidden rejection by the nondisabled, occurs at all social and economic levels and in all regions of our country. It is evident in the social, educational, and vocational discriminations that hamper special population members. It is reflected in the very existence of legislation to assist special populations to have the same opportunities as non-

special population members. And lastly, it is clearly manifest in the self-deprecation of the disabled.

Until 1973 no federal law specifically prohibited discrimination against disabled persons. Under pressure from eight hundred various groups concerned with the rights of disabled, and after a much publicized sit-in by disabled people at the Lincoln Memorial, the United States Congress passed the Rehabilitation Act of 1973 (PL93-112). Section 504 of the act prohibits any federally funded institution from excluding disabled persons from programs or facilities on the basis of their disability. However, the regulations to implement the new law were not signed until April 28, 1977—and then only after nationwide protest demonstrations.

Despite the national commitment to improve the social and economic lives of special population members, popular language and thought still confirm the antiquated attitude toward persons who are "different" from the normal. Reference to the disabled as "paraplegics," "epileptics," "mentally retarded," or worse, as "cripples," "deformed," or "abnormal" reinforce the distinction between the disabled and the nondisabled. They are seen as overly sensitive, easily hurt, weak, shy, nonsexual, or sexually perverse. As pointed out in a *New York Times* article, societal attitudes do not reflect the reality of disabled people's capabilities. "Our bodies make us disabled, but society makes us handicapped."[16]

The term *disability* generally evokes thoughts of the permanent paralysis that sometimes results from traumatic injuries or the deteriorating effects of dramatic conditions such as multiple sclerosis; it seldom calls to mind such mundane afflictions as the common cold or the Monday morning hangover, which are undoubtedly among the leaders in terms of the total work days lost they cause. The habit of stereotyping illness according to its most dramatic effect often leads to some poor judgments. Many people think of coronary heart disease as something that causes a quick death;

however, a heart attack disables more often than it kills.

Illnesses vary widely in the degree of disability they cause, and the same illness may produce considerable variation in disability among persons so afflicted. Although the illness condition itself may be an important contributor to disability, many other factors not associated with the illness may influence the extent to which a person feels unable to undertake a variety of activities. Illness is frequently regarded as disabling when a physical or physiological condition makes it impossible for people to perform their usual role obligations. As noted earlier, this is as dependent on the nature of their role obligations and their attitude toward them as it is on their physical condition. It is also dependent on the attitudes and reactions of family members, employers, and society in general.

In considering the social aspects of disability, we must note that the disabled individual's willingness or motivation for retraining plays a crucial role. Individuals who have a keen attitude toward rehabilitation appear to overcome vast difficulties, while others who, by medical criteria, seem handicapped only to a minimal extent are greatly hampered in their rehabilitation by attitudes that encourage their disability. The attitude of family and colleagues can have a similarly substantial impact on the course a pattern of disability takes. To the extent that the family and others value the person, they are more likely to try to impose their own definition of the situation on him or her.[17]

Although improving, attitudes toward the disabled are expressed in consistently negative prejudgments and behavior. It appears to be a stereotyped reaction that emphasizes devaluation and rejection of the disabled. The roots of these negative attitudes are found in our social customs and norms, child-rearing practices that stress normalcy, our personal insecurities, and the kind of behavior by the disabled that provokes discrimination.

Attitude toward Self

Society—conceived of as a pattern of institutions, customs, and interpersonal relations designed to routinize social living—provides preestablished social roles and expectations regarding behavior appropriate to these roles. Cues learned in childhood serve as a guide for distinguishing and differentiating various types of disabilities in accordance with socially accepted norms. Society furnishes, in addition to roles and language, a historical attitude toward the disabled: the Greek belief that the physically impaired were inferior; the preprophetic Hebraic idea that the sick were being punished by God; the early Christian concept that disabled persons acquired more virtue because of suffering; the Darwinian theory of the survival of the fittest; the faith in the progress of mankind through science; and lastly, the concern for human rights that is evidenced in the social and economic legislation enacted by the U.S. Congress during the last quarter century aimed at restoring the physically or mentally disabled individual to a responsible, contributing role in society.

This mixture of attitudes results in a marked ambivalence toward disability. A continuous barrage of advertising that emphasizes health and well-being inculcates the belief that physical or emotional disability or injury results from inadequacy, misfortune, or lack of care. Studies show that the nicknames most commonly used by children refer to physique, such as Four-Eyes, Fatty, Slim, and Freckles. Our comics, our films, and our ads on television, on billboards, and in newspapers have long utilized physical attributes of individuals for comedy effect. As Meyerson pointed out some years ago—and it is still so today—if normal variations in physique, such as being strong or weak, tall or short, handsome or ugly, are important factors in personality development, clearly the pathological variations known as physical disability are likely to be even more potent.[18]

Social attitudes toward the disabled are reflected in the family, which teaches discrimination by example, by custom, and by institutionalized values. Child-rearing practices tend to predetermine adult behavior toward the disabled. Psychologists tell us that most parents live in constant anxiety lest a child of theirs become disabled. The fear of impairment is evident when a parent examines a newborn child. Seeing a physically whole child brings an instantaneous feeling of relief. An impaired child evokes a sense of guilt.

Similar feelings are evident in the reluctance of many parents to permit a close relationship between nondisabled and disabled children. In a recreation setting, it is easy to imagine the reactions of parents who bring their children to a playground program and encounter a mentally retarded youth when they were not expecting it. Or the reaction of individuals who attend a public pool and encounter several amputees or a cerebral palsied individual. What reactions do they experience, and what types of questions are raised? How many of you can recall instances where even passing contact with a physically disabled person was avoided. Why? Because you had undoubtedly learned that the attributes or behaviors of such a person were so bizarre as to be annoying, embarrassing, dangerous, or sufficiently distasteful to warrant avoidance. The barrier that is raised by society's emphasis on conformity and reinforced by the peer group leads both parents and children to avoid physically and mentally impaired children.

The existence of a prejudicial climate conditions disabled persons or former mental patients to accept the role of the disabled. As they assume the pattern of behavior and value deemed appropriate, they prepare themselves to become an object of prejudice. Their appraisal of themselves as inferior reflects the attitudes of those about them. As Mariann Soulek, a recreator with a physical impairment states:

To a degree we are what people think of us. If we are constantly reminded both in words and in actions that we are dependent, we will be dependent. Society has placed the physically impaired in a minority role by its attitudes toward physical impairment; a well-developed stigma has resulted in prejudice and discrimination. We have reacted and, in many cases, performed according to what society has expected.[19]

Physically disabled children at any early age, for example, require an unusual amount of help and attention and thus receive social status and self-esteem. However, as they become older, their reactions to their disability change. They are more expensive in terms of both time and money. Their parents may reject them because of feelings of resentment or guilt. This rejection may then be transferred to the child who, in turn, resents the parents. But being dependent upon the parents, they are forced to suppress this blame, which produces self-hostility, guilt, and anxiety. On the other hand, the parents, either from genuine sympathy or from guilt reactions, may tend to overprotect the child, with equally harmful results. In either instance, the child's ego and social-status needs are frustrated.

The forces that make for a differentiated and segregated social life for disabled children follow them through all phases of their development. During adolescence perceptible differences in appearance, gait, mannerisms, or speech, make dating difficult. As they grow into adulthood, they become categorized as a member of a minority group. In many instances, they are socially ostracized and rejected by normal persons. They are discriminated against in employment, even for jobs that they are physically and mentally able to perform. The disabled person is a marginal person—physically, socially, and economically. The fact that many avenues of normal relationships are blocked for them—whether actually by the disability, by their attitude toward the disability, or by social pressures—then tends to produce more frustration and conflict.

Many disabled individuals, of necessity, seek the companionship of other disabled persons in social clubs or at centers for various disability groups. Here they see themselves as not being different, and therefore groups composed of persons with similar disabilities tend to become self-perpetuating subcultures. Within them, the person becomes acclimated to the role of a disabled person and learns the pattern of behavior prescribed for the disability group and adopts feelings and attitudes consonant with society's perception of the role of the disabled person.

Because of the value society places on the "body-whole" the "body beautiful," and on emotional stability, mental alertness, and other positive concepts, the role individuals must assume carries with it a sense of devaluation. They may feel shame, inferiority, even worthlessness. Not only are they often considered inferior, but they also begin to feel that they "ought" to feel inferior, that they "ought to know their place" much in the manner of some minority-group members. The assumption seems to be that the disabled are perceived as being different and this difference is "bad." The disabled are confronted with a serious situation because two basic psychological needs are the need for self-esteem (high self-evaluation) and the need for social status (high evaluation by others). For optimal adjustment these needs must be satisfied in some way and to some degree. At the same time the disabled expect and become dependent upon preferential treatment and assistance from the nondisabled.

Distinguishable differences, therefore, in behavior and social perception accentuate the impact of the disability. The characteristics ascribed to and accepted by disabled persons exercise a reciprocal influence upon the behavior and attitudes of the nondisabled. However, in the final analysis it is the individual who exhibits prejudice and re-jects disabled persons. It is the "I" rather than the "he" or "she" who commits discriminatory actions. The roots of prejudice come to fruition in the attitudes and behavior of a nondisabled John Doe toward a disabled Richard Roe. According to behavioral scientists, these prejudices appear to be rooted in the prior life experiences of the nondisabled. Whatever the reasons or lack of them, it is undeniable that such attitudes exist and are a deterrent to successful participation in activities of daily living by the disabled.[20]

In summary, there appears to be no question but that American people harbor mixed feelings about special population members, and that these members sense the resistance to their reentry into any functionally useful roles. While the attitudes of the American people cannot easily be changed, it is suggested by Hamilton and others "that positive, informal interaction, away from institutional settings, is effective in producing accepting attitudes." He continues by suggesting "that integrated leisure activities would provide a conducive environment for attitude change."[21]

Regardless of attitudes reflected by society toward special population members or self-attitudes, it is important for you, as a potential therapeutic recreation specialist, to consider the following values and concepts regarding special population members:

Special population individuals are a normal part of today's society and do not exist as a group apart with separate lives. Their needs and rights are the same as those of any other person; their problems are the problems of all people and should be considered as a part of the whole society.

The special population person should be regarded as a whole person—physically, mentally, socially, and emotionally—rather than within the narrow confines of his or her limiting condition.

Leisure programs should be designed with and for special population persons on the basis of abilities, not disabilities, and capabilities, not limitations, to most fully develop their assets.

If these program designs are to be reflected in care and treatment services, teamwork of the highest order is required in association with other professional personnel (and such teamwork includes the patient).

CONCEPTS: HEALTH/DISEASE AND REHABILITATION/PUNISHMENT

Basic to the practice of all health and allied health professionals is the *health/disease concept*. A second basic concept, relating to the field of corrections, is the *rehabilitation (resocialization)/punishment concept*.

Health/Disease

In an earlier time the term health was generally accepted to mean the normal, harmonious function of the body—in other words, the absence of organ disease. Over the years this narrow concept changed primarily because of the added new depth and perspective given to health by the World Health Organization's (WHO) definition of health: "Health is a state of complete physical, mental, and social well-being, and not merely the absence of disease or infirmity."[22]

There are many theories of health existing today. The concept of health has come a long way from its original preoccupation with physical well-being through the thinking and research of such people as Hoyman (an ecologic resultant composed of mental, physical, social, and spiritual dimensions), Dunn, who coined the term *high-level wellness* (a continuum influenced by many environmental factors), Dolfman (a personal behavior perspective), Rathbone (a dynamic process that can be assessed and measured

as one responds to daily situations), Dubos ("... the expression of the extent to which the individual and the social body maintains in readiness the resources required to meet the exigencies of the future."[23]), Salk, Tillich, Maslow, and others.[24] Regardless of the various theories or perspectives, the concept of health today incorporates the wide diversity of individual capacities (physical, mental, emotional, and social), goals and values, and lifestyles. Further, the relationship between these factors differs from person to person. And still further, these factors are constantly being modified or changed as a result of human and natural forces. No one person is absolutely healthy or ill. Health, therefore, is a multidimensional variable.

Like health, concepts of disease (germ, psychogenic, stress, ecologic, and symbolic theories), vary greatly because the standards of normality and dysfunctioning held by investigators and lay persons differ; they may also differ between physicians and patients, and even among physicians. The concept of disease, which at times is used synonymously with illness, usually refers to some deviation from normal functioning that has undesirable effects because it produces personal discomfort or adversely affects the individual. Most people think of disease as an organic illness like cancer or a mental dysfunction like schizophrenia. But the word *disease* means only "not to feel at ease"; *dis*, from the Latin prefix, means "apart" or "asunder," and *ease* is "a state of comfort or rest." Its meaning is not implicitly limited to abnormal or deadly conditions or disorders.

In its most narrow meaning disease refers to a medical hypothesis that implies particular pathological processes underlying a specific clinical syndrome. More generally, the concept is used to refer to physical or behavioral deviations that pose social problems for individuals or the community. Finally, there are occasions in which particular personal problems may be defined as disease although they neither imply underlying pathology nor pose serious problems for the community. In sum, disease may result from (1) heredity, (2) diet, (3) infection, (4) stress, (5) environment, (6) degenerative processes, or some combination of these factors.

If we take into consideration those concepts associated with health and disease, a model as suggested by Hoyman (Table 2.3) can be quite useful in understanding the factors that are health producing and disease producing.[25] However, we must remember that these factors are always changing.

René Dubos, an eminent microbiologist and medical historian, has made this point most elegantly:

> (Man's) self-imposed striving for ever-new distant goals makes his fate even more unpredictable than that of other living things. For this reason health and happiness cannot be absolute and permanent values, however careful the social and medical planning. Biological success in all of its manifestations is a measure of fitness, and fitness requires never-

TABLE 2.3. Health-Producing and Disease-Producing Factors

Health-Producing	Disease-Producing
Good hereditary endowment	Poor hereditary endowment
Healthful, safe environment	Unhealthy, unsafe environment
Adequate service and education	Personal experiences and behavior
Resistance to communicable and noncommunicable diseases	Psychogenic factors
Optimum nutrition, growth, and development	Inadequate standard of living
Organic soundness and functional vigor	Inadequate medical and dental care, public health, and education
Optimum dynamic motor fitness and suitable exercise throughout life	Health fads and fallacies and self-diagnosis and self-treatment
Refreshing rest, relaxation, and sleep	Sociocultural isolation and deprivation
Resistance to stress, fatigue, frustration, and boredom	Abnormal growth and development and pathologic conditions, including neoplasmas
Homeostasis, and optimum metabolism	Poor health practices
Healing, repair, and recovery from injury or illness	Endogenous factors related to homeostasis and metabolic disorders
Resistance to premature aging and death	Defects, disabilities, pain, and decay
Healthy mature personality and healthful living	Aging and senescence
A will to live	Stressors and stress
Healthful attitudes, beliefs, and practices	Excesses of deficiencies and deprivations
Freedom for personal-social fulfillment through significant commitments to ultimate concerns	Pathogenic organisms
Useful, satisfying work and creative achievement	Noxious agents and allergens
Love and affectionate sharing and belonging	Radiation hazards
Heterosexual adjustment	Accident hazards and traumatic injuries
Enjoyable constructive recreation and use of leisure	Motion, noise, vibration, and pressure changes
Enjoyable esthetic experiences including those with nature	Existential "human predicament"
Opportunities for risk, challenges, adventure, and new experiences	
Spiritual faith, ideals, values, and a search for meaning	

SOURCE: Howard S. Hoyman, "An Ecologic View of Health Education," in *Science and Theory of Health*, eds. Herbert L. Jones, Margaret B. Schutt, and Ann L. Shelton (Dubuque, Iowa: William C. Brown Co., Publishers, 1966), pp. 8–10.

ending efforts of adaptation to the total environment, which is ever changing.[26]

Personal Reaction to Disease/Illness. We cannot discuss the concepts of health and disease however briefly without mentioning how people react to a health need or problem for which assistance is desired. The ability to cope with our problem—whether physical, emotional, or social—depends on the way we define the problem, the causes we identified as having brought the problem about, the alternatives we see for reversing the problem, and our resources for making use of various alternatives to the problem. While personal experiences, family composition, peer pressures, age-sex role learning, and knowledge acquired about health and disease in the course of our life are determining factors in the ability to cope with a problem as well as influencing attitudes toward the problem, cultural and social conditioning play a major role, though not an exclusive role.[27]

Many studies in the interdisciplinary field of medical sociology dealing with illness behavior reflect the importance of developmental and cultural experiences in determining reactions to illness. Baumann, in a study of differences in people's attitudes toward illness, identified three distinct ways by which people tend to determine whether or not they are ill. One is related to the presence or absence of pain; if a person has pain of a severe nature, he usually considers himself ill. However, pain is relative; a person may live with a backache for years and not consider this an abnormal condition. The second method is related to how people feel: they feel well, or they feel sick. The third way relates to the individual's ability to carry out daily activities. One person is in good health because she works all day and still has energy to play a round of golf in the evening, while another person doing the same work cannot play golf because she feels exhausted and should perhaps have a physical examination. Baumann concludes that whether a person determines the state of his or her health on the basis of symptoms, feelings, or performance tends to vary with age, education, socioeconomic status, cultural background, and value system.[28]

Rehabilitation/Punishment

Since the beginning of time, punishment has been the penalty inflicted by society on those who have violated its laws. Punishment has been justified on the grounds that it is a deterrent to further criminal behavior by the offender, is a general deterrent to other members of society contemplating crimes, and is a source of revenge or justice. Emphasis on these functions has shifted throughout the years, but the use of punishment, either by itself or combined with treatment techniques (such as vocational training, recreation, school), was a constant until recently.

The Auburn System (named after a New York penitentiary that opened in 1817, and will be discussed in a later chapter) served as the model for American prisons for 150 years. It emphasized discipline designed to break a prisoner's spirit and force him or her to conform. Corporal punishment was used to enforce prison rules. As a result of strong humanitarian ideas, increased confidence in the ability of the behavioral sciences to predict and change individual behavior, and a growing frustration of the prison system in its efforts to reform prisoners, the *punishment model* gave way to the *treatment* or *rehabilitation model* (resocialization or social well-being) in the late 1940s and early 1950s.[29]

By the late 1950s and early 1960s the rehabilitation model gained considerable prominence. Institutions became "correctional facilities." Individual and group counseling were introduced. Educational and vocational training programs were expanded along with recreation programs. Offenders were sentenced to prison for as long as it took to be judged "rehabilitated." Punishment as revenge, justice, and deterrence was deemphasized, and corrections came to represent attempts to remake the individual.[30]

However, by the late 1960s and early 1970s, as a result of the failure of the rehabilitation model and public fear of crime, there was a renewed emphasis on the custody orientation to corrections. What is left of the rehabilitation theme today exists in the concept of community-based corrections—probation and parole, halfway-house residential centers, and release and furlough programs.

The concept encourages conventional values and behavior from offenders.[31]

In sum, the correctional system today remains multioriented. In some prisons a punishment framework exists, in others a rehabilitation one, and in still others, a custody framework is found. Some agree that the various frameworks may be a blessing, for they allow the system to begin anew and reconstruct a more realistic approach to rehabilitation.[32]

CONDITIONS AND DISORDERS

As we begin this section it should be reemphasized that acute and chronic conditions may be physical, emotional, social, intellectual, or any combination thereof in nature. Furthermore, whatever the nature of the condition may be, individual differences exist. The following two examples will give you some idea of what is meant by individual differences. Cerebral palsy, for example, may require one child to walk only with a cane, a second to walk with the aid of leg braces and a Canadian crutch, and leave a third child helpless. Dianne, whose IQ is 85, manages to struggle along in the regular grades, though her marks are usually poor; her sister, Sharon, whose IQ is 60, attends an educable class for the mentally retarded; Marie, a neighbor's child with an IQ of 20, has to be sent to a state institution for the mentally retarded.

There is another important characteristic that must be taken into consideration, and that is the time factor. How long has the condition existed? What was the individual's age at the time the disorder originated? What can be inferred with respect to its probable duration? The child who becomes blind at the age of ten is in a very different position from the one who has been blind from birth. That which can be accomplished with relative ease at one age may become difficult at another, for growth proceeds inexorably and ceases when maturity is reached. Correction of a physically disabling condition or behavior deviation often depends on the stage that the difficulty has already reached. Thus, the nature of the deviation may require services and/or devices anywhere from a short period of time to a lifetime.

The potential therapeutic recreation specialist should also be aware that all diseases are not detected early in life. Some are unmistakable as soon as the child is born; *cleft lip* and *palate, clubfoot, spina bifida,* and *Down's Syndrome* are among them. Other conditions that are invisible to the layperson are readily recognized by the physician. Within a minute of birth a physician usually calculates an infant's *Apgar score,* based on heart rate, respiratory effort, muscle tone, reflexes, and color. A low Apgar score and extremely low birth weight are considered immediate danger signals of a possible internal defect. Some defects are not apparent until thirty days after birth or later during the first year of the child's life. Others do not appear until adolescence or adulthood. A child may be in his teens before he shows symptoms of *Wilson's disease,* a metabolic malfunction that results in a deficiency of copper and consequent brain damage—although the condition can now be detected and corrected at three months with a family history of the disease. *Huntington's chorea,* a degenerative nervous system disease,

strikes in the victim's late thirties and for-
ties. The inborn tendency to *diabetes melli-
tus* may not cause disease until the victim is
fifty or older.

Still another factor to consider is that
many of the diseases that kill also cause
varying degrees of disability among the survivors. In addition, a number of diseases not
usually fatal disable large numbers of persons. For example, the large majority of elderly persons who suffer a stroke survive
with a wide range of disabilities over varying
intervals of time. Likewise, the extent of disability in cases of heart disease is highly variable. Some patients are bedridden, unable
to work, and often even unable to carry on
activities of daily living. Other patients may
be only minimally disabled, their disease
well controlled by medication, and their disability scarcely evident to the casual observer. The various types of arthritis and the
rheumatic diseases do not usually kill; however, they rank high in national frequency
as a cause of chronic disability. Mental retardation is a very common cause of chronic
disability but is an insignificant cause of
death. On the other hand, the functional
disabilities it produces interfere with an individual's capacity to work, take care of himself, and get along in our competitive society.

We could continue to consider many
other disorders that produce chronic conditions; however, you probably get the message. It is important to point out that considerable progress has been recorded in
reducing the impact of a number of serious
chronic diseases. Consider, for example, the
reduction in the number of individuals confined to institutions for mental and emotional disorders. By far the most important
reason for the reduction over the past two
decades has been the development of new
drugs that effectively control two of the
most critical problems of mental hospital patients: the agitation and the depression that
often necessitated incarceration for long periods of time. Tranquilizers and antidepres-
sants now make it possible for the large ma-

jority of patients with mental illness to be
treated at home or to require only brief periods of hospitalization.

CONDITIONS FOUND
IN SPECIAL POPULATIONS

The following pages present some of the
major types of acute and chronic conditions
found in special populations. The material
has been prepared primarily to assist potential therapeutic recreation specialists in developing an awareness of those conditions
that affect people's ability to engage in recreative activities, particularly those conditions therapeutic recreation specialists are
more likely to encounter in offering recreation services to special populations. In this
regard, various disorders and their appropriate therapeutic recreation process or programming will be considered through case
studies in later chapters.

This section presupposes the reader's
knowledge of some medical terminology derived from various courses in the social and
behavioral sciences that are required for national therapeutic recreation certification.

Mental Retardation

Mental retardation is not an immutable concept. Rather, it means different things to different people. It is not a disease in the sense
that we usually define a disease. It is a condition, a description of behavior. Estimates of
the percentage of individuals who could be
considered mentally retarded have ranged
from .05 percent to 23 percent.[33] The current definition by the American Association
on Mental Deficiency (AAMD) suggests
that the potential pool of mentally retarded
is 2.27 percent of the general population.[34]
This is in accord with a prevalence estimate
of 2.3 percent to 3 percent of the population
that has been widely accepted by a number
of authorities.[35] However, not all authorities
agree with the 3 percent estimate. They
point out that the requirement that both
low measured intelligence and failure in

adaptive behavior are necessary for a diagnosis of mental retardation reduces the actual prevalance to roughly 1 percent.[36] This 1 percent has been supported by actual community studies conducted by various investigators.[37]

While the above statistics are interesting, the reader should keep in mind that there is no method currently available to determine either the true incidence or the true prevalence of mental retardation. Why? First, sex-linked *recessive syndromes* are more likely to occur in males than females; according to some investigators, the incidence of mental retardation has been found to be higher among males than females.[38] Second, society holds different expectations for males than for females.[39] Third, differing demands made by various communities affect diagnosis of mental retardation (rural areas and urban areas, low socioeconomic class and middle class).[40] Fourth, different tests are used to determine or diagnose mental retardation.

Causes.   A vast range of conditions and diseases can cause or contribute to retarded intellectual development. There are more than 250 known causes of mental retardation, or diseases and conditions so associated with the later development of retardation as to be considered probable causes. The causes cover the range of hereditary, biological, psychological, and sociological determinants of life conditions and development. They include chromosomal-genetic influences derived from heredity or physiology. They include diseases, infections, accidents, and the physical neglect and mistreatment of children. And they include the slow, sometimes subtle, influences of the physical, psychological, and social environment that may influence the development of mental retardation through deprivation.

In addition to cause and probable cause of mental retardation, the reader should also be aware that mental retardation is frequently associated with other types of problems. A large percentage of the mentally retarded have speech and language problems, which restricts them from engaging in effective communication with others. Other problems that occur with a high frequency include impaired hearing and vision, seizures, and ambulation and perceptual motor disorders.

Definition.   The problem of defining mental retardation is made difficult because so many types of specialists are interested in the totality of its psycho-socio-medical implications. Obviously, each type of specialist focuses on the specific dimensions in which he or she is trained and interested. Representatives of the medical profession, for example, view mental retardation in terms of pathology or sickness, which differentiates individuals in their physical makeup and function from the characteristics of the "normal" individual. Educators, on the other hand, become concerned when the mentally retarded individual does not respond to the usually successful methods of instruction in use in the schools. This has led to the statistical focus, which attempts to classify individuals according to intellectual potential and thereby predict the limits of future success or achievement.

As important as scientific concerns are, societal attitudes have been just as important in recent years in the development of any definition of mental retardation. As evidence mounted that more retarded persons were found in certain ethnic or income groups and in certain geographical areas, pressure was exerted to reexamine definitions of retardation to determine whether the consequences of deprivation were being confused with constitutional disability.

It is enough to say that there have been problems for some years in defining mental retardation. Definitions of mental retardation have included reference to such variables as causation, curability, age of onset, intelligence quotient, mental age, educability, and social adequacy. In 1973 the American Association of Mental Deficiency (AAMD) adopted the following definition:

Mental retardation refers to significantly sub-average general intellectual functioning existing concurrently with deficits in adaptive behavior and manifested during the developmental period.[41]

This definition refers to an IQ cutoff at 2 standard deviations below the mean (approximately 3 percent of the general population). The upper developmental period is at eighteen years of age. The definition emphasizes the relationship between intellectual functioning and adaptive behavior by specifying that deficits in the two must exist concurrently. Adaptive behavior was defined as the "effectiveness or degree with which the individual meets the standards of personal independence and social responsibility."[42] The 1973 *Manual on Terminology and Classification in Mental Retardation* suggests that deficits might exist in sensorimotor skills development, communication, application of basic academic skills, social skills, and vocational performances, to name a few.[43]

Classification. Defining, classifying and labeling are necessary to provide a common basis for communicating about mental retardation, designing interventions, and assessing the effectiveness of these interventions. Although a sophisticated classification system based on the etiology of mental retardation has been developed, it is of little value in determining treatment options. Therefore, two education and habilitation classifications have been developed that focus on the continuum of behaviors and abilities. One such system used for educational placement includes three categories: *educable mentally retarded* (EMR), *trainable mentally retarded* (TMR), and *profoundly mentally retarded* (PMR). The other, put forth by the AAMD, is the result of criticism based on the concept that the classification focuses on program development and not on the child. The AAMD considers the following levels of retardation: mild, moderate, severe, and profound.[44] The estimated distribution

TABLE 2.4. Estimated Distribution of Retarded Persons by Degree of Retardation

Degree	Number	Percent
Total	6,500,000	100
Mild	4,875,000–5,850,000	75–90
Moderate	390,000	6
Severe	195,000	3
Profound	65,000	1

of the mentally retarded in the United States by these levels is found in Table 2.4.

A final note regarding labeling. Some mentally retarded people have what appears to be unusually superior abilities in a narrow area of functioning. These individuals have been described by the term *idiot savant*. Examples of their special abilities include the ability to calculate the day of the week on which any date in recorded history fell, the ability to play on the piano any tune they have heard, and the ability to engage in complicated mathematical computations.

Learning Disabled

Other individuals who have been considered mentally retarded, although they are not, include those with a variety of conditions that are categorized as *learning disabilities*. Some have difficulty connecting the printed word with something that makes sense to them. They may have difficulty distinguishing *b* from *d*, *saw* from *was*. Such children may hear a spoken word or sound adequately but be unable to remember the word or interpret the sound accurately. They may not remember how to spell a word from one day to the next. They may gaze out the window rather than listen to their teacher or wander aimlessly about the classroom. They may be hyperactive, continually drumming their fingers or shuffling their feet, or they may act impulsively with sudden rages. These children continually cause frustration—for their parents, for their teachers, and most important, for themselves.

Children with learning disabilities show a discrepancy between expected and actual achievement in written language or mathematics. This learning disability does not appear to be primarily the result of sensory, motor, intellectual, or emotional handicap or lack of opportunity to learn. *Learning disabilities* refers to those children of average or above average intelligence who have a disorder of one or more of the basic psychological processes involved in understanding or using language—spoken or written.

Professionals are skeptical about estimating the number of children who might have a learning disability, though they do know that the majority of children with this problem are boys. Estimates range from 1 to 15 percent of the school population, although some state that as many as 35 percent of all children may have a learning disability that will cause them some kind of school problem. In addition, they come from all economic and social levels. Environment does not appear to be a direct cause. For example, Thomas Edison, Woodrow Wilson, and Sir Winston Churchill were just a few of the famous people who made significant contributions to society despite their learning disabilities.

It appears that no one really knows the causes of learning disabilities. Theories range from chemical imbalance to genetic heredity. These children may be labeled as perceptually handicapped, hyperkinetic, or learning disabled, or with minimal brain damage, minimal cerebral dysfunction, faulty neurological development, or dyslexia. These labels used by various professionals all overlap. None of them totally explains the cause.

Difficulty in evaluation of the percentage of learning-disabled youngsters may be caused, in some respects, by the fact that there are children who become unknown victims of the educational process but are never classified as learning disabled. Early in life these children might be marked by teachers as troublemakers or attention-getters or as lacking motivation. There appears to be a correlation between delinquency and learning disabilities. Surveys of juvenile delinquents have shown that as many as 80 percent may have learning disabilities.

According to pediatricians and psychologists, children with learning disabilities don't socialize well with their peers because their peers realize they are different. They don't play the same way—often they are clumsy and have quick tempers. Often learning-disabled children play with children who are a year or so younger because they get along better with that age group.

Nonsensory Impairments

Human efficiency is dependent upon the smooth function and integration of bodily parts and the various systems, including the musculoskeletal, cardiovascular, respiratory, digestive, genitourinary, endocrine, nervous, and reproductive systems. When an accident or a disease interferes with bodily parts or systems, a disabling condition may result. Furthermore, it is impossible to alter one organ or body system without producing changes in the other. The causes of disabling conditions may be hereditary (for example, hemophilia), congenital (spina bifida), traumatic (severance of the spinal cord), infectious (osteomyelitis), glandular (Addison's disease), metabolic (diabetes), neoplastic (cancer of the bone), circulatory (arteriosclerosis), respiratory (emphysema), myogenic (rheumatoid arthritis), or neurogenic (cerebral palsy).

Precise information concerning the numbers and types of physical disorders is not available. Further, the definition and classification of individuals with physical impairments is far from an orderly process. However, since the early 1960s various individuals and associations (for example, the American Medical Association) have been working toward the development of a system of classification of physical disorders of children that would be equally useful to medical, educational, mental health personnel. While no specific classification has been found satisfactory for all involved, the schema that has been most favorably discussed by various specialists and incorporates medical concerns as well as educational, psychological, and social needs is found in Table 2.5.

A difficulty encountered when considering nonsensory impairments is determining what to include. This problem is further compounded because it is impossible here to identify and describe the variety of even

TABLE 2.5. Classification of Children's Physical Health Disorders

Type of Disability

Motor: a condition that interferes predominantly with motor function either directly or indirectly (e.g., cardiac condition or orthopedic impairment)

Sensory: a condition that interferes with vision, hearing, or speech (e.g., blindness, deafness, or cleft lip)

Cosmetic: a condition that predominantly affects social interaction (e.g., eczema or craniofacial anomaly)

Duration of Disability

Permanent: a condition that is present at age fifteen and whose natural history suggests that it will continue indefinitely (e.g., heart disease)

Indefinite: a condition that is present at age fifteen but whose natural history suggests that it may terminate at a later date (e.g., asthma)

Temporary: a condition that terminated prior to age fifteen (e.g., eczema)

Severity of Disability

Mild: a condition that only prevents the child from engaging in strenuous activities (such as competitive athletics)

Moderate: a condition that interferes with normal daily activities appropriate for age and sex (such as quiet play or school attendance)

Severe: a condition that requires prolonged periods of immobilization, eighteen weeks or more continuous absence from school, or attendance at special schools

SOURCE: I. B. Pless and J. W. B. Douglas, "Chronic Illness in Children: Part I, Epidermeological and Clinical Characteristics," *Pediatrics* 47 (1971), 407–8. Copyright 1971. Reproduced by permission.

the major diseases and conditions that result in disabilities. We have, therefore, selected for mention only those diseases associated with various organs and systems that are of greatest significance in terms of special population numbers, with a brief description of a few specific diseases.

Musculoskeletal Impairments. Bones, joints, and muscles make up the musculoskeletal system. *Bones* form the framework of the body. The places of contact of bones are called *articulations,* or *joints. Muscular tissue* is specialized for contractability; its functions are exceedingly numerous and varied. Disease or injury to any part of this system may cause a disabling condition that in turn may affect the capacity to work or to move. However, human movement is not dependent upon bones, joints, and muscles alone. It is also dependent upon the function of motor nerves, the cells in the spinal cord from which these nerve fibers arise, and the impulses from the motor areas in the cerebral cortex of the brain. In addition, other systems, such as the cardiovascular and respiratory systems, are also involved. Thus, when damage affects the stability of the musculoskeletal system and interferes with the normal function of bones, joints, and muscles (specifically, abnormalities in locomotion), we consider the individual to have an orthopedic problem.

The term *orthopedic* is derived from two Greek words: *orthos,* meaning "right, correct, true, straight," and *pairdeia,* "the rearing of children." Orthopedic is defined by many as "the straight child." In modern usage, the term refers to persons with muscular or skeletal impairments—those impairments associated with the proper function of bones, joints, muscles, tendons, and peripheral blood vessels and nerves. In many instances individuals with orthopedic impairments may require an appliance for body and limb support. The causes of orthopedic impairments may be congenital, infectious, osteochondritic, and traumatic. The term is also applied to a medical specialty concerned with the preservation and restoration of motor and locomotor functions.

Major disabling conditions of the musculoskeletal system associated with the site of the disturbance include the following:

Bone. A bone may become infected, and the resulting inflammation of the bone and its marrow is called *osteomyelitis.* A bone may be the seat of infections such as *tuberculosis of the bone.* Malignant tumors are by no means rare and usually require surgical procedures. If a tumor affects the limb, as it did the son of Senator Edward Kennedy, amputation is required. *Osteoporosis* is a metabolic disorder of the bone common in older persons that leads to excessive risk of fractures. This disorder usually starts early in adulthood, with more women being susceptible than men. In fact, 15 percent of white females over sixty-five have significant osteoporosis. Up to 30 percent reaching seventy-five have sustained fractures related to the problem. The bones most commonly involved are the hip, spine, pelvis, upper arm and wrist. A most interesting side point is that the lack of exercise is included in causes of the condition.[45]

Sometimes bones that should unite before birth fail to do so. One such failure leads to *spina bifida,* in which there is a defect of closure of the body spinal canal. As a result, there is usually a protrusion of the spinal cord through this gap, causing varying degrees of paralysis in the lower extremities. Another such congenital malformation is *clubfoot,* either single or bilateral, in which the front part of the foot is inverted and rotated, accompanied by a shortening of the Achilles tendon and contracture of the fascia in the sole of the foot.

Joints. Among all chronic diseases in the United States, arthritis may be the most prevalent. More than seventeen million persons suffer from arthritis and related rheumatic diseases. Arthritis, which includes over one hundred disorders of the joint and connective tissue, affects one in six Americans of all ages and one in two sixty-five

years of age and older. For unknown reasons, arthritis affects twice as many women as men.[46]

According to the Arthritis Foundation, arthritic Americans and their insurance carriers spent an estimated $1.3 billion on physician visits in 1982. In that year, they spent $1.4 billion more on hospitalization. For the more severely crippled, another $679 million went for nursing home care.[47]

The three most common types are *infectious arthritis, osteoarthritis* (degenerative), and *rheumatoid arthritis;* the latter two are most prevalent. In osteoarthritis, the most pervasive and the one usually associated with old age, the joint cartilage breaks down, with bony outgrowths in the knees, hips, spine, and ends of fingers. In rheumatoid arthritis, which generally strikes between forty and fifty years of age and can be the most debilitating variety, the inflammation (heat, swelling, and pain) is found in both large and small joints. It is estimated that over 6.5 million people suffer from this form of arthritis, and about one-half of them are partially or totally disabled.[48] Another form of this disease found in children is *juvenile rheumatoid arthritis;* however, the prognosis for this condition is more favorable than for the adult form.

Scoliosis (lateral curvature of the spine) is a joint deformity that may involve the entire length or only one portion of the vertebral column. A progressive disease, it can lead over the years to pain, disability, and cardiopulmonary and other complications. Lastly, joints may be dislocated, in which case there is a displacement of one of the bones or a derangement of the parts that compose the joint.

Muscles, Tendons, and Bursae. Skeletal muscles may undergo atrophy from unknown causes. A particularly distressing disease because it strikes children and teenagers, weakening and gradually shriveling the voluntary muscles, is *progressive muscular dystrophy.* As the disease progresses, it may incapacitate so completely that the person cannot stand or sit. In fact, *muscular dystrophy* (MD) is a group of diseases that are for the most part genetically determined and that cause gradual wasting of muscle with accompanying weakness and deformity; there are various forms of MD. Other muscular diseases that produce a disabling condition are *progressive muscular atrophy* and *myasthenia gravis*. While diseases of the tendons and bursae do not produce disabling conditions, they do cause limitations for a period of time in the more severe cases.

Two conditions associated with musculoskeletal dysfunction are *adhesions* and *contractures*. Both can be either acquired or congenital. An adhesion is a pathologic band restricting the normal movement between two adjacent tissues. It is caused by serous or hemorrhagic exudate from the blood vessels, which is either inflammatory or traumatic in origin. When a joint is stiff it is generally because of the presence of adhesions that may be found in or around it. Contractures are caused by structural changes in the soft tissue. A *contracture* is a fixed state of muscle, tendon, fascia, or ligament that does not disappear under anesthesia except in hysterical cases. Contractures are frequently seen following the removal of a cast and in individuals who have suffered a stroke or damage to the spinal cord.

It was indicated earlier that when musculoskeletal stability is disturbed, function is lost. It is well to consider the effect of disease and traumatic injury upon the musculoskeletal system. Traumatic injuries include fractures, dislocations, strains, sprains, lacerations of every type, and thermal injuries. There are many traumatic injuries and, to a lesser degree, diseases that are accompanied or followed by temporary or permanent disability. In some instances the injury or disease is so severe that a brace or an amputation is required. Causes for amputation include the following: (1) accidents, (2) uncontrollable chronic infections, (3) malignant tumors, (4) circulatory insufficiency from peripheral vascular diseases, (5) uselessness of a deformed limb that is objection-

able to the person, (6) thermal injuries, (7) congenital absence, and (8) other conditions that may endanger the life of the individual.

As a result of an amputation or other orthopedic impairment, an individual may be fitted with a prosthesis, brace, or orthopedic appliance. The amputee does not always have a prosthesis prescribed. Some are not motivated to learn how to use the prosthesis; others may be too young or too old; and still others may lack the potential skill for the proper control and function of the prosthesis. Braces and splints are used mainly to render mechanical support to weak or paralyzed limbs and to prevent deformity.

Nervous System. The human brain and central nervous system are awesome instruments, far more advanced than the most sophisticated man-made computer. At the same time, however, disturbances of the brain and central nervous system have historically been among the most tragic, disabling, and intractable scourges of humankind. Not only do these disorders claim lives, but they sentence many to a lifetime of total or partial disability and sap medical and financial resources far out of proportion to the number afflicted.

The nervous system is divided into a central part consisting of the brain and spinal cord, and a peripheral part consisting of the nerves carrying motor messages from the brain and spinal cord to the muscles and those carrying sensory messages from the skin and other parts of the body to the spinal cord and brain. Any infection or injury at any time during the life of the individual or any lack of development of any part of this system is likely to result in disabilities of various kinds.

One of the most tragic disabling illnesses because it strikes at infants, many of whom are treated for the rest of their lives as though they were completely helpless, is *cerebral palsy*. Cerebral palsy may develop during the prenatal, perinatal, or postnatal period. It is estimated that each year about twenty-five thousand babies are born with cerebral palsy—one every twenty-one minutes. About 700,000 people in the United States today have cerebral palsy.[49] Although the cerebral palsied child may present any combination of signs and symptoms that reflect cerebral malfunctions—such as neuromotor disability, convulsions, or vision, hearing, speech, tactile, or perceptual disturbances—the symptom that differentiates cerebral palsied children from others in the syndrome is the neuromotor disability. This disability may be spasticity (about one-half of the victims are spastic) and weakness, either alone or in mixed varieties. Dysfunction may be limited to a single limb or may involve the entire body. Frequently, cerebral palsied children are diagnosed with multiple disabilities such as blindness, deafness, cleft palate, and congenital heart diseases.

While the public has adopted a more open attitude toward many illnesses, *epilepsy* (sometimes called *paroxysmal cerebral dysrhythmia*) still appears to carry a social stigma. This stigma is nothing more than rank discrimination. And though there is less of it now than before, five states still have laws providing for involuntary sterilization of epileptics, and five states permit parents who adopt children to annul the adoption if the child turns out to have epilepsy. In some parts of the world, epileptics are not allowed to marry.[50] The cause of *ordinary epilepsy*, the most common type, also called *genuine* or *idiopathic epilepsy*, is not known; it is not directly inherited, although a predisposition or tendency toward it runs in families. *Acquired epilepsy*, also called *symptomatic epilepsy*, may be the result of brain tumors, diabetes, infectious diseases, toxic cerebral irritations, and psychological disturbances.

The word *epilepsy* is derived from the Greek word *epilepsia*, meaning "a seizure" or "to seize," which includes the idea of being seized by a demon or god and is applied to a type of seizure characterized by loss of consciousness and involuntary convulsive movements. There are different forms of seizures—namely, *grand mal, petit mal, psychomotor,* and *Jacksonian epilepsy*. Today, however, many physicians prefer to use an internationally agreed upon and simplified classification that divides the epilepsies into *generalized* (seizures involving the whole body) and *focal* (seizures affecting just one part of the body and limited to a single identifiable section of the brain). The seizure is due to a temporary disturbance of the brain impulses and abnormal electrical discharges. The student should remember that not all seizures are epilepsy. Seizures can result from a number of things: fever, for instance, hormonal or chemical imbalances, an alcoholic's withdrawal from alcohol, and so on. Generally, only those occurring repeatedly are called epilepsy.

The term *cerebral-vascular accident* (CVA) refers to a stroke. The condition was recognized and described by Hippocrates. In the United States it is the third ranking killer, responsible for over 156,000 deaths in 1983. In addition, it is estimated that it cripples more than 400,000 Americans each year.[51] Like heart disease, stroke is often the culmination of progressive illness. It occurs when blood flow to the brain is interrupted, owing to an obstruction within an artery or to a rupture of an arterial wall. Brain cells served by the affected arteries are robbed of essential oxygen and nutrients. They deteriorate or die, causing a stroke.

Because of the role of the brain in controlling body processes, effects of a stroke can be sudden and far-reaching. When the affected area of the brain governs an arm or leg, that limb weakens or stops functioning. An extensive stroke can paralyze one side of the body (*hemiplegia*). Other cerebral dysfunctions that were mentioned with cerebral palsy may be associated with the stroke. The onset is usually sudden.

The local ischemia responsible for the stroke may be due to: (1) *thrombosis*—a blood clot forms on the arterial wall and obstructs blood flow (most common cause); (2) *embolism*—a bit of arterial wall, tissue fragment, or blood clot carried in the bloodstream gets wedged in an organ like the brain and blocks blood flow; or (3) *hemorrhage*—blood pumps from a ruptured artery into surrounding brain tissue; the pressure exerted destroys the brain tissue. The two major diseases leading to a stroke are atherosclerosis and hypertension.

Paralysis of a muscle or group of muscles is due to pathologic changes resulting from disease or injury in either the upper motor neuron within the brain and brain stem or the lower motor neuron within the spine and its periphery. Specifically, damage to the upper motor neuron causes *spastic paralysis,* and lower motor neuron damage causes *flaccid paralysis.* Furthermore, the degree and extent of the damage to the nervous system will determine the seriousness of movement impairment. There are four classifications, according to the limbs involved: the term *monoplegia* is used if one limb is involved; if half the body (both limbs on one side), *hemiplegia* is used; if both lower extremities, *paraplegia* is used; if all four extremities, *quadriplegia* is used.

Prior to World War II, a broken neck or back with severance of the spinal cord meant death, if not immediately from respiratory failure, then certainly within a short time from secondary infections. According to recent estimates, today there are thousands of paraplegics and quadriplegics. An estimated 125,000 persons have survived spinal cord injuries, and more than 10,000 are added to this population each year. The majority are young men and women; approximately 62 percent of spinal cord injuries happen to adults between sixteen and thirty years of age, with the greatest number of injuries (53 percent) occurring during the summer months. The apparent cause is high-velocity or high-risk activities such as fast driving, skiing, diving, and contact athletic events.[52]

Multiple sclerosis (MS), another neurological disease surrounded by myths, strikes people between the ages of twenty and forty. Almost twice as many women as men get the disease. It is a chronic, often disabling disease of the central nervous system affecting an estimated 250,000 Americans. It is not to be confused with muscular dystrophy. The course of the disease is unpredictable and varies from one MS person to another. For unexplained reasons, MS strikes most often in the world's colder regions. It is not fatal, it is not contagious, it is not hereditary, and in many instances it is not painful.

While the cause of MS is unknown, it generally progresses in a series of exacerbations and remissions, although it sometimes progresses rapidly, producing severe disability within a few years of onset. Exacerbations, attacks during which symptoms get worse or new symptoms appear, often last less than six weeks and are followed by periods of remission, sometimes lasting many years, during which symptoms remain the same or improve spontaneously. Motor symptoms are less likely to improve than sensory (touch, sight) symptoms.

Other disabling neurological diseases include poliomyelitis; meningitis, of which there are many forms; tumors of the brain and spinal cord; Parkinson's disease; Alzheimer's disease; and multi-infarct dementia. The latter two are discussed under emotional disturbances.

Circulatory System. There are three parts to the circulatory mechanism—the heart, blood vessels, and blood. The heart is the center of the circulatory system, pumping blood throughout the body. Since food is delivered and waste removed by the blood stream, the nutrition of the body depends upon the efficiency of the circulatory system. Interference with any part of this system therefore impairs the function of the body.

Three main conditions may result in cardiovascular (*cardio* = heart, *vascular* = blood vessel) disease: (1) endocarditis, an inflammation of the valves; (2) narrowing of the coronary arteries; and (3) high blood pressure. Examples of heart diseases due to these conditions include *rheumatic fever, bacterial endocarditis, coronary artery occlu-*

sion (heart attack), *hypertension, congestive heart failure, angina pectoris, atherosclerosis,* and *congenital heart disease.* Regarding the latter, each year more than forty thousand children are born with defects in the structure of the heart or of the large blood vessels connected to the heart.[53]

Of the above conditions, the commonest is *hypertension.* Approximately thirty-five million Americans are known to have high blood pressure.[54] High blood pressure may actually be a mild condition and in many cases never causes symptoms. However, in others damage results. Hypertension means that there is too much pressure in the bloodstream. It's like a garden hose with a too-tight nozzle. Eventually either the nozzle or the hose bursts, which is exactly what happens to blood vessels when the pressure is too great. If the vessel bursts in the heart, you have a heart attack; if it's in the brain, you have a stroke.

A *heart attack* occurs when the flow of blood is cut off or so severely limited as to cause destruction of cardiac tissue. Without oxygen and nutrients, heart cells die. Sometimes individuals believe they are having a heart attack when in fact they are having an *angina* attack. Chest pains occur during a temporary interruption in or a relative lack of the supply of oxygen to the heart, arising from narrowed coronary arteries. Considered a symptom rather than a disease, angina is a reversible form of ischemia (deficiency in blood supply) to the heart muscle. There is no death of muscle tissue.

Congestive heart failure is the result of the inability of the heart muscle to maintain adequate output, due either to disease of the heart muscle or disease of the heart valve. If the right side of the heart fails, the legs may swell (edema) from blood pooling in the veins. If the left side of the heart fails, fluid accumulates in the lungs. Often both sides of the heart fail at the same time. Symptoms include shortness of breath when exercising, swelling of the legs, poor appetite, weakness, and loss of energy.

The heart is aided in its work mainly by the arteries and, to a lesser extent, by the veins. The arteries are active, contractible organs that not only drive the blood on by a peristaltic contraction, but also control the pressure by narrowing or widening the vessel walls. The most common disease of the arteries, and one that causes much disability in middle age and later life, is *arteriosclerosis,* or hardening of the arteries. This is a physiological process of wear and tear that produces degeneration, calcification, and decrease in elasticity of the tissue. The changes in function that follow such changes can cause angina or a heart attack.

Varicosity is the most common disease of the veins. Women are affected more often than men. Causes include heredity, pregnancy, and obesity. In individuals who stand a great deal of the time, the valves of the leg veins wear out and eventually are unable to resist the pressure of the long column of blood that they are called upon to support. In these instances, the veins become tortuous and dilated, and we speak of them as *varicose veins.* Varicose veins may be unsightly but generally are not serious. If ignored, they can lead to other difficulties, such as phlebitis or ulcers at the site.

The function of the blood is to circulate constantly through the vessels, bringing to all tissues their needed supply of chemicals and bearing away the waste products of their metabolism. The blood cells originate in the hematopoietic system—namely, the bone marrow and lymphoid tissue. There are a number of blood and lymphatic diseases that cause disability. Blood disorders of importance here are pernicious anemia, sickle cell anemia, and hemophilia. *Sickle-cell anemia* results in chronic and severe anemia, jaundice, pain, and swelling of the abdomen and joints, with frequent infections. The disease may also cause damage to bones, kidney, heart, and lungs. *Hemophilia,* "the bleeding disease," is characterized by excessive repeated hemorrhages, both spontaneous and following light trauma, usually into muscles and joints, causing pain, swelling, and crippling affects. The condition is inherited, being transmitted only to males, but the gene is transmitted by females of the family. Hemophilia affects the knee joint more frequently than any other region.

Difficult and distressing lymphatic diseases are the leukemias. In spite of its name, leukemia is not a disease of the blood but essentially a generalized proliferative neoplastic disorder of the blood-forming tissues that usually results in a great increase in the white cells of the blood. Of the four types, two are common: *myelocytic leukemia* and *lymphocytic leukemia*. Either type may be acute or chronic. Children are more apt to be afflicted with *acute lymphocytic leukemia,* while adults more often contract the chronic form. Prognosis in both types is grave; however, chronic cases may live for ten or fifteen years.

Respiratory System. The respiratory system is responsible for taking oxygen into the body and giving off carbon dioxide. The organs concerned with this action are the nose, the pharynx, the larynx, the trachea, the bronchi, and the lungs. Of importance to us are those diseases that affect the bronchi and lungs.

Chronic bronchitis and *emphysema,* frequently grouped as chronic obstructive pulmonary diseases, result in an increasing number of disabilities each year. Individuals with chronic bronchitis and emphysema are partially or completely disabled for many years. Chronic bronchitis is a persistent or recurrent inflammation of the bronchial tubes. Emphysema is a disease in which the lungs lose their elasticity and cannot expand and contract normally to draw in and force out air. *Asthma* is another chronic obstructive respiratory disease, characterized by recurrent attacks of difficulty in breathing and a feeling of suffocation. Most attacks of asthma result from allergies, the individuals being hypersensitive or allergic to substances in the air they breathe or, less frequently, in the food they eat.

Although *tuberculosis* is not as prevalent as it once was, the number of new cases is declining only slowly. The most striking change in incidence is the shift from the young to the old. Some years ago a tuberculosis sanitarium resembled a college dormitory; today it is more like an old folks' home. A few generations ago it could be found in all socioeconomic classes. Today it is associated primarily with low-income groups, and black persons. It should be kept in mind that tuberculosis is not restricted to the lung but may involve every organ of the body. However, it is found more frequently in the lung since its chief method of spreading is coughing.

Cancer is the second leading cause of death in the United States, affecting every age group and almost any part of the body. It has been included here because cancer of the lung is the leading cause of death. Although lung cancer is much more common in men than in women, the rate of increase has been greater in recent years among women than men. The causes of cancer are varied, although there appears to be a link between cigarette smoking and cancer of the lung. Although the death rate from cancer has increased steadily over the years, many do not die immediately as a direct result of the disease.

The future seems to be more encouraging as a result of the discovery by genetic engineers of cancer-causing genes called oncogenes (*onkos* is Greek for "mass," as in the massing of malignant cells in a tumor). In the past, doctors believed that cancer was not one disease but many different diseases. Today they know that most cancers are probably caused by one or more of the twenty known oncogenes.[55]

The most common chronic lung disease in children is that accompanying *cystic fibrosis* of the pancreas. The crippling effect is due to the almost regular appearance of a chronic infection and an obstructive process in the lungs. The condition usually becomes manifest at birth or shortly thereafter. The majority of children with this disease appear thin and chronically ill. The thick secretions in the lung cause paroxysms of severe coughing. Exertion quickly leads to shortness of breath, and thus participation in more than mild exercise is difficult. Eventually the heart will be affected by lack of oxygen, and heart failure with general dropsy will slowly develop. By this time the child is bedridden.

Endocrine and Metabolic Disorders. A *gland* is an organ that secretes one or more substances serving the chemical or physiologic needs of the organism. Glands of internal secretion have no ducts but discharge their secretion by way of the veins and lymphatics with which they are abundantly supplied. They are called *glands of internal secretion, ductless glands,* or *endocrine glands.* They govern metabolism. A person cannot have a serious disturbance of one gland of internal secretion for any length of time without other glands becoming affected. Disturbances of endocrine glands may play a major or minor part in producing a disabling condition such as arthritis, certain epiphyseal disturbances, and various disorders of bone growth and development. For example, *hypothyroidism,* an underactivity of the thyroid gland, causes the individual to be sluggish and overweight. *Hyperparathyroidism,* an overactivity of the parathyroid glands, causes pain in bones and joints, weakness, and loss of muscle power and tone. *Addison's disease,* another glandular disabling condition, in which there is weakness, low blood pressure, darkening of the skin, and weakness of other systems, is the result of a deficiency of hormones from the adrenal glands.

Metabolism refers to all the changes in foodstuffs from the time they are absorbed from the small intestine until they are excreted as waste products from the body. The processes of metabolism are carried out by means of enzymes within the cells. Many of the cellular enzymatic reactions depend on the presence of vitamins and are regulated by hormones.

Two of the more common metabolic problems are *phenylketonuria (PKU)* and *dia-*

betes. In the former, an enzyme deficiency apparently prevents the proper metabolism of phenylaline, one of the essential amino acids. Its subsequent buildup causes irreversible brain damage if the condition goes untreated and results in mental retardation. Treatment consists mainly of special dietary measures throughout the early years of childhood.

Diabetes, a chronic disease, is a serious and common condition characterized by excess sugar, or glucose, in the blood. The high blood sugar stems from the inability of body tissues to use insulin. It is estimated that approximately 5 percent of the population—ten million Americans—have diabetes, and three million of these are juvenile diabetics. Diabetes is a major health problem in that it is increasing by 6 percent a year, is the direct cause of more than 38,000 deaths per year, and is a factor in perhaps 260,000 more.[56] It is the third leading cause of death by disease in the United States and the leading cause of blindness. There is no cure at present for this metabolic disorder, but it can be controlled once it is detected. Most diabetics can lead full, active lives.

There are two forms of the disorder: *insulin-dependent* or *type I,* often called *juvenile diabetes,* and *insulin-independent* or *type II,* also called *adult onset.* Type I affects children and young adults and is the more extreme though less common form of the two. It comes on more suddenly, is usually more difficult to control, and tends to run in families. *Insulin-independent* diabetes is characterized by a decrease in insulin receptors and an intracellular defect. As a person becomes overweight, the number of insulin receptors decrease. This form often strikes people over forty years of age who are overweight and affects more women than men. Because this type of diabetes develops gradually, symptoms often go unnoticed for many years before it is diagnosed. Heredity is a factor; overweight is the major risk element.

Serious complications may develop fifteen to twenty years after the disease begins regardless of form. The eyes, kidneys, nerves, and blood vessels are most affected. Problems include atherosclerosis, blindness, kidney failure, peripheral neuropathy, circulatory disorders, and increased incidence of infections.

All diabetics must eat meals on schedule and may be advised to have between-meal snacks. Strenuous exercise can decrease the need for insulin, and therefore onset of the illness may increase the need for such exercise. The therapeutic recreation specialist should always be on the lookout for symptoms suggesting the onset of a diabetic coma—irritability, pallor, trembling, blurred vision, perspiration, fatigue, confusion, and headache. The symptoms may be overcome or halted by quickly consuming sugar, fruit juice, candy, or a sweetened carbonated beverage (not diet). If the diabetic faints, get medical help promptly.

Another diabetic condition, which is just the opposite of diabetes, is *hypoglycemia* (low blood sugar). However, with proper diet and rest, this disease presents no major problem.

Allergic Conditions. The term *allergy* denotes an altered reactivity or a hypersensitiveness, natural or artificial, of an individual to a variety of substances introduced into the body. Allergens may be classified generally as follows: inhalants, foods, drugs and biologicals, infectors, contactants, and physical allergens.

It is estimated that thirty-five million Americans have some form of allergy. Allergies attack both men and women, young and old.[57] Individuals can develop an allergy at any time in their life. Fortunately, allergies are not contagious, but they can present problems and reduce activity, including recreative experiences.

Sensory Impairments

Sensory impairments are disorders of perception and communication. Special populations so affected include the visually impaired (blind and partially sighted) and the hearing impaired (deaf and hard of hearing).

Visual Impairments. Sight is the most important special sense that an individual has. According to the American Foundation for the Blind, it is estimated that about 6.4 million individuals in the United States have some type of visual impairment even with corrective lenses. They are categorized as having partial sight, residual vision, partial blindness, low vision, or reduced central vision. Of the 6.4 million, about 1.7 million are considered "legally blind"—having central visual acuity that does not go beyond 20/200 in the better eye with correcting lenses. Of these, nearly 450,000 are totally blind or have no usable vision at all. As a result of increased life expectancy, nearly 65 percent (one million) of the severely visually impaired are sixty-five years of age or older.[58]

Generally speaking, most of the severely visually impaired can perceive light and motion, and many can count fingers at arm's length. Some see only a portion of an object because their visual field is limited. Some can spot a pin on the floor but fail to see a moving van on the road.

The precise causes of blindness and severe visual impairment are unknown, although diseases, accidents, and heredity play their part. Individuals who are born blind are considered to be *congenitally blind;* those who become blind as the result of disease or accident are referred to as being *adventitiously blind.*

Some of the major causes of blindness in this country are as follows:

Glaucoma, which is caused by an abnormal accumulation of fluid in the eyes, produces elevated intraocular pressures that seriously impair vision. One out of every eight blind persons is a victim of this disease, and the percentage of black citizens with glaucoma is higher than in the general population. Glaucoma is responsible for much of the blindness after forty years of age, and the incidence may be as much as 17 percent higher in blacks than in whites between the ages of forty-five and sixty-four, according to the American Academy of Ophthalmology.[59]

Diabetes of long duration results in *diabetic retinopathy*. Despite insulin therapy, it is present in about 6 percent of people with diabetes. Diabetic retinopathy is the leading cause of blindness in the United States.[60]

Cataracts are opaque areas that develop on the lens. They develop chiefly in older individuals and represent part of the aging process.

Detached retina can interfere seriously with vision and may eventually cause blindness. The retina, which is essentially an extension of the optic nerve lining the interior of the eyeball, receives the light rays and transmits the impulses to the brain, where they register as sight. Injury or inflammation can cause a detached retina.

Retrolental fibroplasia, a form of blindness that formerly occurred among premature babies, has been virtually eliminated since physicians stopped administering oxygen in high concentrations to these babies.

Hereditary defects are the result of an inherited predisposition.

The causes of partial sight include not only the above but also refractive errors (*myopia* and *hyperopia*), developmental abnormalities of structures, defects in muscle function, and defects and injuries of the eye.

Hearing Impairments. In popular parlance, the term *deaf* is used to designate any type of auditory impairment, ranging from slight to profound. Actually, there are various categories of hearing impairment. For both educational and social purposes, the major classifications of hearing disabilities are *deaf* and *hard of hearing*. The division between the deaf and hard of hearing is a hearing loss of 75 to 80 dB in the better ear.[61]

The designation *deaf* represents a unique situation. Its singular quality stems from the fact that individuals so affected are the only ones of all the population for whom the major portion, if not the whole, of life development takes place without benefit of effective auditory contact with the environment. The *hard of hearing* are those whose hearing ability is significantly less acute than the normal individual but still great enough to be used for the understanding of verbal communication and contact with the environment.

At present, about one out of every ten, or twenty million people, in the United States has some form of hearing impairment, and over 200,000 cannot hear human speech.[62] The most recent figure given for the incidence of hearing disabilities among children suggests that 52,000 deaf children and 350,000 hard-of-hearing children under nineteen years of age are served in special education programs, and another 500,000 are in regular classrooms.[63] Impaired hearing may come on suddenly or gradually and may manifest itself in many ways.

A hearing disability present at birth is referred to as a *congenital hearing impairment*; one acquired after birth is referred to as an *acquired hearing impairment*. There are two basic types of hearing loss: *conducive type (conduction deafness)*, where there is some disturbance in the passage of sound through the outer or middle ear to the inner ear; and the *sensorineural type (nerve deafness)*, resulting from disease of the auditory nerve. The latter impairment may be partial or total, and it is irreversible. Infection is the major cause of both types; however, in the sensorineural type, aging and noise are contributing factors. *Otosclerosis* is a fairly common cause of conduction hearing loss. This condition prevents movement of the bones of the middle ear that transmit vibrations. Nerve deafness is often noticed in people sixty years of age and older, resulting from degenerative changes in the auditory nerve.

In addition to the obvious derangements of the ear that might ensue from a variety of physical traumas, acoustic trauma from loud and sustained noises can cause hearing loss.

Depending upon a person's needs and circumstances, hearing aids can be fitted in a variety of ways: behind the ear, in the ear canal, in the earpiece of eyeglasses, or elsewhere on the body. The most exciting development in recent years is *cochlear implants:* mechanical substitutes for defective hair cells in the ear that can translate incoming sound vibrations into electrical signals that are sent to the brain. Hearing aids today are also lighter and smaller, some small enough to fit into the outer ear canal. Furthermore, it now has been realized that the fit of the ear mold can be critically important to how well a hearing aid works.

The most widely used aids for the hard of hearing are devices that amplify the vibrations reaching the inner ear. Although hardly perfect, hearing aids have been improved in recent years; some can now compensate for specific insensitivities rather than amplifying all sounds equally, which would make some sounds too loud. Acoustical filters in the newer hearing aids amplify only those sounds the wearer has difficulty hearing, resulting in greater auditory comfort. The newer models are also equipped with directional microphones that screen out much of the background noise and produce sounds with much higher fidelity than in the past.

Speech and Language Disorders. Although they are not sensory impairments, it seems important to mention speech and language disorders. Recent estimates suggest that the incidence of these disorders among children is between 1.9 million and 2.5 million.[64] The American Speech and Hearing Association roughly estimates that phonological disorders (lisping, lalling) are the most frequent disorders, followed by disorders of speech flow (stuttering), language disorders, and voice disorders.[65]

In older persons deterioration of speech may be associated with a number of systemic diseases and toxic states, such as *Parkinsonism, multiple sclerosis, Huntington's chorea,* and *nutritional encephalopathy.*

Mental Disorders

Mental illness is probably the oldest and most baffling of human afflictions. The problem was first met, as one might expect, with sorcery and witchcraft, then with cruelty and incarceration, and until recently, merely with custodial care.

A recently completed study (1984) by the National Institute of Mental Health, found that 29.4 million Americans have some kind of mental disorder during any six-month period, although some of these problems may be mild or transient. The study also found that about 19 percent of all adults over the age of eighteen suffer from at least one psychiatric disorder, but fewer than 20 percent of them seek help. Men, contrary to previous studies and beliefs, have as many emotional disorders as women.[66] Mental illness accounts for a substantial percentage of divorces, crimes, work absenteeism, unemployment, and other personal troubles. According to one investigator, mental illness costs this nation $37 billion in direct expenses and lost wages annually.[67]

The problems connected with mental illness or disturbances were dramatized in 1972 by the controversy surrounding the nomination of Senator Thomas Eagleton as the Democratic vice-presidential candidate. When it was revealed that Eagleton had been treated for emotional problems, the issue grew so heated that he was forced to withdraw his candidacy.

It is often stated that half the beds in all hospitals are for the emotionally disturbed. In 1981, according to the American Hospital Association, there were 205,003 beds in psychiatric hospitals, of a total 250,892 beds in long-term hospitals. Further, psychiatric hospitals had the highest bed occupancy rate of all long-term hospitals.[68] These statistics, the reader should note, do not include individuals or beds in general medical and surgical hospitals or extended-care facilities (nursing homes).

Causes. Like many physical illnesses, mental illness includes not a single disorder but a host of them, and their classifications are far from clear-cut although this has dramatically changed in recent years, as we will note shortly. While the causes of mental illness are open to question in a technical sense, there is general agreement that mental illness involves both the body and the mind. In other words, some causes may be physical in nature (biological), some predominantly mental (emotional), and some a combination of the two. These disorders may range from mild and temporary to chronic and severe. Regardless of the causes, the result is a personality that behaves in an abnormal way. In fact, mental illness can encompass virtually any departure from what is considered normal or socially acceptable behavior. All of us behave abnormally, irrationally, and unrealistically at times; it is only when unusual behavior persists that mental illness may be indicated. In a stricter sense, mental illness generally describes mental or emotional disturbances that cause so marked an alteration in thought, mood, or behavior that the individual finds it difficult or impossible to meet the everyday requirements of living.

Individuals suffer emotional conflict whenever anything interferes with their adjustment to demands or pressures. These demands are usually of two kinds. One is primarily social or interpersonal, resulting from having to live interdependently with other persons. The second is primarily internal, arising in part from biological needs and in part from having learned from personal experience to desire certain kinds of social conditions, such as approval and achievement. The external demands are closely related to the internal ones, and usually excessive demands from one side produce a counteraction from the other. To live successfully requires coming to terms with external pressures as well as satisfying internal ones.

The study of mental disorders is typified by considerable uncertainty and in some cases profound disagreement. Experts differ among themselves in their appraisal of the nature and character of mental disorders, especially those of a psychological nature, even though more is known about all disorders than ever before. Considering the many explanations of abnormal behavior, Bootzin and Acocella have identified four major theories or perspectives resulting in abnormal behavior:

1. *The psychodynamic perspective,* which assumes that abnormal behavior issues from unconscious conflicts within the psyche, originating in childhood.

2. *The behavioral perspective,* which holds that the cause of abnormal behavior is inappropriate conditioning, whereby maladaptive behaviors are rewarded and adaptive behaviors are not rewarded.

3. *The humanistic-existential perspective,* which maintains that abnormal behavior results from a failure to accept oneself, to take responsibility for one's actions, and to pursue personal goals.

4. *The neuroscience perspective,* which analyzes abnormal behavior in terms of its biological components.[69]

The neuroscience perspective may also be referred to as the biogenic, resulting from malfunctioning within the body. In many respects the biogenic theory is associated with what is sometimes called the medical model. That is, the abnormal behavior is like a physical disease, and each abnormal behavior has a different disease, has specific causes, and has a set of symptoms. Therefore, treatment is of a physiological, organic, or medical nature, as opposed to a psychological approach, that is, psychotherapy.

Classification. The varieties of adjustive failure must somehow be classified and described, although a heated controversy has ranged for years over the role of diagnostic labels.[70] The classification of psychological disorders was initiated by German psychiatrist, Emil Kraepelain, in 1883. As described in his *Textbook of Psychiatry*, the disorders were primarily biological in nature. Some years later two French physicians, Ambrose Liebeault and Hypolytle-Marie Bernhein, through their work with hypnosis concluded that some psychological disorders might be due to emotional states rather than to organic states. In recent years, as a result of research, it has been suggested that some kinds of abnormal behavior thought to have an emotional base may very well have a biological base.[71]

During the past fifteen years the nosology (classification) of psychological disorders has undergone a significant evolution in the United States. The most recent and ambitious effort to revise the classification of psychological disorders is the revised third edition (1987) of the American Psychiatric Association's *Diagnostic and Statistical Manual of Mental Disorders (DSM-III-R)*. The manual includes more than two hundred mental disorders grouped in seventeen categories.[72]

The new edition improves upon earlier editions in several ways: the term *mental disorder* is carefully defined; diagnostic criteria are given for each disorder to increase the reliability of diagnosis; and new diagnostic entities have been created (and others deleted) to take into account discoveries in the last twenty years regarding the causes, natural history, and treatment responsiveness of many forms of mental disorder. Finally, and perhaps most important, the diagnostic criteria have been based for the most part on actual research-derived data, including longitudinal follow-up studies to establish validity and reliability, rather than simply being fashioned from the fabric of a particular theory structure.

A unique feature of the Manual is the introduction of a multi-axial descriptive system involving the use of five major *axes*, or areas of assessment. Axes I and II include all of the mental disorders. Axis III refers to physical disorders that relate to Axes I and II diagnosis or are felt to be relevant in some other way to the assessment or management of the patient. Axes IV and V are designed to provide the clinician with an enhanced view of a patient's individual needs and vulnerabilities regarding treatment and other management issues. Axis IV rates the magnitude and contribution of the stress factors to which the patient has been exposed during the year proceding onset or exacerbation of psychological dysfunction. Axis V consists of an assessment of the individual's highest level of psychological, social, and occupational functioning during the preceding year and currently as rated on a scale from 1 to 90.

The major components or diagnostic classes in DSM-III-R, Axes I–V are as follows:

AXES I AND II CLINICAL CONDITIONS

1. *Disorders usually first evident in infancy, childhood, or adolescence:* including intellectual, behavioral, emotional, physical, and developmental disorders.

2. *Organic mental disorders:* disorders caused by or associated with impairment of brain tissue function

3. *Substance use disorders:* including alcohol, drugs, and tobacco

4. *Schizophrenic disorders:* disorganized, catatonic, paranoid, undifferentiated, and residual

5. *Delusional (paranoid) disorders:* paranoia, shared, acute, and atypical paranoid disorders, respectively

6. *Psychotic disorders not elsewhere classified:* psychotic disorders that do not meet the criteria for organic, schizophrenic, paranoid, or affective disorders

7. *Mood (affective) disorders:* mood disorders with manic, depressive, or mixed (bipolar) symptomatology

8. *Anxiety disorders:* including panic phobias and obsessive compulsive disorders

9. *Somatoform disorders:* physical symptoms suggesting physical disorders

10. *Dissociative disorders:* including multiple personality and psychogenic fugue and amnesia respectively, and depersonalization disorders

11. *Sexual disorders:* including those paraphilia disorders associated with acting on or distressed by sexual urges and arousing fantasies involving either " . . . nonhuman objects, the suffering or humiliation of oneself or one's partner . . . , or children or other nonconsenting persons," as well as disorders of a sexual dysfunction and other psychosexual disorders

12. *Sleep disorders:* chronic disorders associated with disturbances in the amount, quality, or time of sleep and those which focus on an abnormal event that occurs during sleeping or between full wakefulness and sleep

13. *Factitious disorders:* disorders deliberately simulated by the individual for psychological gain (malingering is excluded because it aims at environmental gains)

14. *Disorders of impulse control not elsewhere classified:* including pathological gambling and kleptomania

15. *Adjustment disorders:* maladaptive reactions to psychosocial stress

16. *Personality disorders:* enduring, maladaptive patterns of relating to, perceiving, and thinking about the environment and oneself that cause significant impairment of social or occupational functioning or subjective distress

17. *Psychological factors affecting physical condition*

18. *Conditions not attributable to a mental disorder:* including academic problems, malingering, adult antisocial behavior, marital problems, occupational problems, and other life and circumstance problems

AXIS III
Physical Disorders and Conditions

AXIS IV
Severity of Psychosocial Stressors (boyfriend/girlfriend problems, marital problems, divorce, death of spouse, retirement, victim of rape, etc.)

Severity Rating Scale: none, mild, moderate, severe, extreme, catastrophic, and no information, inadequate information, or no change in condition.

AXIS V
Global Assessment of Functioning: associated with an individual's psychological, social, and occupational functioning on a numerical scale or continuum of mental health/illness at the present or current time and over the past year respectively.

Rating levels: Current GAF, 1 (serious) to 90 (absent or minimal symptoms), and Highest GAF, past year 1 to 90.[73]

Treatment. Just as there is no single accepted cause of mental illness, there is no accepted or preferred means of treating it. In some forms of therapy patients are helped to understand the psychological origin and meaning of their problems and apply this insight to their solution. In other forms, patients are taught new behaviors to replace the pathological behaviors that made them unhappy or ineffectual. In still other forms, patients are first treated medically so that their overt symptoms of behavior pathology are reduced or eliminated; psychotherapeutic treatment may proceed from that point.

The term *psychotherapy* embraces a multitude of treatment techniques and procedures carried on by a number of different professions. It may be defined as a form of treatment for problems of an emotional, behavioral, physiological, or environmental nature in which a person is assisted in removing, modifying, or retarding existing symptoms or disturbing patterns of behavior and in promoting positive personality growth and development. Since body, mind, and environment are so thoroughly intermeshed, psychotherapy must take into account all the important dimensions of human functioning—thought, emotion, behavior, and interaction with the environment.

There are four major types of psychotherapy:[74]

1. *Cognitive therapies.* These therapies seek to change, modify, or strengthen the thought processes in ways that are functional for the patient. Therapists usually do not deal with unconscious motivations and processes but rather with the thoughts that the patient is able to verbalize, based on the assumption that human beings strive to avoid unpleasant experiences and devise ways to explain traumatic-like experiences. Studies indicate that cognitive therapies are effective in treating depression, phobias, and some kinds of neurotic behavior. Types of cognitive therapy include rational-emotive therapy, cognitive behavior modification, psychoanalysis, transactional analysis, and person-centered therapy.

2. *Behavioral therapies.* The aim in these therapies is to change the person's behavior—with the expectation that feelings will change as a result—and focus on observable change. Techniques are primarily action focused, with the patient interacting with the therapist and others in the environment. Behavior therapy has been found to be effective in the treatment of maladaptive behavior and psychotics whose symptoms are in remission or controlled by medication. Types of behavioral therapies include behavior modification, assertion training, play therapy, reality therapy, modeling, role playing, and relaxation exercises.

3. *Affective therapies.* The aim in these therapies is to change the expression of feelings and emotions. Although cognitive and behavioral therapies talk about feelings and their change, such therapies do not direct their specific techniques to the identification, quality, or handling of feelings. Feelings are considered a byproduct, important but not central to therapy. Affective therapies are based on the assumption that, with a change in feelings, the person's behavior and thinking will change. The therapist is interested in facilitating emotional growth that will enhance the quality of life for the patient. Homeostasis and self-actualization are basic concepts. Treatment is terminated when the patient determines that desired solutions have been achieved. The treatment process requires time and effort, and the mode is a group approach. Gestalt therapy, psychodrama, encounter groups, and guided group interaction are some of the therapies that focus on affective change.

4. *Environment (milieu) therapies.* Direct intervention in the patient's environment is referred to as milieu therapy, environmental manipulation, environmental support, or therapeutic milieu. It is a viable methodology that focuses on changing or modifying the patient's environment, thereby effecting changes in thoughts, feelings, and behavior. Supportive group therapy, therapeutic recreation, vocational and social skill training, self-care training, behavioral therapies, affective therapies, and cognitive therapies represent a few of the specific techniques utilized in milieu therapy. The latter three techniques may be introduced into the milieu process by a therapeutic team or used in individual sessions. Some of the modes of treatment include foster home care for children and adults recently released from institutions, day-care treatment centers, halfway houses, group homes, and hospital or institutional placement. (Further con-

sideration of this approach will be given in Chapter 9.)

Another form of treating mental disorders is by *medically based therapies.* The student should not assume that a sharp line exists between treating individuals through psychotherapies when the abnormal behavior is considered psychological in nature, and medically based when the behavior is thought to be biologically or organically based. Many psychiatrists employ drugs as a way of calming the patient down so that a particular psychotherapy can be employed. Psychotherapeutic drugs are probably the most common treatment approach to mental disorders today. Of the three forms of medically based therapy two are used quite frequently, while the other one is mentioned only in passing.

1. *Psychopharmacology.* The introduction of effective psychotherapeutic drugs has been a significant factor in shaping mental health care and treatment since the 1950s. Of course, psychotherapeutic drugs are neither curative nor a panacea. In some cases they are totally ineffective or produce only minor symptom reduction; in other cases they cause adverse effects that outweigh any benefits obtained. Nonetheless, their existence has immeasurably advanced psychiatric treatment. When skillfully and judiciously used, psychotherapeutic drugs have an enormous potential for enhancing the quality of life, markedly improving global functioning, and improving the effectiveness of other concurrent modes of psychiatric treatment. (See Appendix B.)

2. *Electroshock, or electroconvulsive therapy (EST or ECT).* Not as popular as it once was as a result of the introduction of tranquilizing drugs, EST involves a brief period of unconsciousness following induction of a convulsion. The convulsion is produced by passing an electric current across the frontal portion of the ce-

rebral cortex for a fraction of a second. The current is delivered by means of electrodes attached to the patient's forehead. EST has been found to be most effective with patients suffering from depression, although positive results have been noted with other forms of mental disorders. In the opinion of many psychiatrists, its value is in treating psychotic patients. In most cases, EST is effective only when used in conjunction with other forms of psychotherapy.

3. *Psychosurgery.* The surgical procedure on the intact brain to relieve symptoms of mental disorders is rarely performed any more. There were many different forms of the procedure; however, their effectiveness has always been debatable and debated. We are reminded that ancient man also performed a version of psychosurgery called *trephining,* in which a hole in the brain was cut to permit the demons that presumably occupied the brain to be released.

   Other organic therapies—such as insulin coma, hydrotherapy, cold packs, and physical restraints—are seldom if ever used today; they have almost passed into history.

You may ask whether mental illness can be cured. This is a difficult question to answer. Some professional workers would say yes, while others would hedge, responding that the individual's ability to deal with the requirements of everyday living can be improved. Yet it goes without saying that recovery from mental illness, as from any illness, is dependent on many variables. How soon treatment is administered is one of them, the severity of the condition is another, and the type of illness is a third factor.

But the time has passed when people entered mental hospitals with little hope of ever leaving, and almost anyone suffering from a mental illness can expect to benefit measurably from treatment today. Several large health insurance companies report that the average stay for their policyholders is only sixteen days. Growing recognition of the problem, increased knowledge, better staffed hospitals, and advances in treatment have all helped to improve the outlook for the mentally ill.

Alcoholism and Drug Abuse

Chemical agents that alter consciousness have been widely used in many different societies throughout human history. They have served sometimes to facilitate socializing or celebrating among members of the tribe or community, and other times as an acceptable means of relaxation or escape for the individual from the problems and anxieties of daily existence. Until 1930 a liquid extract of marijuana could be found on many pharmacy shelves in the United States. It was a popular remedy with doctors and was prescribed for many complaints, including loss of appetite, "nerves," and depression. In addition, some religions have used beverages or drugs in their rituals as a means of achieving a closer union with their deities. It is not difficult to see all three of these aspects reflected in our society today.

Alcoholism. The suffix *-ism* means "excess." Alcoholism is a condition resulting from excessive indulgence in alcoholic beverages. It is a disease of addiction not really profoundly different from the craving for narcotic drugs. Alcoholics usually evolve gradually from social drinkers to excessive drinkers to alcoholics. In some cases alcoholics proceed to a stage where their brains or their bodies have been physically damaged by alcohol. This stage is called *chronic alcoholism.*

Alcoholism is one of this country's major medical-social-economic problems. It affects men and women, young and old, rich and poor, the urban person and the rural person. In short, alcoholism has no boundaries.

Who is and who is not an alcoholic is difficult to define since no studies exist that clearly differentiate an alcoholic from a nonalcoholic. Further, there is by no means a clear definition of what constitutes alcoholism. Alcoholics, in the opinion of some authorities, tend to be people who experience greater extremes of psychological discomfort than most other people; they have deep-seated feelings of inadequacy or are frequently anxious and depressed and, as a result, they drink to obtain temporary relief. On the other hand, there are those who find the alcoholic to be no different from the nonalcoholic, that alcohol provides little real symptom relief, and that it is the alcohol which causes the anxiety and depression. Still others believe the cause to be hereditary.[75]

Regardless of causes, when intoxication occurs repeatedly, invariably causing problems of personal health or interfering with psychological or social functioning of the individual in family, job, or community, the drinker can be considered a problem drinker. Problem drinkers who have developed a physical dependency on alcohol, or who have lost control over their ability to stop drinking once they have started, or who cannot refrain from drinking in inappropriate situations are usually alcoholic.

The most common statute definition of alcoholic is illustrated by Indiana's commitment law:

> The term "alcoholic" means any person who chronically and habitually uses alcoholic beverages to the extent that he loses the power of self-control with respect to the use of alcoholic beverages, or any person who chronically and habitually uses alcoholic beverages to the extent that he becomes a menace to the public morals, health, safety and welfare of the members of society in general.[76]

The exact number of alcoholics at any given time is impossible to determine. According to some recent investigators, 3 to 10 percent of the population will become alcoholic at one time or another in their lives, affecting one out of three families.[77] This statistic, to some degree, supports the 1972 *Medical World News* estimate that slightly less than ten million, or 4.6 percent of the population, were alcoholics.[78] Alcoholics Anonymous reports that 11.3 percent of its members are under thirty years of age, and that since 1974 the number of members in that age group have increased nearly 50 percent.[79] Among alcoholics, men outnumber women by a ratio of four to one in this country. However, the relative rates for women seem to be rising. Cirrhosis, chiefly a disease of alcoholism, takes roughly 26,000 lives each year.[80]

Drug Abuse. They have been smoked, chewed, injected, sniffed, and mainlined. They are referred to as a *joint, roach, H, coke, grass, smack, boo, meth, hog, super weed, cyclone, cadillac, downers, uppers, Red Devils, crack, horse, Dolly, bam, Black Beauties, Yellow Jackets, acids,* and *angel dust.* After they are used, an individual may become *strung out, on a trip, crash,* or *get busted by the narcs.* Strange terms? Not to those people who have experimented with, dabbled in, or abused certain drugs.[81]

The term *drug abuse* refers to drug taking that causes physical damage to the user, impairment of the user's ability to function in social situations or on the job, or behavior that is harmful to others. Such a drug is referred to as a *psychoactive drug,* since it alters a person's experience or consciousness—sensations, feelings, thoughts, or the function of the nervous system.

We are a drug-oriented society. Year after year pharmaceutical manufacturers have sales amounting to billions of dollars to satisfy a national demand for billions of prescription tablets and capsules. While there is no accurate report of the number of people who report having used drugs nonmedically, the cost to the nation according to one report is approximately $200 billion a year.[82] In addition, like alcoholism, there is a problem of definition.

Until 1906, when the Federal Pure Food and Drug Act was passed, there was no control over drugs. It was not until 1914 that the Congress of the United States passed the Harrison Act to control narcotic addiction.

The act did not make addiction illegal, but it did put controls on the production, manufacturing, and distribution of narcotics by imposing taxes. The Marijuana Tax Act of 1937 provided similar controls over marijuana. In 1965 the Drug Abuse Control Amendments extended the Federal Pure Food and Drug Act to control stimulant, depressive, and hallucinogenic drugs that may be subject to abuse.

Cocaine appears to be the latest star among dangerous drugs. Today some twenty-two million Americans have used cocaine. One report indicates that although twenty million Americans use marijuana regularly, it is falling from the best-seller list and cocaine is climbing.[83] American's appetite for drugs creates new products, new markets, new epidemics. The acceptance of these products and epidemics can only be born of ignorance. The experts say the solution is to abolish that ignorance.[84]

Aging

The elderly make up the fastest-growing group in the population. The number of people sixty-five and older increased 28 percent between 1970 and 1980. Every day some 5000 Americans celebrate their sixty-fifth birthday.[85] As of 1983, 27.4 million passed that mark; that's 11.7 percent of the population. A projected population estimate of people over age sixty-five by the year 2000 is from a low of 33.6 million to a high of 36.2 million.[86] The rapid increase in the number of older Americans will certainly affect their economic, social, and political roles and will bring about changes in their position in American society.

The dramatic increase in the size of the elderly population doesn't mean that people are living longer than they used to; in fact, today's sixty-five-year olds live only 4.4 years longer than their predecessors in 1900.[87] An infant girl today has a fifty-fifty chance of reaching age eighty, according to the *Journal of the American Geriatrics Society.*[88] A sixty-five-year-old man today can expect to live another fourteen years, while a woman the same age can expect to live another eighteen years.[89] If the number of deaths from heart disease, cancer, and stroke—major causes of death—can be reduced, the nation's elderly population will live significantly longer and will represent an even greater portion of the population.

The majority of older Americans are women. In the oldest age brackets, most women are widows, and many of them live alone. As of 1983, 50.3 percent of women over the age of sixty-five were widowed, compared to only 13.3 percent of the men; 40.9 percent of the women and 15.4 percent of the men lived alone.[90] By contrast, most elderly men lived with their wives. Men are less likely than women to face the disruption caused by a spouse's death and to live alone in a house that is more and more difficult to maintain.

The imbalance between the number of older men and older women becomes more pronounced as their ages increase. One result of this is seen in nursing homes, where three out of four patients are women. In addition, while only 5 percent of the elderly—about one million—are found in nursing homes and similar institutions, most elderly who enter nursing homes die there; the average stay is 1.1 years.[91]

Health is a major concern of the elderly. The elderly are particularly susceptible to respiratory infections; generally, aging contributes to the weakening of the body's protective responses to infection agents. Certain ailments—heart disease, cancer, and arthritis, for example—are more prevalent among the old. Alzheimer's disease and multi-infarct dementia are becoming major causes of death.

Elderly people spend more time in hospitals, fill a third of the nation's hospital beds, and visit physicians more frequently than the young and middle-aged adult. The 1985 House Select Committee on Aging reported that this country's elderly will spend approximately $2500 annually on health care by 1990—up from $1500 in 1984. The report

TABLE 2.6. The Changing Health Picture from 1983 to 2003

Life expectancy will increase from 74.5 years to 80 years.

An older population will mean 318 million more doctor visits each year.

The number of people with chronic health conditions will increase from 31.2 million to 45.8 million.

The number of days spent in hospitals will jump 48 percent to 406.8 million; hospital bills will rise 43 percent to $105 billion.

Nursing home residents will more than double to 2.8 million; costs for care will soar from $14.5 billion a year to $30.3 billion.

SOURCE: Joanne Poindexter, "Elderly, Sick, Not Synonymous: Most Feel Healthy," *Roanoke Times and World-News*, Oct. 19, 1983, pp. B1, B2.

also indicated that elderly Americans now spend 15 percent of their income on health care. In 1977 the figure was 12 percent. Further, it was estimated by the committee that by 1990 the nations' total nursing home bill will be more than $75 billion annually. As a result of the continued increase in health-care cost, it was projected by the committee that 63 percent of Americans age sixty-six and older who live alone on a set income would be impoverished after just thirteen weeks in a nursing home.[92] A capsule view of the future elderly health picture is given in Table 2.6.

SOCIAL-OFFENDER DISORDERS

Theories about the causes of crime are many, varied, and not definitive. Attempts to pinpoint a single or simple cause or even a constellation of causes are more likely to illuminate the bias of the investigator than to illuminate the behavior in question. Crime has been attributed to original sin, to possession by evil spirits, to mental disorders, to heredity, to alcohol and drugs, and to a "social predisposition." Such physical causes as endocrine imbalance, somatotypes, the double-Y chromosome, and "constitutional defects" are adduced by biological determinists. Sociologists emphasize ecological factors in delinquency areas, the concepts of role and status, the differing value system of subcultures, and the shifting roles of the family. Psychology and psychiatry call attention to emotional maladjustments and imperfectly controlled aggression.

According to Joseph Sheley, a well-known criminologist, sociologists have softened their view in recent years regarding the biological and psychological explanations of criminal behavior. It is now thought that, to a high degree, some physiological and psychological conditions may predispose some persons to violent behavior. However, the question of how nonsocial factors influence behavior has yet to be addressed.[93]

Whatever the theories, they fail to explain behavior deemed criminal by society. These societal theories may illuminate factors such as poverty, slum residence, membership in a minority group, low intelligence, or poor impulse control, but they do not adequately explain those who "get away with it" as a result of protection by influence or simply because they are never caught.

In sum, the question: What causes crime? is still unanswered, although there is considerable literature that studies criminal behavior.[94] Criminal behavior is not caused simply by biological or psychological disorders. Nor is it simply the result of such factors as poverty and lax parents. Better education or better this or better that will not eliminate crime or many other like problems. Complex problems rarely have simple solutions.

SUMMARY

This chapter considered a number of factors associated with special populations: the prevalence of special populations, the attitude of society toward special populations, the attitude of some special population members toward themselves, and the concept of health/disease and rehabilitation (resocialization)/punishment. The bulk of the chapter discussed in brief various biological, emotional, mental, and social conditions and disorders found in or associated with special population members.

Readers need to keep in mind that the onset and subsequent severity of most diseases typically depends on the combined effects of several factors. Within the pattern of causes related to any given disease, one may commonly find genetic, physical, emotional, and social factors. The typical coronary thrombosis provides the clearest example, as it often involves a genetically acquired deficiency of fat metabolism that is aggravated by socially derived eating habits, lack of sufficient physical exercise, and undue emotional stress resulting from family or job tension. Neurotic problems provide another fine example. By definition, neurotic conditions involve inappropriate reactions to emotional stress; however, social conflicts provide a common source of this stress. The potential effects of such physical factors as fatigue and poor nutrition are well known, and the contributing role of genetic factors is a widely supported possibility.

Regardless of the causes, these pathogenic activities involve either a direct attack upon tissue structure or an interference with the functioning of physiological or psychological processes.

What has just been stated about the combined cause of physical and mental diseases can also be stated about social disorders and the rehabilitation (resocialization) of the offender. The causation of crime is complex. It is influenced by the individual as well as the group, by biological factors as well as environment factors, and by the crime as well as the criminal.

NOTES

1. National Center for Health Statistics, *Chronic Conditions Causing Activity Limitations*, Public Health Service, U.S. Department of Health, Education, and Welfare, series 10, no. 51 (Washington, D.C.: U.S. Government Printing Office, 1969); and Lawrence D. Haber, *Social Security Survey of the Disabled: 1966*, U.S. Department of Health, Education, and Welfare Reports no. 2, 3, and 6 (Washington, D.C.: U.S. Government Printing Office, 1968–69).

2. Bureau of Census, *Disability, Functional Limitations and Health Insurance Coverage: 1984–85* (Washington, D.C.: U.S. Government Printing Office, December 1986).

3. "3 percent of Men in Correctional System in '85," *Columbus Dispatch*, Jan. 2, 1987, p. 9A.

4. Bureau of Census, *Statistical Abstract of the United States, 1985*, (Washington, D.C.: U.S. Government Printing Office, December 1984), p. 173.

5. Lois B. DeFleur, "Male Criminal Stereotype Fading," *South Bend Tribune*, Oct. 2, 1983, p. 8.

6. "Where Business Is Booming," *Parade*, Jan. 11, 1987, p. 18.

7. Joseph F. Sheley, *America's "Crime Problem"* (Belmont, Calif.: Wadsworth Publishing Co., 1985), p. 304.

8. *Statistical Abstract, 1985*, p. 182.

9. Cited in "Crime Study Says Juvenile System Is Found Ineffective," *Athens (Georgia) Banner-Herald*, July 9, 1978, p. 7.

10. Bernard G. Suran and Joseph V. Rizzo, *Special Children* (Glenview, Ill.: Scott, Foresman & Co., 1983), pp. 470–99.

11. E. H. Muth, "Prison Recreation in 1990," *Parks and Recreation*, 9, no. 9 (1974), 27–29.

12. U.S. Bureau of the Census, "Characteristics of the Low-Income Populations: 1973," *Current Populations Reports* (Washington, D.C.: U.S. Government Printing Office, 1975), pp. 159–62.

13. *Statistical Abstract, 1985*, pp. xxi, 430.

14. Clara G. Schiffer and Eleanor P. Hunt, *Illness among Children* (Washington, D.C.: U.S. Government Printing Office, n.d.).

15. M. A. Caliendo, *Nutrition and Preventive Health Care* (New York: Macmillan, 1981).

16. "Handicapped No Longer Act Like It," *New York Times*, Oct. 2, 1977, p. F6.

17. David Mechanic, "Stress, Illness, and Illness Behavior," *Journal of Human Stress* 2 (June 1976), 2–6.

18. Lee Meyerson, "Physical Disability as a Social-Psychological Problem," *Journal of Social Issues* 4, no.4 (1948), 2–10.

19. Mariann Soulek, "A Look at Stigmas and the Roles of Recreators and Physical Educators," *Journal of Physical Education and Recreation* 46, no.5 (1975), 28.

20. Beatrice A. Wright, *Physical Disability: A Psychological Approach* (New York: Harper & Row, Publishers, 1960).

21. Edward J. Hamilton, "An Examination of the Effects of Selected Integrated Leisure Activities on Able-Bodied Persons' Attitudes toward the Physically Disabled" (Master's thesis, University of Maryland, College Park, 1978), p. 28.

22. World Health Organization, "Constitution of the World Health Organization," in *Chronicle of the World Health Organization* 1 (1947), 3.

23. Cited in James H. Price, Nicholas Gali, and Suzanne Slenker, *Consumer Health: Contemporary Issues and Choices* (Dubuque, Iowa: William C. Brown Co., Publishers, 1985), p. 493.

24. An excellent review of the various theories of health and disease is given in James H. Price, Nicholas Gali, and Suzanne Slenker, *Consumer Health: Contemporary Issues and Choices* (Dubuque, Iowa: William C. Brown, Publishers, 1985), chap. 15.

25. Howard S. Hoyman, "An Ecologic View of Health and Health Education," in *Science and Theory of Health*, ed. Herbert L. Jones, Margaret B. Schutt, and Ann L. Shelton (Dubuque, Iowa: William C. Brown Co., Publishers, 1966), pp. 8–10.

26. René Dubos, *Mirage of Health: Utopias, Progress, and Biological Change* (New York: Harper & Row, Publishers, 1959), p. 25.

27. Judith G. Rabkin and Elmer L. Struening, "Life Events, Stress, and Illness," *Science* 194 (Dec. 3, 1976), 1013–20.

28. Barbara Baumann, "Diversities in Conceptions of Health and Physical Fitness," in *Social Interaction and Patient Care*, ed. James K. Skipper, Jr., and Robert C. Leonard (Philadelphia: J. B. Lippincott Co., 1965), pp. 206–10.

29. D. Rothman, *The Discovery of the Asylum* (Boston: Little, Brown & Co., 1971).

30. Ibid; also George G. Kassebaum, David A. Ward, and D. M. Wilmer, *Prison Treatment and Patient Survival* (New York: John Wiley & Sons, 1971).

31. Ibid; also Sheley, *America's "Crime Problem."*

32. Ibid; also Ronald J. Waldron, *The Criminal Justice System* (Boston: Houghton Mifflin Co., 1984).

33. The first estimate is from Jerry E. Wallin, "Prevalence of Mental Retardation," *School and Society* 86 (1958), 55–56; the second is from Henry B. Birch et al., *Mental Subnormality in the Community: A Clinical and Epidemiological Study* (Baltimore: Williams & Wilkins Co., 1970), p. 31.

34. Cited in Patricia T. Cegelka and Herbert J. Prehm, *Mental Retardation: From Categories to People* (Columbus, Ohio: Charles E. Merrill Publishing Co., 1982), p. 15.

35. L. M. Dunn, "Special Education for the Mildly Retarded—Is Much of It Justifiable?" *Exceptional Children* 35 (1968), 5–22; President's Committee on Mental Retardation, *The Six-Hour Retarded Child* (Washington, D.C.: U.S. Government Printing Office, 1970); and Nancy Haring, *Behavior of Exceptional Children,* 2nd ed. (Columbus, Ohio: Charles E. Merrill Publishing Co., 1978).

36. J. Mercer, *Labeling the Mentally Retarded* (Berkeley: University of California Press, 1973).

37. Ibid; also Harry B. Birch et al., *Community: A Clinical and Epidemiological Study* (Baltimore: Williams & Wilkins Co., Publishers, 1970).

38. D. L. MacMillan, *Mental Retardation in School and Society* (Boston: Little, Brown, 1977); and D. L. Mumpower, "Sex Ratios Found in Various Types of Referred Exceptional Children," *Exceptional Children* 36 (1970), 621–22.

39. American Association on Mental Deficiency, *Sociobehavioral Studies in Mental Retardation,* Monographs of the American Association on Mental Deficiency, no. 1 (b) (Washington, D.C.: the association, 1973).

40. Ibid.

41. Herbert Grossman, ed., *Manual on Terminology and Classification in Mental Retardation* (Washington, D.C.: American Association of Mental Retardation, 1973), p. 5.

42. Ibid, p. 11.

43. Ibid., p. 12.

44. Ibid., pp. 29–33.

45. L. W. Garnett, "Osteoporosis Becoming Major Medical Problem," *Roanoke* (Virginia) *Times and World News,* Jan. 11, 1987.

46. *Facts on the Major and Crippling Diseases in the United States Today,* National Health Education Committee (1971).

47. N. R. Kleinfield, "Arthritis 'Industry' Derives a Huge Livelihood from Hope," *Roanoke Times and World News,* Sept. 1, 1985.

48. Paula Dranov, "A New Drug that Relieves the Pain of Arthritis," *Family Weekly,* Jan. 21, 1979, p. 23.

49. "Hotline," *Parade,* Nov. 16, 1986, p. 28.

50. Keith Coulbourn, "MCG Helps Epileptics Out of the Closet," *MCG Today,* 8,no.1 (Spring 1979), 3–9.

51. *1986 Heart Facts* (Dallas: American Heart Association, 1985), p. 2.

52. *Consequences—Spinal Cord Injury* (film), sponsored by Regional Spinal Cord Injury Center, University of Washington, Seattle (Aspen, Colo.: Crystal Productions, 1979).

53. American Heart Association, *Cardiovascular Diseases in the United States—Facts and Figures* (New York: the association, n.d.).

54. "The Heart: An Amazing Pump," *For Your Good Health,* (Radford Community Hospital), Winter 1984–85, p. 1.

55. Earl Ubell, "A World without Disease," *Parade,* Jan. 27, 1985, special section.

56. "Detection and Care: Keys to Controlling Diabetes," *For Your Good Health* (Radford Community Hospital), Fall 1984, p. 1.

57. M. Clark, D. Shapiro, and J. J. Lindsay, "Allergy—New Insights," *Newsweek,* Aug. 23, 1982, pp. 40–45.

58. American Foundation for the Blind, *Facts about Blindness* (New York: the foundation, n.d.), p. 5.

59. Paul Donohue, "Your Health," *Roanoke Times and World News,* May 31, 1985.

60. American Foundation for the Blind, *Facts about Blindness,* p. 7.

61. Bernard G. Suran and Joseph V. Rizzo, *Special Children* (Glenview, Ill.: Scott, Foresman & Co., 1983), p. 215.

62. "Deafness Is among Worst of Disabilities," *Roanoke Times and World News,* Oct. 14, 1985.

63. Ibid.

64. P. A. Craig, "Counting Handicapped Children: A Federal Imperative," *Journal of Educational Finance* 1 (1976), 318–39; also Hobbs, *Futures of Children,* p. 561.

65. Cited in Suran and Rizzo, *Special Children,* p. 230.

66. "Mental Illness Afflicts 20%, Researchers Say," *Roanoke Times and World News,* Oct. 3, 1984.

67. Tad Bartimus, "Schizophrenia," *Roanoke Times and World News,* Feb. 6, 1983.

68. Cited in U.S. Department of Health and Human Services, *Health—U.S. 1982* (Washington, D.C.: U.S. Government Printing Office, PHHS publ. no. (PHS) 83–1232, Dec. 1982), p. 111.

69. Richard R. Bootzin and Joan Ross Acocella, *Abnormal Psychology,* 4th ed. (New York: Random House, 1984), p. 8.

70. T. Szasz, *The Myth of Mental Illness* (New York: Harper & Row, Publishers 1961).

71. Bootzin and Acocella, *Abnormal Psychology,* p. 8.

72. American Psychiatric Association, *Diagnostic and Statistical Manual of Mental Disorders,* 3rd ed., Revised (Washington, D.C.: American Psychiatric Association, 1987).

73. Ibid., pp. 3–12. Copyright 1987 American Psychiatric Association. Reprinted with permission.

74. LeNora B. Mundt, "Mental Health Treatment Methods," in *Handbook on Mental Health Administration,* ed. Michael J. Austin and William E. Hershey (San Francisco: Jossey-Bass, Publishers, 1982), pp. 42–47.

75. George E. Vaillant, *The Natural History of Alcoholism* (Cambridge, Mass.: Harvard University Press, 1983), pp. 1–182; E. Mansell Patteson and Edward Kaufman, eds., *Encyclopedic Handbook of Alcoholism* (New York: Gardner Press, 1982); and Donald W. Goodwin, *Alcoholism: The Facts* (New York: Oxford University Press, 1981), pp. 29–130.

76. Indiana State Statutes *Burns,* 22 (Indianapolis, Ind.: Bobbs-Merrill, Inc., 1957), p. 1052b.

77. U.S. department of Health and Human Services, *The Fourth Special Report to the United States Congress on Alcohol and Health* (Washington, D.C.: Alcohol, Drug Abuse, and Mental Health Administration, Jan. 1981), p. 3.

78. "Alcoholism: Age of Enlightenment?" *Medical World News* 13 (March 17, 1972), 6.

79. "Drinking Generation," *Parade,* Nov. 12, 1978, p. 19.

80. Michael Watterlond, "The Telltale Metabolism of Alcoholics," in *Health 84/85* (Guilfork, Conn.: Duskin Publishing Group, 1984), p. 79.

81. For additional terminology, see *Glossary of Terms in the Drug Culture,* Bureau of Narcotics and Dangerous Drugs, U.S. Department of Justice (Washington, D.C.: U.S. Government Printing Office, 1972).

82. John A. Barbour, "What You Don't Know Can Hook You," *Roanoke Times and World News,* Nov. 23, 1986.

83. Ibid.

84. Ibid.

85. John Barbour, "Taking a New Look at Growing Old," *Roanoke Times and World News,* March 14, 1982. Pp. xxii, 27.

86. *Statistical Abstract, 1985,* pp. xxii, 27.

87. Joanne Poindexter, "Elderly Sick, Not Synonymous; Most Feel Healthy," *Roanoke Times and World News,* Oct. 19, 1984.

88. Cited in ibid.

89. Ibid.

90. *Statistical Abstract, 1985,* p. 456.

91. "The Aged: Rising Challenge To A Nation," *Chicago Tribune,* Sept. 24, 1978.

92. Associated Press, "Health Care Still a Burden to Elderly," *Roanoke Times and World News,* July 30, 1985.

93. Sheley, America's *"Crime Problem,"* p. 212.

94. Ibid., p. 213.

SUGGESTED READINGS

ALBRECHT, GARY L., ed. *The Sociology of Physical Disability and Rehabilitation.* Pittsburgh: University of Pittsburgh Press, 1976.

AMERICAN PSYCHIATRIC ASSOCIATION. *Diagnostic and Statistical Manual of Mental Disorders, Third Edition, Revised.* Washington, D.C.: American Psychiatric Association, 1987.

BAROSH, D. P. *Aging: An Exploration.* Seattle: University of Washington Press, 1983.

BATSHAW, M. L., and Y. M. PERRET. *Children with Handicaps: A Medical Primer.* Baltimore: Paul H. Brookes, Publishers, 1981.

BEAN, P. *Mental Illness: Changes and Trends.* New York: John Wiley & Sons, 1983.

BIRKERSTOFF, E. R. *Neurology* (3rd ed.). New York: ARCO Publishing Co., 1982.

BOOTZIN, R. R. *Abnormal Psychology: Current Perspectives* (3rd ed.). New York: Random House, 1980.

BOWE, FRANK. *Handicapping America: Barriers to Disabled People.* New York: Harper & Row, Publishers, 1978.

CHALKLEY, T. *Your Eyes.* Springfield, Ill.: Charles C Thomas, Publishers, 1974.

CRANDALL, R. C. *Gerontology: A Behavioral Approach.* Reading, Mass.: Addison-Wesley Publishing Co., 1980.

"The Crime Wave," *Time,* June 30, 1975, pp. 10–24.

DOLFMAN, M. L. "Toward Operational Definition of Health," *Journal of School Health* 44 (1974), 201–13.

DOUGLAS, J. *The Sociology of Deviance.* Boston: Allyn & Bacon, 1984.

DUBOS, RENÉ. *Man, Medicine and Environment.* New York: Praeger Publishers, 1968.

DUNN, H. L. *High Level Wellness.* Washington, D.C.: Mt. Vernon Publishing Co., 1961.

FEINGOLD, B. A., ed. *Developmental Disabilities of Early Childhood.* Springfield, Ill.: Charles C Thomas, Publisher, 1978.

GOLDENSEN, ROBERT M., ed. *Disability and Rehabilitation Handbook.* New York: McGraw-Hill, 1978.

GOODE, E. *Deviant Behavior* (3rd ed.). Englewood Cliffs, N.J.: Prentice-Hall, 1984.

GROSSMAN, H. J. *Manual on Terminology and Classification in Mental Retardation.* Washington, D.C.: American Association on Mental Deficiency, 1977.

HAMILTON, EDWARD J., and STEPHEN C. ANDERSON. "Effects of Leisure Activities on Attitudes toward People with Disabilities," *Therapeutic Recreation Journal,* 17, no.3 (1983), 50–57.

HARRIS, C. *Fact Book on Aging: Profile of American's Older Population.* Washington, D.C.: National Council on the Aging, 1978.

HESS, B., and E. MARKSON. *Aging and Old Age: An Introduction to Social Gerontology.* New York: Macmillan, 1980.

HOLE, JR., J. W. *Human Anatomy and Physiology* (3rd ed.). Dubuque, Iowa: William C. Brown Co., Publishers, 1984.

HOYMAN, H. S. "Our Modern Concept of Health," *Journal of School Health,* 45, no.9 (1975), 509–18.

JOHNSON, ELMER H. *Crime, Correction, and Society* (4th ed.). Homewood, Ill: Dorsey Press, 1978.

KART, C. S., E. S. METRESS, and J. F. METRESS. *Aging and Health—Biological and Social Perspectives.* Reading, Mass.: Addison-Wesley Publishing Co., 1978.

KERSON, TOBA S. Understanding Chronic Illness, New York: Free Press, 1985.

KOESTLER, FRANCES A. *The Unseen Minority: A Social History of Blindness in the United States.* New York: David McKay Co., 1976.

LAFFERTY, J. "A Credo for Wellness," *Health Education* 10 (1979), 10–11.

MATTSON, P. H. *Holistic Health in Perspective.* Palo Alto, Calif.: Mayfield, 1982.

MONK, C. J. *Orthopedics for Undergraduates.* New York: Churchill Livingston, 1981.

NELSON, W. et al. *Textbook of Pediatrics.* Philadelphia: W. B. Saunders Co., 1979.

STOLOV, W. C., and M. A. CLOWERS, eds. *Handbook of Severe Disability.* Seattle: University of Washington Press, 1981.

STUBBINS, JOSEPH, ed. *Social and Psychological Aspects of Disability: A Handbook for Practitioners.* University Park, Pa.: University Park Press, 1977.

SURAN, BERNARD G., and JOSEPH V. RIZZO. *Special Children: An Integrative Approach.* Glenview, Ill.: Scott, Foresman & Company, 1979.

WRIGHT, B. *Physical Disability: A Psychological Approach,* New York: Harper & Row, Publishers, 1960.

ZARIT, S. H. *Aging and Mental Disorders.* New York: Free Press, 1983.

3

Agencies and Institutions Providing Service to Special Populations

We naturally tend to think of rehabilitation progress as the removal or mitigation of the end effects of disease or injury, the number retrained to work and participate in activities of daily living, the rapid numerical growth of education programs for handicapped children, the individuals who go straight after serving prison sentences, or the recognition of the needs of the disabled and disadvantaged. However, the key contributors to this progress are the organizations, facilities, personnel, and services that assist the individual in reaching the maximum physical, emotional, social, intellectual, and vocational potential. Concerted action for rehabilitation can be attained only through a quality care delivery system designed to overcome the effects of the problem.

This chapter considers those contributors to rehabilitation, first, from a health and health-related perspective, thereafter, from a correctional view. In addition, the quality of the contribution is also discussed.

HEALTH AND HEALTH-RELATED FIELDS

ORGANIZATIONS

The past four decades have seen more publicity, more legislation, more money appropriated, and more community campaigns related to meeting and serving the needs of special populations than at any other period in our country's history. Over the years many organizations have been established in response to the obvious need for service and rehabilitative action, of either a governmental or a nongovernmental nature. Furthermore, they are usually directly concerned not with rendering a specific service but rather with the social and political incentives for planning and organizing specific services to special populations.

Governmental Organizations

The national government has only certain limited powers granted to it by the Constitution. The protection and welfare of individuals are responsibilities reserved for the states by the Constitution. The various state legislatures meet these responsibilities by establishing departments or boards at the state level through appropriate legislation and by

47

encouraging and supporting the development of local departments, when necessary, for delivery of direct services to individuals.

Government at all jurisdictional levels (federal, state, and local) in the United States is involved in health-care services to a much greater degree now than in the late 1940s. Even so, our government is less involved in health care than the governments of most other industrialized countries. Among the many reasons for this difference, perhaps the most important is the strength of the private sector and its opposition to "government control and interference" except in select areas, such as care of the sick poor and care of the mentally ill and mentally retarded. Restricted as the government's role is, however, on an absolute scale it looms rather large. This role has developed and expanded as the result of such initiatives as Medicare and Medicaid, planning acts, new regulatory powers, and support of various kinds of biomedical research and health profession education.

Most of this section deals with the three jurisdictional levels of government as they relate to those agencies providing service to special populations and the legislative acts within which the services function. The federal government generally provides service to specific categories of persons: merchant seamen, American Indians, veterans, members of the uniformed services and their families, and so on. State governments generally provide service for categories of disease: mental illness, mental retardation, and diseases of a long-term or chronic nature. Local governments generally provide service to the lower socioeconomic class and the medically indigent, although there are a large number of local governmental hospitals that provide service to people regardless of socioeconomic class. There is some overlapping: the federal government does provide service to those afflicted with leprosy and drug abusers and operates St. Elizabeth's Hospital, a mental institution in the District of Columbia; governments at all levels provide health service for prisoners, but the distinction holds for the most part.

On the other hand, certain activities are shared with the private sector. In public health education the voluntary agencies—for example, the Cancer Society and the Heart Association—are very important. Private institutions, of course, play a vital role in health sciences education and research through grants and contracts given by governments. Lastly, governments pay providers on an item-of-service basis for the delivery of care to third parties under Medicare and Medicaid.

Federal. Because of its constitutional authority, the federal government has gradually developed a formidable array of agencies and bureaus. The development of field health services began in the eighteenth century, when the thirteen colonies depended on the seas for both protection and trade. To encourage enlistments and expansion of the small merchant marine, the government established a Marine Hospital Service within the Department of the Treasury to provide medical care for seamen when they came ashore. As our frontiers moved westward, extension of public health services soon became necessary because of widespread epidemics of yellow fever, smallpox, and cholera. With the evolution from a rural to an urban civilization, it became apparent that some public health organization would have to be responsible for studying and regulating the relationship of people to their total environment.

In 1912 the Marine Hospital Service (established in 1798) was disbanded, and the U.S. Public Health Service was established. It is interesting to note that this branch of government still fulfills its historic function, controlling the marine hospitals for the benefit of members of the merchant marine. In 1939 the government's activities in the fields of health, education, and welfare were transferred to the Federal Security Agency. In 1953, under President Dwight D. Eisenhower's administration, most of the health activities were brought together as part of the newly created Department of Health, Education, and Welfare (HEW). However, HEW went out of existence in 1980 as a result of being labeled unmanageable by many critics and was replaced by two departments: the Department of Health and Human Services (HHS) and the new Department of Education.

Within HHS there are many divisions, agencies, institutes, bureaus, and offices. Of note is the National Institutes of Health (NIH) at Bethesda, Maryland, which is responsible for supporting and carrying out health research through its eleven institutes. It has an intramural research program on its campus and supports research through extramural grants and contracts. NIH also fosters research by supporting training, resource development, and construction. At Bethesda patients participate in research in cancer, heart, lung and blood disorders, mental illness, arthritis, metabolic and digestive diseases, neurological diseases, eye disorders, allergy and infectious diseases, dental diseases, child health and human development, and aging. Other agencies and offices include the Health Service Administration, Bureau of Quality Assurance, Bureau of Health Planning and Resource Development, and National Institute on Alcohol Abuse and Alcoholism.

Apart from HHS, other government agencies carry on important activities related to health and health protection. Ten million people are eligible to receive their health care under the auspices of the Department of Defense; these are military personnel on active duty and their dependents, survivors of active duty personnel, retirees, and dependents and survivors of retirees. The Veterans' Administration (VA) is another independent agency reporting directly to the President. The VA operates the largest centrally directed hospital and clinic system in the United States. The origins of the VA can be traced back to a 1776 report

of a committee of the Continental Congress that recommended establishing provision for those persons wounded or disabled "in the land or sea service. . . . " By 1789 the federal government took over such responsibilities.[1]

Legislation. Health-care legislation as it has developed in our democratic society over the past 196 years has been an interesting and many-faceted process. It has involved vested interest groups that have reflected the climate of the times and the various forces that act and react on a particular environment. Social legislation originates with a specific need and, given the legislative process and the influence of political forces, often requires decades for completion. Legislation does not just happen; it is a result of the relationship of six elements at work in the total process—conceptualization of an idea, political support, leadership, negotiation, public debate, and finally, decision making. The political process in a democratic system is founded on laws that represent the collective decisions of the community. Our discussion of legislation will focus on health-related legislation as such, the legislative process, and the role of the lobbyist. The latter two, as will be pointed out shortly, are important for the therapeutic recreation specialist to know as a special population advocate and change agent.

It was not until 1918 that Congress enacted the first nationwide rehabilitation act: the Smith-Sears Veterans Rehabilitation Act. This act provided vocational training and placement for disabled veterans of World War I. This act for disabled veterans was destined to play a major role in the establishment and development of services for the civilian disabled, including recreation services.

In 1920 Congress passed the Vocational Rehabilitation Act, which provided vocational training, counseling, and job placement for disabled civilians through federal grants to each state. Since then there have been many amendments to this act. Of special note was the 1963 revision, which incorporated training and research funds in the area of recreation for the disabled. This was the first recognition by a federal agency of the importance of recreation services for the disabled. As a result of these funds, specialized training programs in therapeutic recreation were implemented at the graduate level in several colleges and universities.

The Vocational Rehabilitation Act was revised considerably with amendments in 1973. The 1973 amendments included retitling the law to the Rehabilitation Act, which focused on the total rehabilitation of *all* disabled not just on vocational rehabilitation. It provided for a study of services for individuals for whom vocational rehabilitation is not a feasible goal because of their severe limitations, but who can improve their ability to live independently through rehabilitation. The act continued the authorization for funding of recreation services in training and research. Of particular interest from a recreation-service perspective was Title III, Section 304 (Special Projects and Demonstrations), Title V, Section 502 (Architectural and Transportation Barriers), and Title V, Section 504 (Nondiscrimination under Federal Grants). The Special Projects and Demonstration section includes the authorization of grants for "operating programs to demonstrate methods of making recreational activities fully accessible to handicapped individuals."[2] The Architectural and Transportation Barriers Compliance Board was created through this act to insure compliance with the Architectural Barriers Act of 1968 (PL 90–480). In addition, the act asked the board to "investigate and examine alternative approaches to ... barriers confronting handicapped individuals, particularly with respect to public buildings and monuments, parks and parkland. ..."[3] In 1978 the board ruled and won a court action against the National Park Service regarding the accessibility of the National Visitors Center in Washington, D.C.[4]

A major effort to provide greater opportunity for individuals with disabilities and impairments to enjoy and participate in recreation and leisure programs and services was afforded through Section 504, which required that federal-fund recipients make their programs and activities accessible to the handicapped. Section 504 of the act states:

> No otherwise qualified handicapped individual in the United States . . . shall, solely by reason of his handicap, be excluded from the participation in, be denied the benefits of, or be subjected to discrimination under any program or activity receiving federal financial assistance.[5]

Section 504 covers all grant programs from general revenue sharing to categorical grants. It also defines handicapped individuals broadly, including physical and mental disabilities, diseases such as cancer, diabetes and heart ailments, and conditions such as alcoholism and drug abuse. It includes individuals who have a record of a handicap and those who are regarded as disabled even if they are normal.

Since the passage of the 1973 Rehabilitation Act, amendments to Section 504 have further guaranteed rights to persons who are disabled. The amendment to the 1974 Rehabilitation Act (PL93–516) authorized the planning and implementation of the White House Conference on Handicapped Individuals. Recreation was one of sixteen major areas of concern when the participants met in 1977. The 1978 amendment (PL95–602) to the act contained six separate sections which addressed recreation and leisure services. Three of these sections were a carryover of 1973 programs, but the other three were newly authorized programs. One considered the inclusion of recreation as a service to be provided in rehabilitation facilities; another, grants to public and nonpublic agencies for special project demonstrations and evaluations; and the last, making funds available for the development of comprehensive services to disabled individuals not served by other titles of the law. This includes the elderly, blind, and severely disabled who are not eligible for vocational rehabilitation. Recreation and leisure services were included within the intent of comprehensive services.[6]

Equally as important as the Rehabilitation Act, if not more so from a recreation-service recognition and funding perspective, is the enactment of education legislation. The Education for Handicapped Children Act of 1967 (PL90-170) created funds for the development of training programs in adapted physical education and therapeutic recreation under a provision titled "Research and Training in Physical Education and Recreation Programs for Mentally Retarded and Other Handicapped Children." This provision also established the Unit on Physical Education and Recreation for Handicapped Children within the Bureau of Education for the Handicapped.

In 1975 the Education for Handicapped Children Act was amended by PL94-142 (Education for All Handicapped Children Act). This act required that all handicapped children ages three to twenty-one starting in 1980 be provided a free appropriate public education and included recreation as a related service area. Recreation services must be provided as a support service in schools, institutions, or the child's home to assist the handicapped child to benefit from special education. According to many educators, this act was by far the most significant education law passed in the last two decades. Recreation professionals felt the law had great importance to the field of recreation. It was the first time recreation had been included in education legislation.

Other Significant Legislation. A legislative act that has marked social and economic significance for the disabled or those with specific health-related impairments by providing sanctions and support for services of a recreation and leisure nature is the Social Security Act (SSA) of 1935. Despite its limitation to the aged and to certain carefully defined categories of needy or medically needy persons, its impact on every aspect of the provision of health or medical care has been tremendous.

What may have been the first government health insurance program in the United States was established by Congress in 1798, when merchant marine personnel were required to contribute a few cents a month to pay for hospital care provided by a new marine hospital. It was not until the early twentieth century, however, that the idea of compulsory health insurance for the general public gained serious attention. Various attempts to enact government-sponsored health insurance programs from 1917 until 1965 were met with considerable opposition, even though the Social Security Act provided a broad range of social insurance and public assistance programs.[7]

As finally passed by Congress July 28, 1965, the amendments (PL89-97) to the SSA provided for two additional titles: Title 18 (Medicare) and Title 19 (Medicaid). Initially, Medicare provided hospitalization and medical insurance for those age sixty-five and over who were eligible for Social Security or railroad retirement benefits. Since 1972 this coverage has been extended to disabled Social Security beneficiaries and persons afflicted with chronic kidney disease, regardless of age. Medicaid, on the other hand, is a public assistance program that uses state and local tax money as well as federal funds to provide medical care to the poor.

The importance of both Medicare and Medicaid to therapeutic recreation is that the programs authorize payment for a wide range of services, including therapeutic recreation service in psychiatric facilities, extended care facilities, and others.

Major amendments to the Medicare and Medicaid program were included in the Social Security Amendments of 1972 (PL92-603). One, the Professional Standards Review Organization (PSRO), mandated an evaluation system to improve the quality of health care and monitor health costs under Medicare, Medicaid, and Maternal Child Health programs. As a result of this amendment, statewide PSRO councils were established to develop criteria and evaluate the effectiveness of health services. The councils were also responsible for establishing advisory groups consisting of health-care practitioners other than physicians.

In 1983 a new Medicare hospital payment system was established with the intent to save money for both patients and hospitals by setting flat fees for each illness. The new system breaks down all illnesses into 467 diagnosis-related groups (DRGs). Hospitals receive the same fee for each DRG they treat. The system is intended to save money by giving hospitals an incentive to send patients home sooner.

Currently, many legislative proposals concerning health issues are being debated. One of the most controversial is national health insurance. Although several bills have been introduced to help consumers deal with the rising cost of health care, no consensus has been reached concerning the type of system to adopt. Some of the proposals favor strict governmental-control responsibility, while others support control by private insurance groups like Blue Cross and Blue Shield. The inclusion of direct payment, or third-party payment, is a major concern for all health-care providers, including therapeutic recreation specialists. Without this provision, these health-care providers would have decreased control over health-care costs. This could result in a decrease in quality of patient care since the major control of care would not rest with the entire health-care team.

The Legislative Process. During each two-year congressional term literally thousands of legislative proposals are introduced by members of the House and Senate. Any member of either house can submit a bill for consideration by his or her house on any subject. These bills can be written by the member, his or her staff, lobbyists, members

of the executive branch, constituents, or anyone else designated by the member.

Most legislative time is spent renewing expiring legislative acts, except on the Appropriations Committee. Authorization measures establish programs and provide for spending goals; appropriations, which require separate votes, specify exactly how much money is to be made available for a particular authorized program. Almost all authorizing legislation is written with a time limit, usually two or three years. The renewal process gives Congress a chance to review programs, collect testimony, and consider changes.

After introduction, each bill, whether for a new program or a renewal, is assigned to the appropriate committee or subcommittee that has jurisdiction over the subject area of the bill. If the committee leaders consider it important, public hearings are held. Interested organizations and individuals, including executive-branch officials, will be invited to express their opinions. After hearings, a subcommittee "mark-up" session will be held during which the bill is rewritten by the members, taking into account testimony heard in hearings. The bill next will be considered by the full committee, which may also hold hearings. Then, if it is favorably endorsed by the committee, it is reported to the floor of the respective house.

Often problem areas will be the subject of similar but not identical bills passed by each house. In that case, what is called a conference committee will be necessary to reconcile differences. If agreement is reached, the conference committee report, essentially a revision of the bill passed in each house into a mutually acceptable version, must be resubmitted to both houses for approval. If no agreement can be reached, the bill "dies in conference." Once the final common bill has passed both houses, it is sent to the President for signature. He may sign it, allow it to become law without his signature, or veto it within ten days.

After legislation is passed, it must be implemented, and the first step is generally the development of what are called *regulations,* which describe how the law is to be administered. During the early stages of regulation writing, personnel in the designated agency generally consult with the groups involved, including congressional members and staff, officials of state and local governments, and lobbyists. In effect, this is a legislative process with all the forces contending, but it is a hidden process compared to the rather open congressional operations. Draft regulations are published in a daily official publication called the *Federal Register.* Final regulations are then published, usually ninety days after the appearance of the draft regulations. They have the force of law.

The Role of Lobbyists. Why, the reader may ask, does the potential therapeutic recreation specialist need to be concerned with the legislative process and the role of the lobbyist? The answer is quite simple. Initially, the specialist should be aware of how legislation affecting recreation service for handicapped individuals is enacted, since Congress is becoming increasingly involved in the delivery of services. Secondly, it is critical that therapeutic recreators have some understanding of the legislative process, since they will be asked to participate more and more in the process whether it is at the federal, state, or local level.

Many interest groups set up their own offices to lobby the Congress and the executive branch; sometimes they hire a professional lobbying firm. In the health area two better-known lobbying groups are the American Medical Association (AMA) and the American Hospital Association (AHA). The National Recreation and Park Association (NRPA) and the National Therapeutic Recreation Society (NTRS) are not strangers in the lobbying business.

There are two kinds of interest groups. One kind are special-interest groups (AMA, NRPA/NTRS) whose interest is shared by only a few members of society; the other are public-interest groups, whose interest is shared by a substantial number of citizens of the community and nation.[8] Sometimes these groups work in harmony, and at other times they disagree. Where both have worked together, much has been accomplished. National hearings involving disabled individuals, advocacy groups, therapeutic recreation providers, and NRPA/NTRS personnel have played an important role in promoting legislation that focused on the delivery of recreation services to special population members.

Interest groups are aware that the important work of Congress takes place in committee, and they focus their attention accordingly. Besides seeking to influence votes directly, they supply valuable information; they may draft bills and contribute to research and other technical committee work; they may appear at public hearings; and they may serve as a bridge from committees to administration experts, who might not be experts without such help.[9]

State. At the state level, the responsibilities of the various departments concerned with public health, mental health, rehabilitation, welfare, and correction vary considerably among different states, depending largely on their wealth and the progressiveness of their administration. In the main, their responsibilities are in the general area of planning, coordinating, and offering supportive service. Most state departments establish standards of service and personnel quality, and provide educational opportunities. Standards of service and personnel may be the single most important element in determining the character of the health-care delivery system in the state. This matter of quality will be discussed later in this chapter.

States also have the responsibility for the disbursement of federal funds and the development of new and improved methods for the provision of health and rehabilitation service. Direct services are limited to state institutions for the mentally ill, mentally retarded, chronic-disease hospitals, and general and medical teaching and research hospitals.

Local. At the local level, health responsibilities are primarily restricted to community public health departments. They vary from small rural county departments to large departments responsible for the health needs of populated metropolitan areas. In general, they provide a variety of services. Some county and city health departments have responsibilities also for the operation of public hospitals, clinics, and outpatient services.

Nongovernmental Organizations

Nongovernment organizations are perhaps even more diverse in their origins and functions than their government counterparts. In this country, however, a vast amount of health, rehabilitation, and social welfare work is being done by these organizations. Some of them are voluntary organizations supported by contributions or membership dues; others are endowed philanthropic foundations; others are professional organizations; others are large business enterprises, such as insurance companies and industrial corporations. Still others are local organizations for various types and purposes, such as educational institutions, labor unions, and community chests. They have the largest investment in health, social, and welfare problems.

Voluntary. National voluntary health, rehabilitation, and social welfare organizations are composed of individuals, both lay and professional, whose primary purpose is either combating a particular disease, disability, or social problem (or group of diseases, disabilities, or social problems) or improving the health or social welfare of a particular group of people. The movement for voluntary organizations began with the Anti-Tuberculosis Society of Philadelphia in 1892. Three-quarters of a century later over thirty thousand voluntary agencies had

been organized. They have been supported largely by voluntary contributions from the public at large rather than by government sources or endowments. They engage primarily in programs of research, education, and service to individuals and agencies or institutions in their particular spheres of interest.

Prominent among the organizations that operate in this country are the National Association for Mental Health, the American Lung Association, the American Cancer Society, the American Heart Association, the American Red Cross, the National Association for Retarded Citizens, the United Cerebral Palsy Association, the Muscular Dystrophy Association, the American Foundation for the Blind, and the National Easter Seal Society for Crippled Children and Adults.[10]

Philanthropic. Most of the philanthropic foundations, of which there are over twenty-one thousand, have been established and endowed by wealthy individuals. They have interests that are broader in scope than any particular health, rehabilitation, or social welfare problem. Some operate in local areas or special fields; some are national or even international in scope. Their main source of financial support is often the investment earnings resulting from securities provided by the philanthropic individual or family. The Ford Foundation, the Rockefeller Foundation, the Commonwealth Fund, and the Kellogg Foundation are prominent examples. They often support new lines of research, training of personnel, and pilot programs. In this manner they often open up new approaches that government agencies may have overlooked or cannot provide.[11]

Professional. Various groups of professional workers have formed organizations to promote their professional interests. These national organizations usually have affiliates at the state level, and some may also have local chapters. Such organizations strive to improve the social and economic welfare of their members, keep their members informed of changes and developments in professional practice, set standards of ethical conduct and of professional practice and aid in the enforcement of these standards, engage in research to improve practice and utilization of professional services, speak for and on behalf of the profession in planning and action groups, monitor government activities in relation to their profession, represent the profession in the determination of public policy, mediate for the profession with the various governments and their agencies, and provide the public with information relative to their profession. Examples of such organizations are the National Rehabilitation Association, the National Therapeutic Recreation Society, the American Therapeutic Recreation Association, the American Physical Therapy Association, the American Medical Association, and the American Nurses Association.

Becoming a member of a professional association or society usually implies that the individual has met certain qualifications of education and/or experience. Associations usually maintain records on current and past members. In turn, members may receive the journal of the association, listings of employment opportunities, and other informational items.[12]

As health organizations developed in this country, the need to provide for an exchange of ideas and for the coordination of certain services became obvious. This led to the formation of the National Health Council. All major voluntary health agencies, professional associations concerned with health, and major units of government concerned with health are members of the National Health Council. Among its activities the council conducts an annual forum devoted to the consideration of major health issues, the improvement of community health services, and the promotion of careers in the health fields.

Some people ask whether these nongovernment organizations are needed since federal, state, and some local governments are appropriating money for similar types of work. The answers to such questions are: (1) voluntarism is an essential element of a free, democratic society; (2) nongovernmental organizations are better able to deal with many controversial problems and to experiment with new ideas and programs; and (3) research people should have more than one possible source of support. No one speaks more positively about this subject than those who administer federal research programs.

In concluding this section it is fair to say that government operates no piece of the health-care system in its entirety. On the other hand, government is closely involved in one way or another in everything: collecting and disseminating information, training personnel, operating institutions, providing services, participating in financing, supporting and carrying out research, planning, evaluation, and regulation.

FACILITIES

The spectrum of health and social rehabilitation services in a community ranges from preventive and health maintenance services, through primary-care facilities, to inpatient services for the sick, and home-care and restorative and rehabilitative services for those who require them. A wide variety of agencies provide these services, and many agencies combine a number of them. Mental health centers, for example, often have outpatient services for diagnosis and treatment as well as in-patient facilities for the acutely ill. In many instances two or more agencies combine to provide a more complete range of services for individuals. For example, a special school for the mentally retarded may work with a vocational training center to provide vocational training and with the municipal recreation department to provide recreation service.

In this section we will briefly consider the history, classification, and governance of health and health-related facilities.

History

Although Chapter 4 considers the historical development of many health and health-related facilities, it is well to note here that hospitals for the most part began in the Middle Ages as places of refuge for the sick, the weary, and the poor. Most were church sponsored. In the American colonies the earliest hospitals were actually infirmaries in poorhouses: Henricopolis in Virginia (1612); Blockley in Philadelphia (1732); Charity Hospital in New Orleans (1736); and the Public Workhouse and House of Corrections in New York City (1736).[13] Private voluntary hospitals go back to the eighteenth century in the United States. These institutions also cared for the poor; since hospitals could do little for their patients, there was no reason for the self-supporting to go to them.

The first voluntary hospital in the American colonies was the Pennsylvania Hospital in Philadelphia (1751).[14] Although a number of other such hospitals developed, there were only an estimated 178 voluntary hospitals by 1873. By 1909 there were more than 4300 general hospitals with more than 421,000 beds.[15] As hospitals grew, the types of patients treated changed with each medical discovery and treatment as well as with the development of specialty hospitals. However, in recent years because of fiscal exigencies, considerations of efficiency, and medical advances, specialty hospitals have now closed or admit a full range of patients. The rapid advance of medical science in the middle of the twentieth century accounted for the expansion of hospitals, which began to assume their role as the center of the medical-care system.[16]

Classification

Health and health-related facilities can be classified, even though there is some overlap, according to their size, type, mode of ownership, and length of patient stay (see Figure 3.1). Hospital size is determined by the number of beds, excluding bassinets for newborns. They may range from twenty beds in a small rural community general hospital, to over one thousand in an urban/university teaching hospital, and to over two thousand in some state institutions for the mentally ill. The type of hospital may be general or special. A *general hospital* is one wherein individuals of all ages and health-care needs are admitted; it offers a diversity of services, such as medical, surgical, urological, orthopedic, obstetric, pediatric, and psychiatric. Hospitals or institutions admitting only patients of one sex, people with a particular illness, or people of a specific age group are *specialty hospitals*. Hospitals that

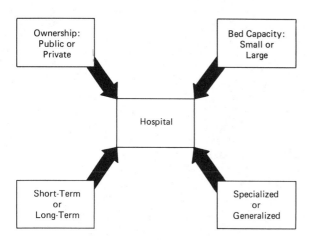

FIGURE 3.1. Types of Hospitals

treat only female diseases and children's hospitals are examples of the first and the last, respectively. Hospitals or institutions for the mentally ill and hospitals for individuals with orthopedic disorders or cancer are examples of specialized hospitals concerned with a specific disorder or impairment.

There are two principal modes of ownership, private and public. Private hospitals are categorized by the use to which they put their surplus income. They may be investor owned, for profit (proprietary), or not for profit (voluntary). Some of the facilities that are part of the former (proprietary) are specialized hospitals and skilled-care facilities (nursing homes). During the past decade there has been an increase in the number of general for-profit hospitals. Many of these for-profit hospitals represent corporations such as American Hospital Corporation, Republic Health Corporation, and Humane Health Care. The not-for-profit hospital is usually supported by fees and charges, donations, gifts, and grants and is associated with religious denominations. Public hospitals are supported primarily through taxes and are categorized by the level of government jurisdiction that owns and operates them: federal, state, county, or local.

Length of stay recently has become another basis on which to classify an institution. There are two types: short term and long term. Short term refers to a length of stay of thirty days or less and is associated with acute-care institutions, namely, general medical and surgical hospitals. Long term refers to a length of stay of thirty days or more. Chronic-care institutions—rehabilitation centers, extended-care facilities, and nursing homes—are examples of long term institutions.

Characteristics of Short-Term and Long-Term Facilities

It is important that we briefly highlight a number of these highly visible short- and long-term health and health-related facilities since it is important for the therapeutic-recreation specialist to be familiar with these various facilities. Some of the facilities mentioned here will again be considered in more detail in later chapters when considering case studies.

Short Term. Of the facilities housing and caring for acute patients on a short-term basis, general community hospitals are the most numerous. In the United States as of 1982, there were nearly seven thousand hospitals with more than 1.5 million beds.[17] They are the institutional center of the health-care delivery system, according to many observers. Because of its complexity, the hospital has been described as a city whose major enterprise is the restoration of its citizens' health; and indeed, all the major services, resources, and social forces of a city have parallels in a hospital.

Like cities, the hospital has changed dramatically in character in the past century. The hospital has evolved from a place of refuge where people went to spare their families the anguish of watching death approach to a multiservice institution providing interdisciplinary medical care to ambulatory as well as bed patients. Aside from delivering health and medical services, the hospital is a center for training both graduates and undergraduates in many health-related fields, and it conducts health and medical research. It is a highly organized, complex institution with many departments and health-care providers. And lastly, the hospital has a symbolic importance: being the most visible component of health care, the hospital *is* the health delivery system in the minds of many laymen.

Hospitals are licensed through the state and must meet minimum standards. In addition to licensure, hospitals may participate in voluntary accreditation through the Joint Commission on Accreditation of Hospitals (JCAH). This accreditation indicates the attainment of high standards with eligibility for federal funding and affiliation with education programs.

In these health facilities the major focus

is on the patient with a potential or identified illness or disorder. While preventive and rehabilitation measures may take place in these settings, their main function is to treat illness or disorder.

While community hospitals are the major short-term facility, there are a number of other short-term facilities, including those considered to be outpatient:

Neighborhood health centers: There are many types of neighborhood health centers—prenatal, well-child, and birthing centers. For the most part they concentrate on providing and coordinating comprehensive care, including preventive care and early diagnoses, and physical, social, and vocational rehabilitation of those with residual disabilities. For example, in a prenatal clinic an expectant family might receive education concerning growth and development of the unborn child, financial planning, nutritional requirements, physical changes of the mother, birthing, child care, and psychosocial responses to a new family member. Well-child centers assist the mother and family in the care of their growing child. Many neighborhood health centers are found in nontraditional settings (churches, schools, homes).

Clinics: Clinics may be affiliated with a hospital but may be independently operated. As an ambulatory-care facility, the clinic provides service to consumers who require short-term health care or follow-up care after hospitalization. Clinics span all levels of health-care needs; however, a large proportion of them provide treatment and diagnosis of disease for ambulatory care. They are usually organized to meet potential and actual health care needs of specific groups of consumers— psychiatric, eye disorders, internal disorders, minor surgical procedures, or follow-up after surgery in the hospital.

Hospital outpatient services: These are very similar in nature to clinics and may very well be same except for the "term" reference. They concentrate on services of a medical or psychiatric nature for those individuals who are generally ambulatory and who do not require or presently receive services as an inpatient.

Mental Health Centers: The federal Community Mental Health Centers (CMHC) program was established to improve the delivery of mental health services to the entire U.S. population. Some two thousand centers were established, and each was made responsible for providing services to all residents of a geographic area (catchment area). These services included inpatient hospitalization, partial hospitalization, twenty-four-hour emergency care, outpatient care, and community consultation and education. There is no accurate count of centers today since some are independently operated and others are associated with communities and/or hospitals. Individual CMHCs vary widely in staffing patterns, financial arrangements, population served, and administrative organization. Their catchment areas range from inner city ghettos to rural areas and affluent suburbs. Since 1975 (CMHCs amendments, Title III, PL94–63) the centers have established services for children, the elderly, drug addicts, alcoholics, and chronically and severely impaired patients. Although the centers are generally organized as outpatient services, they may refer for additional diagnosis and treatment to psychiatric inpatient units of general hospitals. In general, the aim of the centers is to help consumers with emotional dysfunctioning to function within society while participating in treatment.

Community health agencies: Community health agencies are established to meet health needs of individuals, groups, and communities. They include public health departments, home health services, visiting nurse associations, and other types of nursing clinics and centers. The home health services concentrate on providing services in the home to those individuals who may have chronic diseases or impairments. Services may range from programs offering one type of health care, such as nursing care or Meals on Wheels, to physician-directed medical, social, and related services including therapeutic recreation service. The type and extent of care is dependent on the health needs of the client.[18]

Long Term. We will discuss a number of long-term facilities here. Sometimes these long-term facilities are referred to as *tertiary health-care facilities.* The goal of tertiary care is *rehabilitation*—the restoration of a person to an optimal level of functioning. Individuals are encouraged to attain their maximum ability of function and to develop a realistic view of their strengths and limitations. The success of tertiary care depends upon the person's willingness to progress through the stages of rehabilitation. The patient usually enters tertiary facilities by a referral from a health specialist, another agency, or the court.

One of the more common long-term facilities is the *psychiatric facility,* public and private. These institutions include state and county mental hospitals, private (profit and not-for-profit) mental hospitals, and residential psychiatric facilities for children and adolescents, which may or may not be associated with the adult public or private institution.

In many respects, the public and private psychiatric hospitals are like community hospitals in that they are like a city. In fact, until the late 1940s and early 1950s, many mental hospitals, but specifically state and county hospitals, had their own farms, which made them self-supporting to a large degree. These institutions evolved from attempts to classify the mixed population of prisons and almshouses. From special institutions of terror, they became special institutions where humanitarian treatment was provided. And like community hospitals,

they provide clinical training and continued education and conduct research. The reality of life in an institution has been presented in books such as *One Flew Over the Cuckoo's Nest, The Snake Pit* and others.[19]

Another mental health facility that must not be overlooked is the *psychiatric inpatient unit of the general community hospital.* Since World War II such units have increased dramatically as a result of insurance coverage for treatment of mental disorders and federal funding for construction of psychiatric units (beds), training, and coverage for mental illness under Medicare and Medicaid. Patients in these units are usually treated by their personal physician or psychiatrist and participate in psychotherapy, occupational therapy, and therapeutic recreation service.

Residential psychiatric facilities for children and adolescents provide inpatient services primarily to moderately or seriously disturbed children under eighteen years of age. Some facilities may contain a unit for heavy drug users. The programs and physical facilities are usually designed to meet patients' daily living, schooling, recreational, socialization, and routine medical care needs. Because of the larger number and variety of staff needed, costs are high. Treatments include milieu therapy, psychotherapy, behavior modification, psychotropic drugs, and special education.

Other long-term facilities are the public and private *institutions for the mentally retarded.* Like state mental hospitals, these institutions for many years sought to provide little more than custodial care, although a more professional sensitivity toward the mentally retarded did develop during the 1930s. Even though the 1950s brought about extensive changes as a result of the concerns parents had for their retarded child or children and the expansion of special education programs in the communities, it was not until the 1960s and 1970s, with the expanded recognition of human and civil rights and substantially increased federal funding for human services and programs, that changes really took place. For example, institutions had to make a concerted effort to increase the independence of their retarded residents, preparing them for community placement and, if possible, independent living. Thus, the basic goal of programming for retarded individuals consisted of maximizing their human qualities through education and training. And the physical arrangement of the institution changed from dorm living to cottagelike so as to promote small-group living in a home-like atmosphere.[20] According to many, more changes took place in attitude and treatment from 1960 to 1980 than in all previous years put together.

A final note regarding institutions for the mentally retarded. During the 1970s there was considerable debate over conflicting ideologies and research findings regarding the abolishment and replacement of institutions with a variety of community-based, normalized residential alternatives. Thus, as the decade of the 1970s ended, the future of residential services for mentally retarded people remained uncertain. Certainly there had been a major shift in attitude and opinion away from institutions and toward decentralized community-based alternatives. Yet opinions continued to remain divided on whether institutions should remain a viable component of the continuum of residential services.[21]

Another long-term facility is the *skilled nursing facility*, sometimes referred to as a nursing home. Skilled nursing facilities have increased in number since the Medicare/Medicaid enactment of 1965. Patients no longer needing acute care in a hospital setting but still needing skilled care (not to be confused with intense rehabilitation) are transferred or referred to a skilled nursing facility for continued treatment at a lower cost. Other patients, on their physicians' referral, may be placed directly in the facility from their home. The majority of these facilities are operated under proprietary auspices. The preponderance of private, profit-making ownership is the most important

characteristic of residential facilities for the aged in the United States.

The last long-term facility we will consider is the *physical rehabilitation center*. Rehabilitation facilities provide extended care for patients who no longer require the acute-care service of a general hospital but who do need intensive care and training to cope with their illness or change in functioning. Rehabilitation facilities operate under a variety of auspices. They range from those that are an integral part of hospitals and medical schools to those that may be independent, free-standing facilities within the community and serve any number of health-care facilities. Regardless of sponsorship or administration, type of patient or client served, or specific purpose or goal, hospital and medical school rehabilitation programs tend to be directed toward inpatient medical and physical restoration, with some psychosocial service, whereas the independent, community-oriented centers tend to be directed toward functional therapy and vocational preparation with possible sheltered workshop association. Like hospitals, rehabilitation centers may participate in a voluntary accreditation program through the Commission on Accreditation of Rehabilitation Facilities (CARF).

Governance

Hospitals are bureaucratic, highly organized, complex institutions with many departments, as we have noted. All hospitals receive their authority to operate from the government of the state in which they are located. Although many different governance structures are found among hospitals, we will be concerned here with the governance of voluntary hospitals in general and also with traditional public hospitals and institutions.

Voluntary Hospitals.   A majority of hospitals in this country, as noted, are voluntary. These hospitals were originally established by the upper class in America to provide for the welfare of the sick and poor in cities by financing the buildings and operations of hospitals through philanthropic contributions. Some of the individuals involved in the establishment of these hospitals became members of the governing body of the hospital, which was called a board of trustees. Making and soliciting philanthropic contributions today is not a major activity of hospital trustees. However, hospital trustees have now become legalized in all states.

The typical voluntary hospital is organized according to a constitution and bylaws that invest in a board of trustees the legal responsibility for the operation and financial maintenance of hospital services. The board has the ultimate responsibility for the medical care delivered in the hospital. It acts as an organ of review, appraisal, and appeal in a judicial manner and assures the physical integrity of the hospital. Trustees are very cognizant of the administrative and medical appointments made to the hospital, especially physician appointments. They also review the short- and long-range objectives of the hospital and review and approve the various departmental budgets.

Some changes are imminent in the membership of hospital boards. A professional trustee may develop in the future, with expertise in a specific area and with experience on boards of several hospitals.[22] Another change that is about to take place is the addition of community representatives to hospital boards. Many argue that boards, which are usually made up of representatives of the upper and middle classes, do not understand the wishes and value systems of the poor and lower class. One reorganization occurring on hospital boards that does reduce the control of trustees over administrators is adoption of the corporation model: integrating the board of trustees and the administration of the hospital. The board of the future will have full-time presidents and salaried vice-presidents covering the specialties of management.[23]

Public Hospitals. There are a variety of governance forms for public hospitals. At the federal level the Department of Defense, the Veterans Administration, and the Public Health Service operate their hospitals without boards of trustees or their equivalent. The hospital directors are directly accountable to their administrative supervisors and indirectly responsible to the President and the Congress. State hospitals are also overseen directly by government departments, usually departments of mental health or hygiene for psychiatric and mental retardation facilities. These hospitals usually do not have boards of trustees, although the government department may be in part responsible to a board of mental health or of hygiene, which may exert some board-of-trusteelike influence on individual hospitals as well as have contact with state legislators. As at the federal level, state hospital directors are mainly accountable to their administrative superiors and indirectly to the governor and the state legislature.

At the county level, a department within county government is responsible for the county hospital, which is managed by a board of managers appointed by the chief executive officer of the county. At the local level, governance becomes more complex, with a variety of approaches used. In some cities hospital directors are directly accountable to a commissioner and indirectly accountable to the mayor and city council. In other cities a semi-independent health and hospital corporation is established.

PERSONNEL

The health-care field has enjoyed a long period of expansion with continuous growth in funding of services and programs by both the private and public sectors. Since World War II, but especially during the past three decades, both the number and types of health-care workers have increased greatly.

Overall, the health industry is labor intensive. Many new health services require a large number of personnel, which significantly affects costs. Furthermore, health-care personnel have a tendency to create a demand for their own services. Increases in the personnel pool and the development of new specialties tend to increase the total supply of services. More therapeutic recreation specialists mean that more therapeutic recreation services will be available. It is interesting that since health personnel may very well create their own demand by prescribing the use of services for patients, increases in supply may well increase the demand for services.

In 1984 approximately six million people were employed in the health-care industry.[24] The total does not include the large but unknown number of housekeeping, kitchen, and maintenance personnel who work in the health-care industry, primarily in long-term institutions. The range of skills required in the industry is vast and overlaps those of many other industries.

In terms of mode of functioning, health-care providers may be divided into three major groups: independent practitioners (physicians, etc.), dependent practitioners (nurses, psychologists, various therapists), and supporting staff (clerical, maintenance, housekeeping workers, researchers, aides, assistants, technicians).

The independent practitioner is allowed by law to deliver a delimited range of services to people who want them without supervision or authorization of the practitioner's work by third parties.[25] The dependent practitioner is allowed by law to provide a range of services under the supervision and authorization of independent practitioners, often of a particular type specified by law. However, in certain situations and in relation to certain patients, many dependent practitioners may assume the role of independent practitioner. The definition of the line between the independent and dependent groups is the source of many conflicts at present.[26]

Supporting staff, rather than providing a range of services to patients, carry out specific tasks authorized by and under the supervision, directly or indirectly, of independent and/or dependent practitioners. The work of supporting staff may or may not be regulated by laws directly pertaining to them, but if there are no special laws, they work under the legal sanctions provided for their supervisors.[27]

Regardless of mode of functioning, the term *allied health discipline* is used to encompass the large and rapidly growing family of occupational groups (excluding physicians) that are involved in providing health services.

Kinds of Personnel

A complete listing of personnel in the health and social rehabilitation field has increased so greatly that it is hard to enumerate them all, let alone describe their responsibilities here. Also, it is not possible to include the hundreds of interested people who participate indirectly in rehabilitation programs—volunteer groups, fund-raising groups, parent groups, service and fraternal organizations, and others. However, it is important to identify some having a more significant role in the rehabilitation process as well as those who may work closely with the therapeutic recreation specialist. They are as follows:

1. *Administration of health services*
   a. *Health officer, commissioner, or public health administrator of state health department*: with few exceptions, a physician with specialized professional education and training in public health, psychiatry, or other specialty.
   b. *Hospital administrator, executive director, superintendent, or director of hospital, nursing home, or related institution (rehabilitation center, training school, sheltered workshop, or similar facility)*: may or may not be a physician with specialization; recently individuals with professional education and training in administra-

tion as a specialty have been employed.

c. *Administrator or executive director of voluntary health agency* (the National Easter Seal Society for Crippled Children and Adults, the National Association of Mental Health, and the like): administrative professional education and training vary; however, the administrator usually has some sort of professional or technical health skill, such as physician, psychologist, social worker, physical therapist, nurse.

2. *Correctional therapist*: uses assistive, resistive, and active exercises designed to strengthen and coordinate functions and to prevent muscular deconditioning.

3. *Educational therapist (special educator)*: administers medical treatment through the use of educational activities and materials designed to develop the mental and physical capacities of the patient.

4. *Library services*
   a. *Medical librarian*: provides library services to meet the needs of professional staff and professional schools. May be assisted by a *medical librarian technician*.
   b. *Patients' librarian (hospital librarian)*: develops library facilities to meet interests of bedridden and ambulatory patients, provides book-cart service, and encourages reading as part of therapeutic program.

5. *Medical records administrator (librarian)*: is responsible for planning, organizing, directing, and controlling medical record services; for developing, analyzing, and evaluating medical records and indexes; and for cooperating with the medical and administrative staff in research projects utilizing health-care information. May be assisted by a *medical records technician* who performs the technical tasks associated with the maintenance and use of medical records.

6. *Medicine and osteopathy—M.D. (Doctor of Medicine) and D.O. (Doctor of Osteopathy)*: both are concerned with the prevention, cure, and alleviation of disease and may use surgery, drugs, and other accepted methods of medical care. While not restricted to any specialty, of which there are over thirty, all doctors contribute to rehabilitation. Of the various medical specialists, therapeutic recreation specialists most frequently interact with internists, cardiologists, orthopedists, neurologists, psychiatrists, and physiatrists. (The latter is a specialist in physical medicine).

7. *Manual arts therapist*: administers a program of actual or simulated work situations through the use of industrial arts activities to help prepare the patient to become a productive member of the community.

8. *Music therapist*: uses instrumental or vocal music to bring about changes in behavior that can serve as a basis for improved mental and physical health.

9. *Nursing services*
   a. *Registered Nurse (R.N.)*: is responsible for rendering nursing care to patients, carrying out physicians' instructions, and supervising personnel who perform routine care and treatment of patients.
   b. *Licensed Practical Nurse (L.P.N.)*: provides nursing care and treatment of patients under the supervision of a licensed physician or registered nurse.
   c. *Nursing aide*: assists R.N. or L.P.N. by performing less skilled nursing tasks in the care of patients.
   d. *Orderlies and attendants*: usually men, they assist in performing a variety of duties associated with male patients and certain heavy duties in the care of all patients.

10. *Occupational therapist*: uses a variety of activities in a therapeutic manner to evaluate learning and performance abilities in relation to physical or emotional conditions so as to improve social well-

being and ability to function independently. May be assisted by an *occupational therapy assistant* and/or *aide* and *noncertified assistants* who have received on-the-job training.

11. *Orthotist and/or prosthetist:* the orthotist makes and fits orthopedic braces; the prosthetist makes and fits artificial limbs.

12. *Physical therapist:* is responsible for the restoration of function and the prevention of disability following disease, injury, or loss of bodily part through the use of exercise, heat, cold, electricity, ultra-sound, and massage. May be assisted by a *physical therapy assistant* and/or *aide.*

13. *Psychology*
    a. *Clinical psychologist:* engages primarily in the diagnosis and treatment of mental illness.
    b. *Counseling psychologist:* is responsible for helping individuals understand themselves so that they can utilize their own strengths to deal effectively with their own problems.

14. *Social worker:* is responsible for helping patients and their families cope with problems related to severe or long-term illness, recovery, and rehabilitation. Assists physicians and other personnel in understanding the social and emotional factors related to a patient's health problems. Social workers may specialize in social welfare, medical, and psychiatric services.

15. *Speech pathologist and audiologist:* identify persons with disorders in the production, reception, and perception of speech and language as well as determining the etiology, history, and severity of the disorders through interviews and special tests.

16. *Vocational rehabilitation counselor (rehabilitation counselor):* is concerned with evaluating the vocational potential of the patient or client, thereafter matching the abilities of the client with a suitable job. Counselors may specialize in

services to the blind, mentally ill, and others.[28]

All of the above careers require educational preparation at the baccalaureate level or above; however, as noted earlier, occupations have evolved because of the need for people with specific skills or as a result of the delegation of certain functions to assistants. The amount of education and training varies for these assistant positions from a few weeks of on-the-job training to two or more years of education or an associate degree. Attempts have been made to standardize the titles in relation to the level of training. The distinction is as follows:

1. *Technician or assistant:* educational preparation at the associate degree level (two years of college education or other formal preparation beyond high school).

2. *Aide:* specialized training of less than two years' duration beyond high school or on-the-job training.

Human-Service Teams

Perhaps one of the most important developments in recent years, resulting from the tremendous advances in scientific knowledge and technology and the trend toward specialization throughout our entire society, has been the creation of teams. No one person can be expected to be knowledgeable about the whole person, but by bringing together experts from various professions, the agency or institution can give the individual who is receiving service the advantage of their combined knowledge and skills.

Generally speaking, the team is usually composed of a variety of personnel representing professional disciplines concerned with the health and welfare of people. The membership varies with the needs of the individual. Each member of the team possesses knowledge and skills specific to his or her discipline. In many situations the members of the team confer regularly about the care and treatment of the individual. In this way, each member augments the services of the others in orienting their functions toward goals that will assist the individual.

As an example of a team meeting, the physician, the nurse, and the dietitian may pool information relative to the diet of the patient in a general hospital. Or the psychologist, social worker, vocational rehabilitation therapist, and therapeutic recreation specialist may be members of a team planning the discharge needs of an educable mentally retarded adult in a residential institution for the retarded. The team and the function of the therapeutic recreation specialist on the team will be discussed in later chapters.

SERVICES

Rehabilitation services are numerous, varied, and broad in nature, and are offered for the direct benefit of the individual. Services may be rendered in any one of a variety of facilities. However, this does not mean that all kinds of rehabilitation services are offered in the same facility. One facility may provide only one kind of service, while another facility may render any number of services. Also, one individual may provide one service, while another may render more than one kind of service.

Kinds

The services provided in the health rehabilitation process are as follows:

Clergy-medic services

Corrective therapy

Dentistry and allied services

Dietetic and nutritional services

Health aide services (directed primarily toward various ethnic and socioeconomic minorities)

Health-care institutional services (inpatient, outpatient, and nonpatient services—hospitals, institutions, day-care facilities, rehabilitation centers, extended-care facilities, etc.)

Health education services (community, public, school, etc.)

Homebound services

Library services

Manual arts or training theapy

Medical services (prevention, cure, and alleviation of diseases)

Music therapy

Nursing and related-care services

Occupational therapy

Ombudsman services

Optometry services

Orthotic and prosthetic services

Podiatric services

Psychological services (diagnosis of mental health problems, testing, counseling—personal and group, etc.)

Social work service (medical, psychiatric, welfare, etc.)

Sheltered employment

Speech pathology and audiology services

Suicide prevention centers

Vocational rehabilitation service (vocational guidance, training, and placement)

Delivery System

We conclude this section by briefly touching upon the system that delivers health-care service. The health services system is one of the nation's largest industries. In fiscal 1982 Americans spent over $322 billion on all health services.[29]

The goods and services made available to special populations by the health-care system involve the participation of a variety of organizations and individuals. To a large degree the major components of the system have already been described in the previous chapter and this one: the people for whom it provides care; the people who provide the care; the services these people provide; the organizations and institutions within which the people work and the services that are provided; and the government under which the system functions. The only factor that was not included was the financial mechanisms that allow the components to interact.

Since World War I our health-care delivery system has evolved from one featuring the general physician and the community hospital to one having an incredibly complicated and bewildering array of providers and institutions. The change from a physician-dominated to a systems-oriented model has brought into being a whole language of health care—for example, health teams—and has made health care a focus of nationwide attention.

Not only have physicians become specialized; they have been subsumed into complex health teams, and the system they work in has become organized into regionalized referral networks of institutions and agencies providing varying levels of specialized patient care. This specialization also extends to other workers in the system. Thus, the health-care delivery system is a complex social organization. It is an interdependent, coordinated system. (Some would disagree with the term coordinated and say the system is a nonsystem.[30]) whose purpose is the maintenance of health and provision of illness care to all persons, families, and groups. The providers in the system are professionals and paraprofessionals with special training in meeting health-care problems and/or needs of special population members.

The health-care system, as a whole, is considered to be an *open system* developed around the health-care needs of society.[31] The system consists of special population members and consumers in general, professionals, paraprofessionals, and various health and health-related agencies. It is influenced by such factors as cost, accessibility, politics, and disease types and distribution. The parts of the system interact in various degrees with one another, and all respond to changes in individuals, society, and health. Figure 3.2 illustrates these interrelationships.

Evaluation of Quality of Service

Health-care services, affecting as they do the lives of all of us, have become a major social issue, and the extent to which health-care services can be evaluated has been a subject of debate for some years. There are many models for evaluation. Donabedian has provided the generally accepted classification of the techniques of quality assessment. He has identified three major approaches to the evaluation of quality—structure, process, and outcome.[32]

Structure

Structure involves the examination of an individual's or an institution's ability to meet established evaluative criteria at a particular time. Individuals are evaluated on the basis of experience, education, and knowledge. Institutions are evaluated on the basis of physical structure, administrative and staff organization, services, and personnel qualifications. The general approach to meeting structure is through accreditation, licensing, and certification.[33] As a whole, these terms are referred to as *credentialing*. The various types of credentialing are defined below, with a brief discussion of that approach to quality care following.

Accreditation. Unlike licensing, accreditation is a voluntary system used only in relation to institutions (educational, health, and health related). Groups of like institutions or organizations with mutual interests get together, set up an organization, establish standards, and proceed to inspect and accredit (or not accredit) themselves or the institution in which they have an interest on a periodic basis.

There are two types of educational accreditation: institutional and specialized. *Institutional accreditation* is concerned with the overall quality of education within the

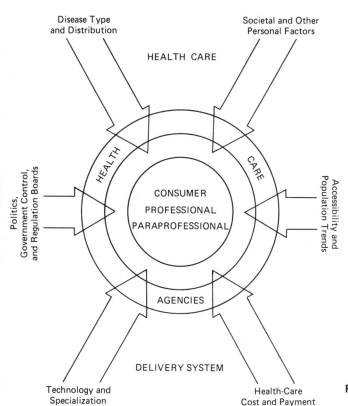

FIGURE 3.2. The Health-Care Delivery System

total institution. It indicates that the total institution is achieving its own specified objectives in a satisfactory manner. *Specialized,* or *program* or *professional accreditation,* is conferred on a national basis by a number of national organizations, each representing a professional, technical, occupational, or specialized educational area. Specialized accreditation applies to an individual curriculum, department, or program within the educational institution and is aimed at protecting the public against professional or occupational incompetence.

Since January 1976 the Council on Accreditation of the National Recreation and Park Association (NRPA), in cooperation with the American Association for Leisure and Recreation (AALR), has been accepting applications for accreditation of recreation, leisure services, and resources curriculum. At present, only baccalaureate programs are being considered. In addition, therapeutic recreation is one of a number of professional options within the total curriculum that the department may request to be accredited. In October 1986 the Council on Postsecondary Accreditation recognized the accreditation process of the NRPA/AALR Council.

Regarding health-care accreditation, which focuses on quality of care, services, and standards, there are a number of accrediting organizations. Two such major organizations are the Joint Commission on Accreditation of Hospitals (JCAH) and the

Commission on Accreditation of Rehabilitation Facilities (CARF). The preferred way to refer to JCAH is "Joint Commission" since not all institutions requesting accreditation are hospitals per se.

Accreditation is not a legal procedure, but there are strong legal incentives for accrediting certain kinds of institutions; for example, the Medicare law restricts payment to unaccredited hospitals.

Licensing. Licensing systems exist for both individual and institutional providers in the United States. As of 1981 approximately forty-five health professions and occupations were licensed by one or more states; approximately twelve types of health facilities were licensed.[34]

Individual licensing is a complex matter. It represents a compact between defined professional groups and state legislatures in which the profession is granted control over individuals' entrance into, maintenance of good standing in, and exit from the profession. Most professions define the content of their own work and thus gain what may be called a monopoly over the provision to the public of that body of work. In return, the profession, in theory at least, guarantees to the state legislatures that the work will be of high quality. The states use the criminal justice system to enforce the agreement. Individual licensing is usually granted for an indefinite period of time. The states of Utah and Georgia have therapeutic recreation licensure acts.

Licensure of health facilities did not become common until the 1940s. Most states require licensing of psychiatric, short- and long-term-stay hospitals, hospitals and institutions for the mentally retarded, skilled nursing facilities, and various kinds of homes for the aged, unwed mothers, and dependent children. Licenses are usually granted on an annual or biennial basis. The evaluation techniques are almost entirely structural. In institutional licensing, unlike individual licensing, state departments usu-ally have more control over the actual licensing process than do the statutory boards.

Certification. Certification combines features of licensing and accreditation. Applied to individuals, it uses standards of education, experience, and achievement on examinations to determine qualifications. However, it is a voluntary system undertaken by health-care provider professions and occupations and is neither directly sanctioned nor backed up by force of law. Nevertheless, like accreditation, there are incentives for individuals to become certified. For example, more and more public and private health-care agencies are requiring therapeutic recreation specialists to be certified with the National Council for Therapeutic Recreation Certification (NCTRC). Some confusion may arise in the use of the word *certification*. Some professions or occupations use *registration* in the same sense as *certification*, while others use the term *registration* instead of *licensing* in dealing with certain health professions. In considering the terms, you should check on exactly how a particular state uses the various terms. Requirements for certification with NCTRC can be found in Appendix D.

Process

Process is the evaluation of the activities of the health professionals in the care and treatment of the special population member. The criterion generally used is the degree to which care and treatment of the special population member conforms to the standards and expectations of the respective professions. These standards and expectations may be derived from what is considered to be good or acceptable practice as formulated by recognized leaders in the profession or through research studies involving actual practice.[35]

Outcome

The evaluation of end results in terms of health and satisfaction is outcome. This evaluation in many ways provides the final evidence of whether care has been good, bad, or indifferent. There is broad fundamental social and professional agreement on what results are deemed desirable. To a large degree, this procedure involves judgment on the part of both the patient and the provider or therapist. However, the assumption is made that the patient-centered goals established for meeting patient needs determine the outcome criteria. Furthermore, there is the assumption that particular elements or aspects of care are known to be specifically related to successful or unsuccessful outcomes or end results; good results are the result of good care and treatment.[36]

An organization using both process and outcome is the PSRO system mentioned earlier. If you recall, the PSRO is required to review services furnished in and by hospitals and other health-care institutions, such as skilled nursing facilities. PSROs represent a distinct departure from the American tradition of quality control. It was the first time a specific approach to quality control was legally mandated.

CORRECTIONS

As we begin our discussion of corrections, it is necessary to clarify what is meant by such terms as criminal justice system, correctional system, and correction. *The criminal justice system* in the United States is a collection of interrelated semiautonomous bureaucracies. The four major social processes utilized in the criminal justice system are law enforcement, prosecution, courts, and corrections. Law enforcement involves a diverse number of agencies, such as local police and sheriff's departments and state and federal police organizations. It is concerned with the detection and arrest of suspected offenders. Prosecutorial agencies, whether state or federal, investigate cases, make decisions about charges against criminal suspects, present cases to grand juries, negotiate pleas, and try cases in criminal courts. The courts supervise the treatment of accused persons, decide bail arrangements and trial dates, conduct trials, and sentence offenders. *The correctional system* is composed of prisons and probation and parole agencies that serve various custody, rehabilitation, and punishment functions. In general, these agencies are responsible for administering the assigned penalties.[37] The term *correction* implies repair or alteration. Relative to offenders, the word refers to changing or correcting an individual's inclination toward, or pattern of, law violation. According to Sheley, it may be defined as "the deprivation of an individual's freedom in order to alter his or her behavior from criminal to conventional."[38]

ORGANIZATION

It is difficult to generalize about the correctional system when it involves all three levels—federal, state, and local—because they present such a diversity of characteristics. For many years the correctional system was concerned only with institutionalization. In more recent years the continuity of the correctional process from arrest to release has been greatly stressed. It has been argued that since probation, institutionalization, and parole are parts of the same process, all should be included in the organizational structure of the respective levels of government. Unfortunately, each governmental level functions somewhat differently, resulting in many different patterns of corrections. In fact, there is considerable diversity among the three levels of government regarding how each handles probation, institutionalization, and parole. This is the result of many factors, some economic, some philosophical, some political, and some administrative. We can conclude that no one administrative or judicial system is best for everyone, and the variety of conditions within the correctional system will continue to require diversity.[39]

Federal

Congress created the Bureau of Prisons in 1930. It is found within the Department of Justice. Before the federal prison system was established, rehabilitation of federal offenders was virtually an impossibility. Administrators of the then seven prisons functioned independently with relative autonomy. Funds were appropriated separately by Congress to each institution. Because of limited space within the prisons and the lack of funds to build new prisons, nearly twelve thousand federal prisoners were held in state and local facilities.[40]

Today the U.S. Bureau of Prisons operates forty-five facilities covering eight correctional areas: youth and juvenile institutions, young adult institutions, adult penitentiaries, adult correctional facilities, short-term camps, female institutions, community treatment centers, and a medical treatment center.[41] The United States Probation Service is under the jurisdiction of the United States Courts, and an independent Board of Parole exists.

In all federal institutions programs for the rehabilitation of the offender are initiated in the first few weeks of commitment. The offender is given a diagnostic workup regarding requirements for education, vocational training, and treatment of physical or psychiatric problems. A rehabilitation program is developed and goals are set.

State

To describe the adult correctional system within fifty-two jurisdictions is an impossible task. Over 350 prisons, reformatories, camps, training schools for juveniles, and the like are operated by state governments.[42] A universe of differences separates one state from another regarding their operations. In varying degrees and with vastly different mixes, all states provide for custody, discipline, health and medical services, nutrition, classification, counseling, education, recreation, religious work, probation, parole, and community-based programming.

The extent to which probation is used also varies widely; likewise, the statutes regarding parole in every state are different. In addition, the line of separation between adult and juvenile is not uniform between states. In some states young children or juveniles convicted of a serious crime may be sentenced to the adult facility; in others intermediate institutions receive both juvenile and adults.

Juvenile correctional services are normally part of a system separated from its adult counterpart and include, at a minimum, the juvenile courts, probation, supervision (aftercare) in community-based programs, and training facilities. Together these services provide resources for the differential treatment required for juvenile offenders committing offenses from various levels of motivation. However, like adult services, juvenile services vary greatly from one state to another, manifesting at present all stages of a complex problem.

Local

Thoughtful practitioners and scholars alike have condemned local government for decades about the functions and conditions of jails. But it is virtually impossible to fix responsibility for the glaring and obvious inadequacies that exist at this level because the resources of the local government are so fragmented that no one can be blamed.

The well-over four thousand jails[43] and juvenile detention centers are designed primarily as holding centers for individuals awaiting trial or sentencing or appealing decisions. Jails are also utilized as short-term correctional facilities for those serving sentences for misdemeanors. According to a United States Department of Justice report in 1982, approximately 210,000 persons were confined in jails.[44]

In view of what has been said about jails, it should be clear that juvenile detention centers are far from satisfactory. While the juvenile court laws provide for the protective custody of children and juveniles prior to final disposition of their case, such laws are frequently violated because those in authority do not know what else to do with them. Although conditions are improving, evidence indicates that the methods and facilities for juvenile detention are still in need of much improvement.

LEGISLATION

Correctional legislation is a recent concern. Correctional institutions and programs have received little attention because the idea of retributive punishment is deeply rooted in human emotions as well as in the administrative fragmentation of our justice system. It was not until prison riots, parole scandals, and correctional maladministration following World War II that the public and political leaders began to give attention to correctional problems. The Ford Foundation in 1959 provided funds for the American Justice Institute to conduct a survey of modern correctional practices in the Western world.[45] In 1963 President Lyndon B. Johnson established the Commission on Law Enforcement and Administration of Justice, which subsequently issued the report *The Challenge of Crime in a Free Society*[46] in 1967. The report recommended "sweeping and costly changes in the administration" of corrective institutions throughout the country. The Congress in 1964, recognizing the deplorable conditions in correctional institutions, appropriated over $2 million to conduct a study of correctional manpower and training.

Although specific legislation directed toward rehabilitation within any correctional system (federal, state, and local) has decreased substantially in recent years, the public has favored the use of a large share of its tax dollar to fight crime. According to one investigator, 74 percent of the American public desire increases in federal funding to fight crime.[47] Government legislators and administrators apparently listened. In 1975 federal, state, and local governments spent $17.2 billion in criminal justice activities, and four years later, in 1979, spending reached $28 billion. Police services consumed the greater part of these dollars at the federal and local levels. Although the Law Enforcement Assistance Administration, which gave technical and financial assistance to state and local correctional agencies, was phased out of operation in 1980, the 1982 federal budget provided $128 million for assistance to local justice systems. Prisons accounted for the major spending at the state level.

In addition to providing funds for fighting crime, state legislatures passed bills designed to make control of criminals easier: lengthening prison sentences, eliminating parole for some offenses, and developing procedures so that sentences of repeat offenders might be doubled or tripled, limiting procedural rights, enacting gun controls, increasing penalties for noncapital crimes, and incarcerating those "likely" to commit crimes if free pending trial (pretrial preventive detention).[48]

FACILITIES

It was not until the late sixteenth century that prisons as places for the reception of ordinary criminals developed.[49] Earlier, prisons were used to confine military captives and those who committed crimes against landowners and the government.[50] Houses of correction were established in colonial America soon after the colonists arrived. The first penitentiary (Walnut Street jail) was established in Philadelphia in 1794. By 1835 America was credited with the establishment of the first genuine penal system in the world, although practices varied widely in the different states.[51] The first separate institution for women was the Indiana Women's Prison, which opened in 1873.

Many of the state prisons and local jails were built during the 1800s and early 1900s.[52]

Goals

Correctional facilities have multiple goals: (1) punishment, (2) deterrence of actual or potential offenders by making them fear prison sentences, (3) incapacitation of known offenders by holding them securely in custody for society's protection, and (4) rehabilitation of offenders so that they will have more interest in and capacity for legitimate alternatives to crime when they are released.

Characteristics

Correctional institutions today reflect a diversity of characteristics. Some have changed little since the early nineteenth century; others, however, have become the most progressive in the world. Between these two extremes are a great variety of institutions in all stages of development. Despite this, it is possible to identify some important elements about our correctional institutions:

They have become increasingly specialized. Separate institutions have been established for males and females, felons and misdemeanants, adults and youthful offenders.

Their administration has become centralized. Most states have some kind of central agency that exercises control over all correctional institutions, with a division of adult and juvenile authority.

Their programs have become more individualized. Programs are directed toward individual needs.

Their living conditions have improved.

Their social activities have been expanded to include athletic events, recreation, educational classes, and inmate councils.

Personnel standards and training have been increasingly recognized.[53]

Despite these positive elements, obstacles stand in the way of effective institutional correction. At present some of the most important obstacles are as follows:

Many facilities are old and antiquated.

Many facilities are too large but nevertheless are overcrowded.

In general, the living quarters are unnecessarily uncomfortable and unsuitable.

There is a lack of adequately trained personnel.

Segregation of offenders is not widely enforced, and so-called hardened offenders mix with low-risk offenders.

There is not enough work to keep offenders busy, and the type of work training provided is not in demand by potential employers.

Discipline tends to become rigid because rules are made to promote operational efficiency, regulate relationships, supervise offenders, and prevent escapes and disturbances.

Parole policies and practices are sometimes unfair or inefficient.

Life tends to be monotonous and oppressive.

Institutional budgets are inadequate.[54]

Classification

There are many types of correctional insitutions for men, women, and juveniles; the more common ones are prisons and penitentiaries, reformatories, correctional centers, farms, ranches, camps, jails, juvenile detention centers, and training and industrial schools for both boys and girls. These institutions can be classified according to control (governmental), length of stay and type of crime (long term or short term, felony or misdemeanor) and type of security.

There are three types of security: (1) Maximum-security institutions are walled, the prisoners are housed in cells, they work and recreate within the walls, and they are guarded. In essence, the prisoner rarely is unobserved wherever he or she is within the prison. (2) Medium-security institutions may or may not be walled, prisoners are usually housed in dormitories, and recreational, vocational, and counseling programs exist in greater number. Although prisoners may work immediately outside the prison and there is less security, prisoners are still supervised, controlled, and under surveillance. (3) Minimum-security institutions are open institutions, usually with no fence. In many instances they are called correctional centers. Prisoners live in unlocked buildings or dormitories and work inside or outside the center. Guards are at a minimum, and rehabilitation programs are an exception, since most prisoners in such facilities are seen as needing not rehabilitation but punishment. In the state prison systems about one-third of the facilities are maximum security, one-third medium security, and one-third minimum security.

PERSONNEL

In the correctional system many of the same personnel found in the health and health-related facilities are also found—psychiatrists, psychologists, social workers, counselors, teachers, and recreation specialists; however, some personnel besides correctional officers (guards) are unique to this system.

1. *Correctional commissioner or administrator of state correctional department*: is an individual with specialized professional education and training in criminology, penology, police administration, or other closely allied specialty.
2. *Warden or superintendent*: is administratively responsible for the function and operation of an institution within the framework of the laws and departmental policies and procedures.
3. *Associate warden*: usually two administrators and separate divisions; one is responsible for custody or security, the other for treatment.
4. *Classification officer*: is responsible for diagnosing and planning the custodial care and constructive treatment program for the offender as well as preparing the preparole report.
5. *Parole officer*: administers a program of supervision and guidance of parolees; may be assisted by specialized parole officers responsible for preparole investigation, employment placement, training, or research.
6. *Probation officer*: is responsible for presentence investigation and supervision of probationers under the administration of the judicial system; probation officers administer to either juveniles or adults.
7. *Parole board*: is responsible for all parole decisions; membership consists of persons usually appointed by the governor of the state, by a panel of government officials, or by a board of corrections where such exists.[55]

Taking into account the type of population found in our correction system, the rate of turnover, and the mission of the various institutions, over 290,000 individuals were employed in federal, state, county, and local correctional institutions in 1983[56] according to the Bureau of the Census. In the field of correctional recreation no accurate figures are available. It can be assumed that at least one recreation specialist would be employed in each federal and state correctional facility.

SERVICES

The scope of correctional system services is limited as compared to that of health and health-related services. The rehabilitation or resocialization services offered are designed to meet the needs of the offender; however, the quality of such services is questionable. According to many observers, daily services and rehabilitation programs provided by the federal government are superior to those of the various state governments.[57] Services found in the correctional system in addition to recreational services are as follows:

1. *Adult probation:* a type of sentence that requires the individual offender to remain in the community under the supervision and jurisdiction of the court.
2. *Furloughs:* temporary release for family visits, especially in family emergencies; interviews with prospective employers in preparation for permanent release; training or medical care; and participation in religious, educational, social, civic, and recreational affairs.
3. *Halfway house:* a homelike residential facility located in the community for offenders who need more control than probation or other types of community supervision can provide.
4. *Institutional training and treatment:* academic and vocational as well as individual and group counseling and therapy, testing, etc.
5. *Juvenile aftercare:* release of juveniles from an institution or training or school facility at the time when they can best benefit from release and from life in the community under the supervision of a counselor.
6. *Parole:* release of adult felon offenders from an institution after they have served part of their sentence under the supervision of the state and under prescribed conditions.
7. *Pretrial intervention:* a program designed to provide a rapid rehabilitation response for young first-offenders following arrest but prior to trial. The court suspends prosecution for a ninety-day period and places the youth into a program of counseling, training, and employment assistance.
8. *Prerelease centers:* supervised program designed to ease the transition from total confinement to freedom by involving people from the community who come to the prison to provide information in areas of vital interest to the inmate who is about to be released.
9. *Work-release:* the offender is confined in an institution only at night or on weekends but is permitted to pursue normal routine the remainder of the time.[58]

There is one other type of criminal justice program that some believe is an answer to corrections: community-based corrections. *Community-based corrections* refers to all correctional activities that occur in the community. They are viewed as alternatives to incarceration and include such programs and activities as pretrial diversion and probation, halfway houses, release and furlough programs, and parole. The major concept behind the community-based corrections approach is not simply moving the offender from prison to the outside world but involving the outside world in the rehabilitation and resocialization of the offender.[59]

EVALUATION OF QUALITY OF SERVICE

Efforts to establish measurable standards of practice have existed since the mid-1940s. In 1946 the American Correctional Association (ACA) developed a Manual of Correctional Standards. In 1974, with the assistance of the LEAA and several private foundations and corporations, the Commission on Accreditation for Corrections was established. The commission has promulgated standards (including recreational standards) for both adults and youth in parole, residential services, probation and parole field services, correctional institutions, local detention centers, training schools, and standards for the correctional system.[60] Since the early 1980s there has been a strong push toward accrediting programs and agencies.

While accreditation is a move in the right direction, it is evident that it has not kept pace with its counterparts in the field of education and medicine. If one considers the recidivism rate as a criterion for measuring success, quality of service has failed. One investigator involved in a long-term study of offenders in correctional institutions found that 35 percent of those exposed to a rehabilitation program violated parole or were convicted of a felony within two years after release, and the figure climbed to 63 percent eighteen years after release.[61] Another investigator came to the general conclusion that *some* rehabilitation programs were found to be effective for *some* types of offenders, but a general formula for rehabilitation has yet to be found.[62]

We noted in Chapter 2 that the rehabilitation (resocialization) model introduced into the correctional system (prisons) in the early 1960s was a failure by the early 1970s, and a renewed emphasis was put on the custody model. A number of reasons have been suggested for the failure: lack of political and economic support, lack of prison administrative support, inmate as well as staff resistance, and lack of knowledge about the cause of criminal behavior.[63] In-depth investigations by Martinson and Lipton noted that skill development programs and counseling programs were ineffective in reducing postrelease failure.[64] Lipton also noted that recreation by itself had only marginal effects and was more of a morale builder within prisons.

Relative to the quality of service for youth, the picture is not much brighter than it is for adults in their respective settings. Even those detention centers reserved for youthful offenders awaiting hearings may be a rude shock for first offenders. They are seldom adequately staffed with house parents, social workers, recreation specialists, teachers, and the like. Seldom are they large enough to segregate first-time offenders from more experienced ones. The problems associated with detention centers appear to be related mostly to their misuse or maladministration by judges and court officials.[65] It is difficult to indicate the success of rehabilitation and preventive programs. A few agencies are effectively involved in quality services; however, there appears to be no genuine commitment at most local, county, or state levels.

SUMMARY

This chapter considered various factors that contribute to the rehabilitation of individuals in health or health-related systems and the correctional system. Successful rehabilitation is broad in scope, practical in purpose, and integrated in practice. Considering the inertia of human thought and established practice, the broadened scope of rehabilitation has been little short of startling. No longer are only a few dedicated individuals and a small group of rehabilitation agencies and specialists concerned. Today the general public, voluntary health agencies, government, and many organized professional disciplines have awakened to the challenge of rehabilitation.

NOTES

1. House Committee Print no. 1, *Operations of Veterans Administration Hospitals and Medical Programs.* 94th Cong., 1st Sess. (Washington, D.C.: U.S. Government Printing Office, 1975), p. 29.

2. Cited in David Park, *Legislation Affecting Park Services and Recreation for Handicapped Individuals* (Washington, D.C.: Hawkins & Associates, 1980), p. 15.

3. Ibid., p. 6.

4. Ibid., p. 16.

5. Federal Programs Advisory Service, *Handicapped Requirement Handbook* (Washington, D.C.: the service, 1978), app. 111:c:1.

6. Park, *Legislation*, pp. 7, 17–19.

7. "Medicare/Medicaid," *Health Policy: The Legislative Agenda* (Washington, D.C.: Congressional Quarterly, 1980), p. 73.

8. Edward Schaltschneider, *The Semi-Sovereign People* (Hinsdale, Ill.: Dryden Press, 1960), pp. 23–25.

9. Ibid., p. 40.

10. A partial listing of voluntary organizations and their addresses is found in appendix E.

11. See Aubrey H. Fine, "Private Foundations: A Need for Further Explorations," *Therapeutic Recreation Journal*, 18, no.4 (1984), 48–55, for an excellent review of foundations and therapeutic recreation.

12. A partial listing of professional health organizations and their addresses is found in appendix E.

13. B. J. Stern, *Medical Services by Government* (New York: Commonwealth Fund, 1946), chap. 6.

14. John G. Freymann, *The American Health Care System: Its Genesis and Trajectory* (New York: Medcom Press, 1974), pp. 22–24.

15. These figures on hospitals are from Richard Stevens, *American Medicine and Public Interest* (New Haven, Conn.: Yale University Press, 1971), p. 52.

16. Malcolm T. MacEachern, *Hospital Organization and Management* (Chicago: Physician's Record Co., 1962), pp. 21–27.

17. Bureau of the Census, *Statistical Abstract of the United States, 1985*, (Washington, D.C.: U.S. Government Printing Office, Dec. 1984), p. 106.

18. Adapted from National Center for Health Statistics, *Health Resources Statistics: Health Manpower and Health Facilities, 1976*, Public Health Service, U.S. Department of Health, Education, and Welfare (Washington, D.C.: U.S. Government Printing Office, 1979), pp. 384–89.

19. See Ken Kesey, *One Flew Over the Cuckoo's Nest* (New York: Viking Press, 1962), or Michael Glenn's *Voices from the Asylum* (New York: Harper & Row, Publishers, 1974), for an interesting and somewhat frightening account of what life can become like in an institution. See also Mary Jan Ward, *The Snake Pit* (New York: Random House, 1940), for a view of what an "enlightened" hospital was like in the 1940s. For contrast, see Morton M. Hunt, *Mental Hospital* (New York: Pyramid Books, 1962), for an account of the experience of New York's Pilgrim State Hospital with large-scale use of tranquilizing drugs.

20. Jerry Zusman and Edward F. Bertsch, eds., *The Future Role of the State Hospital* (Lexington, Mass.: D. C. Heath & Co., 1975); and Milton Greenblatt and Edward Glazier, "The Phasing Out of Mental Hospitals in the United States," *American Journal of Psychiatry* 132 (1975), 1131–39.

21. Fred Redlick and Sam R. Kellert, "Trends in American Mental Health," *American Journal of Psychiatry* 135, no. 1 (1978), 22–28; also Richard Scheerenberger, *Public Residential Services for the Mentally Retarded, 1979* (Madison, Wis.: National Association of Superintendents of Public Residential Facilities for the Mentally Retarded, 1980).

22. Stevens, *American Medicine*, p. 80.

23. "Power to the Coalitions: Experts See New Balance of Health Care Forces," *Modern Hospital* 56, no. 4 (April 1980), 39.

24. U.S. Department of Labor, Employment and Earnings (Washington, D.C.: U.S. Government Printing Office, February 1985), p. 59.

25. Ruth S. Hanft, "Health Manpower," in *Health Care Delivery in the United States*, ed. Steven Jonas (New York: Springer Publishing Co., 1977), pp. 69–70.

26. Ibid.

27. Ibid.

28. Job titles and descriptions adapted from National Center for Health Statistics, *Health Resources Statistics, 1975* (Washington, D.C.: U.S. Government Printing Office, 1979).

29. Census, *Statistical Abstract, 1985*, p. 96.

30. Henry Schwartz, *The Case for American Medicine: A Realistic Look at Our Health Care System* (New York: David McKay Co., 1982), p. 18.

31. Ruth French, *Dynamics of Health Care*, 3rd ed. (New York: McGraw-Hill Book co., 1979), p. 36.

32. A. A. Donabedian, *A Guide to Medical Care Administration, II: Medical Care Appraisal—Quality and Utilization* (New York: American Public Health Association, 1969).

33. Ibid., pp. 2–3.

34. Marcia J. Carter, "State Licensure: Trend or Fad." Paper presented at the National Therapeutic Recreation Institute, Congress of Parks and Recreation, Louisville, Oct. 24, 1982.

35. Donabedian, *Medical Care Administration*, pp. 2–3.

36. Ibid.

37. President's Commission on Law Enforcement and Administration of Justice, *The Challenge of Crime in a Free Society* (Washington, D.C.: U.S. Government Printing Office, 1967), pp. 8–9.

38. Joseph F. Sheley, *America's "Crime Problem"* (Belmont, Calif.: Wadsworth Publishing Co., 1985), p. 296.

39. Cited in Robert M. Carter, Daniel Glaser, and Leslie T. Wilkins, eds., *Correctional Institutions* (Philadelphia: J. B. Lippincott Co., 1972), p. 99.

40. Ibid., 2nd ed. (1977), p. 103.

41. Sheley, *America's "Crime Problem,"* p. 303.

42. Ibid.

43. Ibid.

44. U.S. Department of Justice, *Prisoners at Midyear* (Washington, D.C.: U.S. Government Printing Office, 1983), p. 3.

45. John Conrad, *Crime and Its Correction: An Introductory Survey of Attitudes and Practices* (Berkeley: University of California Press, 1965).

46. President's Commission, *Crime in a Free Society.*

47. Cited in Sheley, America's *"Crime Problem,"* p. 27, as are the other facts and figures in this paragraph.

48. Ibid.

49. Robert G. Caldwell, *Criminology,* 2nd ed., (New York: Ronald Press Co., 1965), p. 493.

50. Thorsten Sellin, "Penal Institutions," *Encyclopedia of the Social Sciences 1934,* vol. 12 (New York: Macmillan, 1935), pp. 12, 57–64.

51. Elmer H. Johnson, *Crime, Correction, and Society* (Homewood, Ill.: Corsey Press, 1964), p. 370.

52. Caldwell, *Criminology,* chap. 20.

53. Sanford H. Kadish, ed., *Encyclopedia of Crime and Justice,* vol. 1 (New York: Free Press, 1983), pp. 143–61.

54. Ibid.

55. Job descriptions adapted from Caldwell, *Criminology,* pp. 572–79, 678–80, 682.

56. Census, *Statistical Abstract, 1985,* p. 176.

57. Harry E. Allen and Clifford E. Simonsen, *Corrections in America: An Introduction,* 4th ed. (New York: Macmillan, 1986), pp. 444–45.

58. Adapted from the American Correctional Association, *Manual of Correctional Standards,* 3rd ed. (College Park, Md.: the association, 1966); President's Committee on Law Enforcement and Administration of Justice, *Task Force Report: Corrections* (Washington, D.C.: U.S. Government Printing Office, 1967); and Elmer H. Johnson, *Crime, Correction, and Society,* (Homewood, Ill.: Dorsey Press, 1978), pp. 553–59.

59. Sheley, America's *"Crime Problem,"* p. 315.

60. Commission on Accreditation for Corrections, *Manual of Standards for Correctional Institutions* (Rockville, Md.: the commission, 1977).

61. Harry Kitchener, "How Persistent Is Post-Prison Success?" *Federal Probation* 41 (1977), 9–15.

62. Thomas Palmer, "Martinson Revisited," *Journal of Research for Crime and Delinquency* 12 (1975), 133–52.

63. Sheley, America's *"Crime Problem,"* pp. 313–19.

64. Robert Martinson, "What Works? Questions and Answers about Prison Reform," *Public Interest* 35 (1974), 22–54; and David Lipton et al., *The Effectiveness of Correctional Treatment: A Survey of Treatment Evaluation Studies* (New York: Praeger Publishing, 1975).

65. John Ortiz Smykla, *Community-Based Corrections: Principles and Practices* (New York: Macmillan, 1981).

SUGGESTED READINGS

ALFORD, ROBERT. *Health Care Politics: Ideological and Interest Group Barriers to Reform.* Chicago: University of Chicago Press, 1975.

ALLEN, A. *Introduction to Health* (2nd ed.). St. Louis: C. V. Mosby Co., 1976.

BEAN, PHILLIP. *Mental Illness: Changes and Trends.* New York: John Wiley & Sons, 1983.

BIRCHINALL, JANE, and MICHAEL E. SREIGHT. *Introduction to Health Careers.* Philadelphia: J. B. Lippincott Co., 1978.

BUTLER, ROBERT. *Why Survive? Being Old in America.* New York: Harper & Row, Publishers, 1975.

CARTER, MARCIA JEAN. "Issues in Continuing Professional Competence of Therapeutic Recreators," *Therapeutic Recreation Journal,* 18, no. 3 (1984), 7–10.

CARTER, ROBERT M., DANIEL GLASER, and LESLIE T. WILKINS. *Correctional Institutions* (2nd ed.). Philadelphia: J. B. Lippincott Co., 1977.

COYNE, PHYLLIS A., and LISA THOMAS TURPEL. "Peer Program Review: A Model for Implementation of Standards," *Therapeutic Recreation Journal,* 18, no. 2 (1984), 7–13.

DOUGLAS, J. *The Sociology of Deviance.* Boston: Allyn & Bacon, 1984.

FREYMANN, JERRY G. *The American Health Care System: Its Genesis and Trajectory.* New York: Medcom Press, 1974.

GREENBLATT, M., and E. GLAZIER. "The Phasing Out of Mental Hospitals in the United States." *American Journal of Psychiatry* 132, no. 6 (1975), 1135.

HATFIELD, DICK. "Selected Bibliography and Glossary on DRG's Prospective Pricing," *Therapeutic Recreation Journal,* 18, no. 4 (1984), 56–61.

HASENFIELD, YEHESKEL, and RICHARD A. ENGLISH, eds. *Human Service Organizations.* Ann Arbor: University of Michigan, 1978.

HOUSE OF REPRESENTATIVES. *How Our Laws Are Made.* Washington, D.C.: U.S. Government Printing Office, 1971.

JEFFERY, CHARLES R. *Biology and Crime.* Beverly Hills, Calif.: Sage Publications, 1979.

MECHANIC, DAVID, ed. *Politics, Medicine, and Social Sciences.* New York: Wiley-Interscience Publishers, 1974.

NATIONAL COMMISSION FOR HEALTH CERTIFYING AGENCIES. *Federal Regulations of Health Occupations.* Washington, D.C.: the commission, February, 1982.

NATIONAL COMMISSION FOR HEALTH CERTIFYING AGENCIES. *Perspectives on Health Occupational Credentialing.* Washington, D.C. U.S. Government Printing Office, DHHS publication no. (HRA) 80–39, April 1980.

OFFICE OF PROFESSIONAL STANDARDS REVIEW. *PSRO Program Manual.* Washington, D.C.: U.S. Government Printing Office, 1974.

PRESIDENT'S COMMISSION ON LAW ENFORCEMENT AND ADMINISTRATION OF JUSTICE. *The Challenge of Crime in a Free Society.* Washington, D.C.: U.S. Government Printing Office, 1967.

PRESIDENT'S COMMITTEE ON MENTAL HEALTH. *Report to the President,* vol 1. Washington, D.C.: U.S. Government Printing Office, 1978.

RILEY, ROBERT, ed. *Evaluation of Therapeutic Recreation through Quality Assurance.* State College, Penna.: Venture Publishing, Inc. 1987.

ROGES, M. "Legislative and Licensing Problems in Health Care," *Nursing Administration Quarterly* 2, (1978), 71–78.

SHAPIRO, IRA G. "The Path to Accreditation," *Parks and Recreation* 12, no. 1, (1977), 29–31, 68.

TALKINGTON, PAUL C. *Delivering Mental Health Services: Needs, Priorities and Strategies.* Washington, D.C.: American Psychiatric Association, 1975.

WHITAKER, GORDON P., and CHARLES D. PHILLIPS, eds. *Evaluating Performance of Criminal Justice Agencies.* Beverly Hills, Calif.: Saga Publications, 1983.

ZUSMAN, J., and E. F. BERTSCH, eds. *The Future Role of the State Hospitals.* Lexington, Mass.: D. C. Heath & Co., 1975.

4

Historical Development of Rehabilitation and Therapeutic Recreation

In the consideration of therapeutic recreation as a helping profession, it is important to devote attention to the development of recreation services in hospitals and in settings of a rehabilitation nature, including correctional settings. In so doing we must consider the historical background and development of health and correctional rehabilitation, since therapeutic recreation service as we know it today was born within the settings concerned with rehabilitation.

The concepts of rehabilitation and therapeutic recreation are not new, although a definitive history of both has yet to be written. The origin of rehabilitation in the history of the human race is dim and is even dimmer as it relates to therapeutic recreation. History does not record an orderly progression of positive trends in relation to the treatment and rehabilitation of individuals who were different in various ways, but rather it displays a highly variable and widely discrepant range of trends during most historical periods.

These trends were determined by nature, irrational and rational beliefs, social and economic conditions, religion, law, and finally by knowledge.

In this chapter we will not only look to other times and places in an attempt to capture the beginnings of rehabilitation and recreation service to those with limiting conditions, disabilities, and social problems in various settings, but we will consider the gains and changes that have occurred. It is hoped that from this historical overview the student will gain a greater understanding of the heritage of therapeutic recreation and an appreciation of the influences that have made it what it is today. To know and understand is to offer a better service.

Initially, this chapter will consider the historical development of rehabilitation and therapeutic recreation from a health and health-related perspective; thereafter, in a similar but limited manner, it will consider the same topics from a correctional perspective.

HEALTH AND HEALTH-RELATED INSTITUTIONS

Disease and disability are as old as life itself. Anthropologists and archaeologists tell us that paleolithic people suffered from the pains of disease. For millions of years before human history, animals too suffered from many conditions we still recognize today. Disease is in reality a part of all life, since it is the reaction of the living organism to abnormal stress or stimulus. We know little about early humans' reaction to disease and disability except what can be pieced together from the study of artifacts and through comparative studies of those remnants of primitive cultures that still exist.

PREHISTORIC PERIOD

The view that humans were savage first and then became civilized and that good treatment of the sick, disabled, and aged is a criterion of higher civilization is contradicted by the facts, so far as primitive societies are concerned. Indeed, we find quite generally that food-gathering, fishing, and hunting communities were inclined to treat their ill and disabled members well. For example, in the 1950s the skeletal remains of several Neanderthal people were discovered in northern Iraq. One appeared to have a variety of severe disabilities, yet the remains indicated that human compassion was well developed in Neanderthal times. The evidence indicated that the people in his group favored him, protected him from undue harm, and found a protective place for him in their society.[1]

Where life was hard, the sick and infirm were sacrificed in special circumstances: when the food or water gave out, when the tribe was starting out on a long migration, or when epidemics caused such fear of the sick that they were abandoned.[2] In general, it appears that the chief cause for the elimination of the sick and infirm was economic conditions. When they were economically useless, there was no point in preserving them.

In the early period of human history it seems safe to assume that only the "fittest" survived. Each person had a role to play in self-protection and self-preservation; if he was not able to do so, he died. Leading a life of hardship surrounded by the hostile forces of nature that they could not understand, humans developed supernatural explanations for the unknowns of life. A great body of religious and magical beliefs and practices developed. It is apparent that many, if not all, primitive people used recreation activities in the forms of dancing and music to drive away the evil spirits of disease. There is also some evidence that the disabled and sick were thought to be agents of a hostile world and were treated accordingly, and that malformed babies were destroyed.

Chanting, dancing, and music were not the only means used by primitive peoples for protection from evil or malevolent forces. *Amulets,* when worn or carried, protected the wearer from evil influences, black magic, and disease. *Talismans* would bring good luck. We cannot help but reflect upon the use of these same articles today. Present-day amulets include copper bracelets or horse chestnuts carried to ward off rheumatism, as well as horseshoes, rabbits' feet, and four-leaf clovers to bring good luck. The carrying of charms and other amulets counteracts the undesirable effects of such things as black cats, broken mirrors, walking under ladders, Friday the thirteenth, hexes, and also the "evil eye."

Medicine stood midway between magic and religion. As the magic lore increased, it became much too burdensome to administer, and a special person was designated to master these skills. Thus the medicine man emerged.

PRIMITIVE PERIOD

With developing civilization, social life became more complex. Families joined to form larger social groups, living and working together and following definite sets of rules. Women played an increasingly important part in the life of the group, doing farm work and attending to the home, while the men took care of the animals and were hunters, fishermen, traders, and also warriors.

At this stage of human history there seem to be some inconsistencies in the beliefs and actions toward the sick, disabled, and aged. There are some indications that while many cultures did not destroy their disabled as a general practice, they subjected them to other types of personal and social abuse and torment. On the other hand, there were groups that considered a disability a mark of distinction that brought special privilege or consideration to the individual. We might speculate that here was the dawn of the new approach to human differences and infirmities—the beginning of a shift from automatically eliminating life to the idea that there might be some worth or value in preserving the disabled.

Practices that hundreds of generations later were to be called *rehabilitation* seem to have started their development here. Archaeological findings reveal that certain mineral and hot water springs were used for special purposes other than drinking. We might speculate again that the water was used for the treatment of ailments, as it is today. It seems reasonable to assume that instinct may have been a source from which other methods of treatment sprang. An individual hurt his leg and spontaneously, without thinking, rubbed it. This rubbing developed into a system and became what we call *massage*. Another individual, suffering from arthritis, crawled to the fire and discovered that the heat relieved the pain. These simple instinctive reactions may then have developed into more controlled methods for the application of heat and cold, using water, steam, sand, or other available materials. Such media are used today by physical therapists.

Before these instinctive acts became a system of treatment of the injured or dis-

abled person, however, another important attitudinal change had to take place—that of mutual aid, of caring for the person involved. The idea that one human being could help to eliminate the suffering of another and thus perhaps prolong or save life appears to have been an early development. For whatever magical or religious reasons this was done, the important consideration here is the fact that care was taken of human life by others.

ANCIENT CIVILIZATIONS

As people invented writing and recorded their traditions and practices, they left explanations of the phenomena of nature, including disease, disablement, and old age. The explanations possess a similarity in all ancient civilizations, based as they are on religious-magical concepts that undoubtedly preceded the oldest written records. Two individuals were primarily concerned with these concepts and practices: the medicine man and the minister of religion, whose function it was to appease the deities. Eventually these two became united in one—the priest-physician who worked in the temple. Medicine as a field of endeavor now began the evolution from witchcraft to craft.

This medicine man or priest-physician was the first "professional." He was not just the forerunner of what we now call the *physician*, but also probably the model for many other professions. He was the wise man, the person who possessed the learning and specialized knowledge of the group. Practices became a blend of superstition and fact, of natural remedies and religious rituals. Yet these practices were logical for these cultures; they were in accord with their philosophy and religion.

Medical practice in ancient Egypt was divided into two schools: the *empiric*, which was costly and reserved for the royal family and the wealthy, and the *magico-ritual*, which was inexpensive and popular. We cannot help but be struck by the idea that even though much early care was purely magical in nature, it nevertheless included elements that are also found in rational therapy. Early Egyptian writings indicate that to receive forgiveness from the gods, one must "walk in the gardens which surround the temple, row on the majestic Nile, and embark upon . . . planned excursions . . . dancing, listening to concerts, and acting in representations. These are the ways required for those possessed by illness."[3] According to Frye, "Priests are said to have been aware that the dispelling of morbid moods was aided by the temple atmosphere, the beauty of lotus gardens, and the ritual songs and dances of the temple maidens."[4] From the very beginning, therapy seems to have been an interwoven combination of empirical, rational, magical, and religious elements.

Paralleling the Egyptian civilization, although not quite as ancient, was the civilization that flourished in the Indus River valley of India, comprising people of unknown origin and the great Aryan migration that peopled India and parts of western Asia and Europe. Some of the most ancient Indian medical texts contain magic formulas against demons. At this time medicine was almost entirely in the hands of the ruling caste of Brahmins. In the Brahmanic period, physicians belonged to a caste lower than the priests. The physician Charaka is considered to be one of the founders of Indian medicine.[5] As noted by Avedon, Charaka not only advocated the use of toys and games but felt that hospitals had the responsibility to provide them for patient use.[6]

In its turn Chinese medicine, influenced by the Buddhist philosophies imported from India and by Confucianist principles, became an extremely intricate art. It also appears that in some parts of China a tradition of kindness and understanding toward the mentally ill existed. Similarly, Confucius admonished that one should be kind and help those of "weak mind."[7] The use of recreative activities as a form of therapy and as an adjunct to treatment was not unknown. Various forms of gymnastics and massage were suggested as prevention to disease.[8]

Other recreation activities were used in association with surgery.[9]

The idea that an individual should be compensated for injury or loss of a part of the body was accepted by most ancient civilizations. The rights of the person injured or afflicted were first expressed in Babylonia in retaliatory terms: "Eye for eye, tooth for tooth, hand for hand, foot for foot."[10] This was the usual compensation between persons of like social status; however, monetary compensation was usual for the injured person who was considered to be of lower status and thus inferior to the injurer. The great code, as given by Hammurabi, provided regulations in regard to fees and compensations for injured persons as well as employment practices.[11] The provisions were mixed with superstition and magic and were harsh, but perhaps for the first time groups or communities were responsible for the individual, both the injured and the injurer.

The Mosaic code given to the Hebrews also provided for individual rights by the group. These were perhaps the first public health regulations, providing rules for sanitation, cleanliness, and reporting and isolating contagious disease, as well as specifying hours for work and rest.[12] The Twelve Tablets of Rome and the Anglo-Saxon codes provided for monetary compensation for injury.[13] Our current concepts and laws of workmen's compensation undoubtedly developed from the same basic ideas embodied in these early regulations.

The Jews, as a result of the strength of their faith in one God, began to stem the tide of superstition and magic. Their God was recognized as the source of health, and the Jews held the extreme view that disease and illness were punishment for sins of the individual and his family. This belief is still held by many people as part of our attitudinal pattern toward disease and disability.

GREEK-ROMAN PERIOD

These beginnings covered a great deal of time in human history, providing the background for the growth of knowledge attained by the Greeks. In contrast to other ancient peoples, the Greeks desired to live according to reason, and they searched for perfection and first causes. Their desire for "a good mind in a good body" seems to have been responsible for a great shift in the philosophy of care for the sick and disabled, if only for a brief moment in history. For the first time the part that a person's mind and feelings play in treatment was recognized. The idea of the whole person, so important in present rehabilitation activities, apparently started at this time.

The healing arts were practiced in temples. These temples were apparently situated in scenic places. It is reported that the temples of Aesculapius were built in healthful pastoral settings, usually with mineral springs at hand; they were equipped with bathing pools, gymnasia, and gardens.[14] At Epedaurus, thirty miles outside Athens, the temples included exercise grounds, a race track, a library, a stadium, and a theater seating twenty thousand persons.[15] On arrival the patient sacrificed an animal to Aesculapius, received a purifying bath in the mineral springs followed by a massage, and then went to sleep on one of the porches, surrounded by sweet odors and soothing music.[16] The effects of the environment and recreational activities on the patient apparently were recognized.

The genius of ancient medicine was a Greek—Hippocrates, the philosopher-physician and "father of medicine." He became the father of medicine by following the prevalent trend of Greek intellectual convictions at the time, by basing his practice of medicine on the study of nature, and by considering disease to be subject to the "natural law" of cause and effect. His oath, defining the ideals, duties, and responsibilities of a physician, is still used today in the medical profession. One of his great contributions was the *case study method* as the approach to medical education.[17] The clinician taught and learned by observation and study at the bedside of his patient. Up to this time

knowledge about illness and disease was handed down from father to son. Hippocrates' fundamental belief was that illness and defects of the body were due to natural, normal, realistic causes and thus removable causes. For example, he dismissed the notion that epilepsy, considered "the sacred disease," was divinely caused. According to Hippocrates:

> It thus appears to me to be in no way more divine, nor more sacred than other diseases, but has a natural cause from which it originates like other afflictions. . . . If you open the head, you will find the brain humid, full of sweat, and smelling badly. And in this way you may see that it is not a god which injures the body, but disease.[18]

His views helped to free the field from superstition and convert it into an empirical art to be studied and mastered by the slow process of trial-and-error learning. For the first time the patient became the center of attention and was studied as an individual; records were kept so that the same signs might be recognized in another person.

Even though Hippocrates, Plato, and Aristotle challenged the common belief that illness was the result of the anger of the gods, powerful forces lingering from the past and beliefs in demons were destined to exert a dominant influence on the scientific approach to treatment. Thus, the conflict over natural versus supernatural causes for physical and mental disorders was to continue for more than a thousand years.

Following Greece, Rome became the undisputed master of the world. Its native system of care for the sick and disabled was very primitive and unscientific compared to that of the Greeks. Rome made few if any contributions to the healing arts. Romans were suspicious of and reluctant to use the medical knowledge they took over from the Greeks. On the other hand, in the story of modern rehabilitation the Romans contributed greatly through their organizational genius in public health measures. They introduced sanitary measures through the issuing of government decrees. One prohibited burials within the city; another ordered officials to look after the cleanliness of streets and the water supply; still another established a public medical service of physicians to look after the needs of the poor. It is reported that a system of semisocialized medicine was organized, with state, circuit, and municipal doctors being appointed.[19] This was probably the first attempt of government to meet the needs of its citizens regardless of class.

During the thirteen centuries of the Roman Empire, treatment of mentally ill and mentally retarded persons varied greatly, often depending upon the changing philosophies and attitudes of the rulers as well as the social class. According to Durant, a special market was established at one time in Rome where one might purchase "legless, armless, or three-eyed men, giants, or dwarfs."[20] At times infanticide was practically nonexistent; in other periods the practice was widespread. Abandonment of children was also a widespread practice. Seneca records that professional beggars often collected such children, deliberately maimed them, and then used them to solicit alms from charitable passersby.[21] Frequently, however, alternatives were available. During the first century A.D., for example, unwanted infants could be placed at the base of the Columma Lacteria, where the state provided wet nurses to look after them.[22]

The greatest of all Roman innovations was the hospital system, although according to some historians, the beginning of a hospital system can be traced back to 1550 B.C.[23] The Roman hospital system was established chiefly by the army, and all early Christian hospitals were modeled after the Roman ones. They were built on the corridor plan, had as many as forty wards, and were supervised by an army surgeon. Infirmaries were built for the poor, and it is reported that physicians' homes were used as nursing homes for better-class patients.[24] Patients were moved outdoors to enjoy the sunshine. A physician named Soranus prescribed music to relieve pain. In a later period of Roman history another physician, Galen, prescribed recreational activities to assist in relaxation of the body and mind.[25]

After A.D. 350 pagan temples were closed in Rome, and the first privately sponsored civilian hospital was founded by a wealthy Roman matron, Fabiola, who dedicated both her wealth and her daily life to nursing the sick. She is reported to have walked the streets of Rome searching out the ill and maimed, even at times carrying them to the hospital on her back. Fabiola may have been the first Mother Terésa. Fabiola's country villa was used as a convalescent home and, as far as is known, was the first rest home annexed to a city hospital.[26]

Jesus, the great teacher of Christianity, in his compassion for those who suffered from physical, mental, and social problems at the hands of their fellow men, emphasized the human, individualized approach to care and treatment. His teachings were based on the Jewish faith in one God and emphasized the dignity of each human life, regardless of race, class, or infirmity—a concept present since the beginning of the recreation movement.

The philosophy that all care and treatment should be based on love and the brotherhood of humankind is directly responsible for much that is included in modern rehabilitation practice. The Christian church as a social organization often failed to live up to these teachings, but it served to preserve the emphasis on the importance of the individual, which is at the heart of Western democratic culture.

THE MIDDLE AGES

The downfall of the Roman Empire left Europe without a single unifying governing structure, and health efforts reverted to a primitive level. What was needed at this time seemed to be a ruling authority under the protection of which some new form of social organization might grow. It was the Christian church—with its excellent organi ation, its strong central authority, and its discipline—that helped make the growth of new Europe possible.

For about eight centuries classical learning and science passed into the church's keeping. This was fortunate for they might have been lost forever. However, the intellectual independence of the individual had to be sacrificed to the authority of the church. The church also took over the role of physician of the body as well as of the mind and soul, and it was again a strange mixture of physical remedies, magic, and ritual that was dispensed. Hippocrates had freed treatment and care from religion and superstition and had taught that illness and disability were not sent by the gods as punishment but rather were natural phenomena to be studied. Under church rule the supernatural origin of disease was revived, partly because to be a physician one first had to be ordained a priest. Very little progress was made in theory and research during the early Middle Ages—the doctrine of the four humors prevailed, and few had the knowledge or courage to question its authority. It was not until the early 1000s that social, economic, and political life began to be revived.

During the Dark Ages in Europe hospitals presented some of the worst environments ever endured by suffering humanity. It was largely dirt and physical abuse that made them houses of death: no bathing, no fresh air, no clean linen, no healthy diets or emotional considerations, and no activities. There was frequent recourse to abusing or flogging patients ill with germ-caused or mental diseases, to drive out the "willfully harbored" demons.[27]

While darkness prevailed in Western Europe, life was brighter in other parts of the world. The idea of the hospital was carried forward by the Arabs and the Christian church. Islamic hospitals became models of human kindness, especially in the treatment of the mentally ill. Cairo's Mansur Hospital cooled its fever wards by fountains; contained lecture halls, a library, chapels, and a dispensary; and was staffed with nurses of both sexes. It employed reciters of the Koran, musicians to lull patients to sleep, and storytellers for their distraction; discharged patients were given money to tide them over during convalescence.[28]

Although the Arabs were not the first to build hospitals, they are supposed to have been the first to perfect them. They are credited with having the first regular medical bedside instruction, outpatient department, and organized inspection of financial and administrative affairs. They were the first to license and examine physicians thoroughly and to require additional licensing for medical specialization.

By the end of the tenth century the excellence of Islamic medical care had become recognized in Europe, and several European centers of learning began to follow their examples of care. In addition, Islamic hospitals so impressed Christian pilgrims to the Holy Land that in the eleventh century a hospital was founded in Jerusalem. This was later expanded by the Crusaders and formed the kernel of the religious Order of the Knights of St. John of Jerusalem, the famous Knights Hospitalers who played a major role in the Crusades. Hospitals were also opened for the care of orphans and the aged, crippled, and blind.[29]

Originally medieval hospitals were built and administered by the church, but after the thirteenth century they began to be considered the responsibility of city government. In most cases the nursing was still done by monks or nuns, but the municipal authorities took over the task of administration. By the end of the Middle Ages hospitals were firmly and permanently established all over Europe. By the sixteenth century and thereafter, city government and wealthy private citizens began to consider it their duty to provide hospital care. Thus the modern pattern for supporting hospitals began to form.[30]

The separation between medicine and surgery lasted throughout the medieval period. In the ancient world the physician traced his art to scholars; he was a man of dignity who served the upper class. The surgeon, who worked with his hands, was of low social status; his professional ancestry was in barbering. It was not until the seventeenth century that surgery was considered a profession fit for men of upper classes. Ambroise Paré brought together in a working relationship the long-robed university physicians and the barber-surgeons whom the people relied upon. He believed in treating the complete person and was known for his ability to inspire his patients. It is reported that he attended to all details of a patient's treatment and recovery, even to methods of relieving boredom through games, music, and reading during convalescence. His practical genius was shown in his construction and development of artificial limbs and the glass eye. He is also credited with the statement: "I treat them, God cures them."[31]

It was during this age that the crippled and the mentally retarded came into prominence as "fools" or "jesters." The greater the deformity, the greater the mirth and laughter it provoked. Courts sought them. It is reported that the demand for jesters created a scarcity, increasing their value to such an extent that parents are said to have crippled their own children in order to enhance their value. For the first time the disabled were able to earn their living, however distasteful the method must have been to some.[32] At other times and places the mentally retarded were considered to be "innocents of God" and as such were not allowed to roam at all. Although they were restricted in their movements, they were not provided for and were often reduced to begging.[33]

The church, in providing custodial care in its monasteries, may have been a forerunner in the development of educational opportunities for those in its care. Up to this time no attention had been paid to the educational or training needs of physically disabled and intellectually handicapped people. With the church serving as the center for both physical care and education, it can be speculated that the idea arose that custodial care alone was insufficient for the individual's needs. Education and training of the handicapped, however, was to occupy a minor role until the eighteenth and nineteenth centuries.

The idea of homebound care was believed to have started in Gheel, Belgium, in the thirteenth century. The program at Gheel placed mentally ill and mentally retarded persons in family settings. Residents had their own bedrooms, ate meals with the family, and engaged in various community activities. This striking approach achieved excellent results and has continued to operate in one form or another in Gheel since its inception. It was not emulated in other parts of Europe until the nineteenth century and not in the United States until the 1930s.[34]

The seeds of knowledge planted in preceding centuries came to fruition in the fourteenth, fifteenth, and sixteenth centuries, initiating the cultural transition from medieval to modern civilization. Some of the forces that changed the existing medieval social order were the Renaissance, the Reformation, nationalism, the discovery of a new world, and the diffusion of knowledge through the printed word. All of these factors influenced the healing arts in one way or another.

MODERN TIMES

With the growth of scientific medicine during the eighteenth century and throughout the nineteenth century, the concept of human dignity was emphasized more and more. Witch burning finally ceased, and the world of demons was gradually overshadowed by a concern with the rights of man. The agents of this movement were rationalism and enlightenment. Although care and treatment did not initially change substantially, society in general began to regard the mentally and physically disabled with pity and to treat them with special care. Also as financial fortunes began to accumulate, the philanthropic concept evolved and was directed toward the medical and custodial care of the poor.

Eighteenth and Nineteenth Centuries

In moving into the eighteenth and nineteenth centuries, we cannot help but speculate about the possible influence of Locke and Rousseau on scientific medicine. John Locke, for example, attempted to distinguish between mental illness and mental retardation.[35] Locke and Rousseau both supported the belief that the mind could be developed through instruction, and they encouraged those attempting to develop the minds of retarded persons. According to some health historians, these philosophers were able to both generate considerable concern for the welfare of the common people and provide general guidelines for their improvement.[36]

We usually think of hospital insurance plans such as Blue Cross, which started in America in 1929, as a twentieth-century idea. However a Parisian philanthropist named Chamousset had a similar strategy. Chamousset's plan, published in 1757, advocated insurance to provide prepaid medical care either at home or in a hospital. The same medical treatment was arranged for everyone, but comforts varied according to the size of one's contribution. Reduced rates were available for workers or domestic servants, who were to be insured by their employers. Private doctors could be retained if patients chose to pay their fees; otherwise doctors were assigned. Hospitals would still be open as usual to noncontributors on a payment of fee. The plan estimated a month of illness for an average of twelve people out of every hundred subscribers.[37]

Phillippe Pinel, in the latter part of the eighteenth century in France, attempted to prove that kind and humane treatment of the insane would do much toward their recovery. According to one source, he was considered a madman engaged in the liberation of animals when he sought and received permission to remove the chains of the insane in the Bicétre Asylum (Paris).[38] He went on to develop the concept of "moral" management, which emphasized a treatment-oriented approach.[39] Likewise, Jean Itard, also in France, initiated the first scientific attempt at training a retarded child. As a result of the concerns of others in France, England, and the United States about the care of those considered insane and feeble-minded, care, treatment, and education in hospitals and residential schools were improved, and a new attitude of optimism was engendered.

The oldest so-called hospital in the United States was begun in a modest poorhouse supported by a church in the city of New Amsterdam. This house and a tiny hospital established by the West India Company in 1658 eventually combined and grew into the city hospital of Bellevue in New York. In 1736 a new building was designated as the Publick Workhouse and House of Correction of New York, and it included an infirmary with six beds. At first, Bellevue was only an epidemic hospital reserved for outbreaks of yellow fever. After the War of 1812 it was enlarged and used to house prisoners, the insane, the destitute, and impoverished sick people. It remained as such until 1848, after which the true hospital era of Bellevue began.[40]

The first general medical hospital in this country was established in 1751. Prior to the American Revolution the Quakers, with the aid of Benjamin Franklin, established the Pennsylvania Hospital in Philadelphia. This was a voluntary hospital designed to provide care for the sick, poor, and "lunatics." Some fifteen years later in this same city, John Morgan is credited with establishing the first medical school in America.[41]

The first American asylum exclusively for the mentally ill, Eastern State Hospital, was built in Williamsburg, Virginia, and opened in 1770.[42] However, mental patients were subjected to treatment that seems incomprehensible today. Dr. Benjamin Rush is known as one of our first gentlemen of medical science, but one of his orders for disturbed patients was to keep them standing and awake for twenty-four hours at a stretch. Mild and humane treatment first became a customary policy at Bloomingdale's sanitarium (now New York Hospital at Westchester), which was built in 1821. The first special-disease hospitals in America were built for the "insane" and for contagious cases, then for eye diseases, and later for countless other distinctions.[43]

It was not until 1817, in Hartford, Connecticut, that the first private school for the deaf was organized, and the first and only college for the deaf, called Deaf-Mute College, opened its doors in Washington, D.C., in 1864. This college was renamed Gallaudet College in honor of the early work of Thomas Hopkins Gallaudet, a teacher of the deaf and mute. Schools for the blind were founded in New York, Pennsylvania, and Massachusetts between 1829 and 1832. In 1899 the first tax-supported school program for physically disabled children was established in Chicago. The first public institution for the mentally retarded was not established until 1848 through legislative action in Massachusetts. The first club for older persons, a forerunner of the senior citizen clubs, was established in 1870 in Boston.[44]

During this period there is evidence of renewed interest in the use of recreational activities as aids in helping those considered to be mentally ill. Physicians were beginning to prescribe physical exercise, handicrafts, reading, and music for their patients. Dr. Benjamin Rush, the first American psychiatrist, wrote a letter to the managers of the Pennsylvania Hospital in 1810 advocating the use of many homely tasks, such as weaving, spinning, and other domestic occupations, for their therapeutic effect. Likewise, he recommended playing chess and checkers, listening to the flute or violin, reading, and making trips to the community.[45]

Patients selected by the physicians on the Committee of the Asylum of New York Hospital in 1821 participated in approved exercises and amusements. In 1822 a doctor at McLean Hospital in Massachusetts described the use of "draughts, chess, backgammon, nine-pins, swinging, sawing wood, gardening, reading, writing and music" as therapeutic in the diversion they provided the "lunatics."[46]

Bockovern and Zilboorg inform us that the moral therapists of the nineteenth century believed that psychiatric hospitals should exist to retrain patients so that they could live more fruitfully in society.[47] So firm was their conviction in the value of planned recreation that they involved all staff members and their children, as well as the patients, in the work of the hospital and in its games, social functions, and intellectual pursuits. For example, at the dinner hour all waited until the superintendent had taken the first bite of food; at the annual ball the grand march was headed by the superintendent and his wife; and in daily living on the wards the patients, attendants, and children of the staff had their recreation together.

Norman Dain, in his investigation of the history of psychiatric thought in the United States, reports that the patients of Friends' Asylum in Frankford, Pennsylvania, beginning in 1830, participated in social gatherings, played ball, flew kites, threw quoits, went fishing, and made trips to places of interest near the asylum. In the late 1830s and early 1840s many asylums had annual fairs that were open to the public. Patients also published weekly newspapers and presented theatrical performances.[48]

It was not unusual for hospital superintendents of the day to assume that activities were the best remedy for functional brain disorders. The "Code of Rules and Regulations for the Government of Those Employed in the Care of Patients of the Pennsylvania Hospital for the Insane at Philadelphia" contains this statement: "It is highly important that patients should, as far as possible, be kept constantly at some pleasant kind of employment—either work of some kind, or riding, walking, or amusements. . . ."[49]

In the first edition of *System of Practical Therapeutics* (1892), the section on the treatment of insanity written by Dr. Edward N. Brush included the following:

> Amusements should not be lost sight of in the enumeration of the remedial measures to be brought into play in caring for the insane. The sane mind enjoys laying aside the cares and perplexities of the hour and being simply amused. In the theatre or opera the outside world is forgotten; the mimic scene becomes real and supplants all else. Many institutions have distinct buildings devoted to the purposes of amusement. Theatrical performances, concerts, negro minstrels, lectures, views shown by the stereopticon, constitute some of the means which may be brought to use. These are of undoubted value and may, with benefit, be enjoyed by all classes of patients.[50]

Although therapeutic recreation activities have been of greatest use in the field of psychiatry until recent years, they have also been used sporadically by some as a muscle builder for those with disabilities of muscles and joints. Dr. Clement-Joseph Tissot of France, in his book *Gymnastique Medicinale et Cherurgicale* published in 1780, recommended "shuttlecock, tennis, football, dancing . . . and the game of barriers."[51]

Florence Nightingale not only led the way toward modern nursing techniques and care but also introduced and provided recreational opportunities for hospitalized soldiers. In her book *Notes on Nursing* she recommended pets for chronically ill patients and commented on the good effects of music upon patients.[52]

Until 1850 the main advances in hospital development resulted from historical changes in social or religious philosophy. While simple decency and humanity should have provided cleanliness, adequate food, sun, air, and water as part of hospital care, the scientific proof that diseases were caused by dirt and germs made hospital reformation inescapable. As innovations came about through an understanding of the role of bacteria in disease, the whole concept of hospitals changed. Sterilizers and daily changes of linen became routine; huge sterile operating rooms became the heart of the hospital. Humanitarianism and love were replaced by social obligations and scientific procedure, and the modern hospital was born.[53]

Industrial growth and urbanization during this same period brought about changes in working conditions and a demand for protection through labor legislation. This period was also marked by increased social consciousness and feelings of social responsibility on the part of the upper class and the educated for the welfare of lower-income groups. This concern resulted not only in social legislation but also in the establishment of settlement houses. The first such house was established by Oxford and Cambridge students in Toynebee Hall, East London, in 1875. The University Settlement, on the East Side of New York, opened in 1886, and Hull House in Chicago, under Jane Addams, in 1889.[54]

The humanitarian outlook was also carried over into a concern for those in special classes—the mentally retarded, the deaf, the blind, dependent children, and others—through federal and state legislation and private interest.[55] The agitation against owning slaves and their eventual emancipation were also aspects of this humanitarian concern. However, it was not until the twentieth century that social and economic conditions for blacks and other minority groups changed for the better.

Building on fragments of knowledge and understanding accumulated over thousands of years while dismantling centuries of cruelty, superstition, and neglect of the disabled, the 1800s firmly established care, treatment, and education as the mandate for the twentieth century.

Twentieth Century

The early twentieth century saw scientific approaches applied to the measurement of individual differences by Binet, the formulation of theories of learning by Pavlov and Watson and others, and the medical investigation of genetic and biochemical factors in mental retardation. In service to the retarded, by 1905 special classes were being introduced into public schools in larger cities.[56] By 1911 nearly one hundred cities had public school classes for the mentally retarded.[57] The 1920s and 1930s saw increased study of the individual variability of the retarded and of statewide coordination of services for their care and treatment. Beginning in 1930 placement of the retarded in families in the community was introduced.

The twentieth century also saw an increased respect for the emotional rights of individuals. Freud and other psychologists made important contributions to the psychological study of individuals. However, it was not until the late 1930s that a consistent effort was made to study the emotional problems of children.[58]

1900–1940. The first four decades of the century witnessed a gradual trend toward the development of organized recreation service for special populations in various institutional settings. This was especially so in the employment of full-time recreation workers to develop and direct recreation programs in federal and state hospitals/institutions serving the mentally ill and mentally retarded and, to a lesser degree, in general medical and surgical hospitals, special schools, and correctional institutions. Likewise, community-based programs were developed to meet the varied needs and interests of the physically disabled, mentally retarded, racial minorities, economically deprived, aged, and other special populations.

Shortly after the entry of the United States into World War I, the Division of Recreation in Hospitals was organized within the American National Red Cross. The function of this division was "to pro-

vide, in cooperation with the Educational Service of the Surgeon General's Office of the United States Army, supplemental recreation for soldiers, sailors, and marines in military and naval hospitals."[59] The Red Cross continued to provide recreation leadership and services to military hospitals and Public Health Service hospitals until 1931. At that time the treatment of ex-servicemen was transferred to the United States Veterans Bureau, and Red Cross recreation personnel were assigned to these hospitals.[60]

Between 1920 and 1930, recreation programs increased in state hospitals for the mentally ill and retarded. Also, shortly after 1931 a recreation service was established in St. Elizabeth's Hospital in Washington, D.C.

Although these programs in most instances were still diversional in nature, psychiatrists and others increasingly recognized the therapeutic value of recreation. As early as 1921 Dr. R. F. L. Ridgway, a psychiatrist at Harrisburg (Pennsylvania) State Hospital, wrote an article on recreation for the mentally ill to arouse interest in providing therapeutic recreation in such hospitals.[61] William Menninger and Isabelle McCall published an article in 1937 describing the value and use of recreation at the Menninger Clinic, a world-famous center for the care and treatment of the mentally ill in Topeka, Kansas.[62]

The White House Conference on Child Health and Protection in 1930 stirred interest in the creative use of recreation with the mentally retarded. As a result, programs based on individual needs and differences of the participants developed. In 1932 Bertha E. Schlotter and Margaret Svendsen at Lincoln State School and Colony in Illinois reported on the two-year success they had obtained in the use of recreation activities in developing social skills in retarded children.[63] Research by others into the play patterns of the mentally retarded during this period fostered recognition of the types of programs necessary to meet both community living and institutionalization.[64]

Although the provision of recreation service to other special population groups—physically disabled, blind, deaf, and the like—during these early years can be traced, such services were scattered throughout hospitals/institutions in the United States. Recreation service to the physically disabled and medically hospitalized was primarily the responsibility of the occupational therapist; teachers and physical educators assumed the responsibility in special schools.

In community services to special populations recreation service has not enjoyed the attention that it had in various hospital/institutional settings. It is interesting to note, however, that according to some historians, the formation of the Playground Association of America (1906) is a direct result of the concern early recreators had for the slum environment and its effects on children. The charter of the Playground Association of America refers, as does the present National Recreation and Park Association charter, to the provision of "broad recreation opportunities to all people regardless of age, sex, and religious faith."[65]

Despite this auspicious beginning, there was a definite decline in the provision of recreation service to meet the recreation needs of special populations, or at least those needs of minority group members, through public recreation agencies until the 1960s. The rationale for this inactivity is summarized by Hutchison:

> . . . it could be said that at its highest point of success, the recreation profession unwittingly allowed the prime focus of its mission to shift from the delivery of specialized human services to professional development and facility management. Unfortunately, it appears that the provision of services to people became a means to broader goals, purposes, and professional status, rather than remaining a vital and satisfying end unto itself.[66]

Despite the shortcomings of municipal recreation agencies in offering recreation services to special populations during the first half of this century, a number of national organizations concerned with various impairments and disabilities, service organizations, and special agencies did provide such services. In 1900, for example, the Association for the Aid of Crippled Children was providing recreation service in homes, schools, and hospitals, as well as operating summer programs for the physically disabled. Camping for physically disabled children was first recorded in 1888, but not until the 1930s did residential camping develop on a national scale. Easter Seal Societies throughout the United States led in this field; many of the state affiliates owned and operated resident and day camps serving children and adults, individuals and families. The Lighthouse, a service center operated by the New York Association for the Blind in New York City, has for many years offered recreation and camping programs. Similar programs for the blind are found in other cities.

It was also during the 1920s and early 1930s that public school systems began to offer recreation programs after school for disabled children. Today one of the nation's most extensive year-round community recreation programs for the physically disabled and mentally retarded is conducted by the Division of Municipal Recreation and Adult Education, Milwaukee Public Schools. A similar program is conducted by the Flint (Michigan) Community Schools. More and more public school systems, in cooperation with municipal recreation agencies, are offering programs for the disabled as the result of federal legislation.

1940–1960. Although World War I had given great impetus to the use of recreation in hospitals, its development was slow until World War II. World War II brought about tremendous expansion and acceleration in the recreation movement in hospitals and institutions. Red Cross hospital recreation workers were again called upon by the military to provide recreation services in military hospitals here and overseas. While medical approval was required for patient participation in recreation activities, the services were not narrow or limited, as indicated by the description below:

> Individualized as well as group activities were conducted indoors on wards, in recreation halls, auditoriums, craft shops, game rooms, and the like; outdoors on lawns surrounding the hospital as well as in other areas such as picnic grounds or small parks often provided on military installations. Offpost trips to nearby communities and to various special events were popular with convalescent patients.[67]

Following the war, recreation services in armed forces hospitals became an established service provided by Red Cross recreation workers.

World War II also brought an expansion in recreation services in veterans' hospitals, although not of the quality found in military hospitals. However, with the increased number of servicemen patients and the expansion of treatment programs in veterans' hospitals at the close of hostilities and thereafter, the Veterans' Administration in 1945 established the Recreation Service as a part of its Hospital Special Service Division.[68] This resulted in the Recreation Services' offering a program of recreation services at each veterans' hospital domiciliary in the United States. In 1960 the Recreation Service was placed in the Physical Medicine and Rehabilitation Service. This organizational change was made, according to Bream, "to add even greater strength to Recreation and improve patient care by placing it under the immediate direction of a physician."[69]

As a result of the importance placed on recreation service in military and veterans' hospitals during World War II, recreation programs and services in state institutions for the mentally ill in the years thereafter were greatly affected. Not only were recreation programs in such institutions expanded, but there was also a shift in the concept of recreation and its value. In the past the objectives of the program were primarily diversion and entertainment. Now, however, recreation service took on a more therapeutic responsibility of assisting the medical staff in treatment, assisting patient adjustment to hospitalization, and assisting the patient in developing skills that could be used for recreative experiences following discharge.[70] Recent years have seen another shift to include the concept of rehabilitation and reintegration of the patient into the community through the use of recreation programs and services. The recreation specialist is no longer saying goodbye to the patient at the institutional door, but instead is offering leisure counseling service prior to discharge as well as following the patient personally or through referral into the community to assist the patient in leisure adjustment. Thus, recreation programs and services for the mentally ill have shifted from custodial services to treatment and to rehabilitation, and today we are talking about recreation services as a preventer of mental illness.

A similar expansion of recreation programs and services since World War II has occurred in institutions for the mentally retarded. There is probably no public or private hospital/institution in the United States today providing care and treatment to the mentally retarded that does not provide recreation service.

In 1946 the World Health Organization its constitution signed by sixty-one nations proclaimed that the highest standard of health is a fundamental right of every human being and that governments are responsible for providing health and social measures. This political idea evolved from Judeo-Christian ethics that had taught for two thousand years that it is not a matter of whether we feel like being charitable—it is our duty to society.[71]

In the early 1950s a small number of cities established special centers to offer recreation services to the physically and mentally disabled. The Recreation Center for the Handicapped in San Francisco, established in 1952 under the direction of Janet Pomer is an excellent example of such a center. In 1955 Kansas City established the Greater Kansas City Council on Recreation for the Handicapped, a citywide council organized to better coordinate recreation service to special population members as well as to establish and develop new services. Since the late 1950s, and especially in recent years, municipal recreation departments in major cities have employed specialists in therapeutic recreation or supervisors of special recreation to initiate and develop comprehensive programs of recreation service for those with physical, emotional, and social limitations. Of special note is the Washington, D.C., Recreation Department, which during the past two decades has developed an excellent community recreation service program for the districtwide needs of the disabled.

Although the first Senior Center opened in New York City in 1943, it was not until the 1950s that municipal agencies began to develop senior citizen centers and golden age clubs for the elderly.[72] Since then, and with the assistance of the government, special residential centers also have been built. The value of centers and clubs is reflected in the 1975 report of the National Council on the Aging on senior centers: "Opportunities that give recognition and status to participants are considered a major potential function of Senior Centers and Clubs."[73]

1960–Present. The needs of the disadvantaged were recognized early in the twentieth century by the National Recreation Association through consultation with various communities.[74] The Cincinnati Park and Recreation Department in 1933 established special centers to conduct programs for the unemployed and their families. In 1941 the San Francisco Park and Recreation Department developed recreation services for those living in public housing developments. However, it was not until the 1960s that a new perspective on recreation service for the socioeconomically disadvantaged and for minority-group members devel-

oped.[75] This new perspective appears to be the result of three factors:

1. The social upheaval and civil disturbances that occurred during the 1960s: The Kerner Commission report and other reports indicate that the lack of recreation programs and facilities was one of the major causes of civil unrest and riots. As early as 1964 municipal recreation departments, with assistance from the federal government, initiated crash programs to relieve the pressure that was beginning to develop in depressed sections of cities. In many instances these programs were restricted to the summer months or were too late in developing to alleviate some of the inadequacies that existed.[76]

2. The financial assistance provided by the federal government to communities and agencies resulting from social unrest: The 1960s witnessed the involvement of recreation service in the "War on Poverty" through the variety of federally funded programs under the Economic Opportunity Act of 1964, such as Head Start, Upward Bound, Community Action Program, and Job Corps. Likewise, recreation service was provided through the Land and Water Conservation Fund Act of 1965, the Housing and Urban Development Act of 1965, the Demonstration Cities and Metropolitan Development Act of 1966, and the Public Health Service Act of 1966.[77]

3. The return to the earlier view on the part of the recreation profession that the recreation needs of all people should be met regardless of their station in life.

In 1959 the New York Service for Orthopedically Handicapped established an integrated program of recreation activities for physically disabled and able-bodied children. Other national organizations and their affiliates that offer recreation services include the United Cerebral Palsy Association, the

Muscular Dystrophy Association, the National Multiple Sclerosis Association, Goodwill Industries, the Kennedy Foundation (which established the Special Olympics in 1968), the American Foundation for the Blind, and the National Association for Retarded Citizens.

Service organizations such as the Kiwanis, Elks, Lions, Moose, Eagles, and Junior Chamber of Commerce have provided financial support and in many instances assumed total responsibility for offering recreation services. Voluntary youth associations such as the YMCA and YWCA, Boy and Girl Scouts, Boys' and Girls' Clubs, the Police Athletic League, and others have either directly assisted or sponsored programs for the disabled or made their facilities available for others to offer programs for the disabled.

In 1979 the federal government took a major step in recognizing the rights of all citizens by assuming responsibility for providing opportunities for special populations to enjoy the programs, services, and facilities of our national parks. In that year the National Park Service of the Department of Interior established the Division of Special Programs and Populations at the Washington office level, with David C. Park being appointed chief of the division. The primary function of the division is to develop a comprehensive and systemwide plan for access to ensure that parks provide full-spectrum visitor services. The division is addressing such issues as historic-site accessibility, wilderness-area experiences, expansion of interpretive programs to enable deaf and blind individuals to participate, exploration of technological approaches to give those with disabilities an opportunity to more fully enjoy outdoor recreation, and accessible transportation systems to and within park areas. In addition, the division formulates policies and guidelines relative to special populations, reviews employment opportunities in the service for disabled individuals, recommends specialized training, provides technical assistance to park areas in eliminating programmatic and physical barriers, and coordinates special demonstration projects.[78]

Although there has been an increase in the provision of recreation service to those with limiting conditions and disabilities, there is still a need for greater community recreation services. While the following statement by David Park is now nearly two decades old, and the 1973 Rehabilitation Act and Education for All Handicapped Children Act is still in effect, Park's comment is still applicable today:

> If the public recreation program is to provide adequate recreation programs and resources for the total population, we must realize that there are significant numbers in our communities who require special programs and it is the communities' responsibility to provide special programs for these special groups.[79]

Other Recent Developments

The twenty-year period from 1960 to 1980 witnessed more changes in attitudes and treatment of the ill and disabled than in all previous years in American history. These gains and changes were the result of a society in which attitudes, sense of responsibility, and human commitment slowly but consistently grew over the centuries and culminated in 1961, when President John F. Kennedy boldly committed the country's resources to the cause of disabled individuals.

Throughout the 1960s and 1970s two trends had a tremendous impact on the ill and disabled citizens: expanded recognition of human and civil rights and substantially increased federal funding for human services and programs. During the early 1960s, as an example, new ideologies emerged as guiding principles of services. Of particular note were the ideologies of normalization and developmental programming suggesting that institutions frequently fostered deviance and impeded development. By the late 1970s considerable support had been generated in favor of deinstitutionalization. Federal statutes and regulations supported the process of deinstitutionalization.[80] Success in this area is reflected in the fact that between 1970 and 1979 the number of residents in state institutions decreased by over fifty thousand persons. In addition, advocates stopped pleading for various services for the disabled and began to insist on their human and legal rights.[81]

Despite the gains made during the 1940s and 1950s in programs and services, many mentally ill and mentally retarded individuals were still not receiving appropriate services. In public schools, for example, large numbers of children were being excluded from educational programs. The landmark case of the *Pennsylvania Association for Retarded Children* v. *Commonwealth of Pennsylvania,* 343 F. Supp. 279 (E.D. PA 1972), in 1970 was the beginning of tremendous change in this area. Such lawsuits paved the way for the introduction of federal legislation concerning the education of all children (i.e., PL94-142). It was also during the 1960s and 1970s that the mentally ill, the mentally retarded and the more severely physically disabled came out of the shadows and became highly visible in society.

We have noted in the previous two chapters as well as this one the involvement of the federal government in the overall health care system. Since the early 1970s more health maintenance organizations, which emphasize prevention, early intervention and treatment, have been set up in place of the curative system, which concentrates on illness and injury. In addition, in more recent years we have noted the growing demands of health-care consumers for a voice in planning and controlling health services.

CORRECTIONAL INSTITUTIONS

As we begin our brief history of corrections, it is well to note that there is little historical comparison between health and health-related developments and correctional developments. The historical development of health and health-related functions is the result of a humanitarian concern for ill and disabled people. While a humanitarian concern also is found in the correctional system regarding sentences, conditions in prisons, and architecture, it is not the same since individuals in the system are in violation of a criminal law. Criminal law is defined conventionally as a body of specific rules concerning human conduct that have been promulgated by political authority and are enforced by punishment administered at the local, state, or federal level. Therefore, the characteristics that distinguish this body of rules regarding human behavior from other rules and regulations are politicality, specificity, and penal sanction.

Corrections, as we noted earlier, is the third and final phase of the criminal justice process. Beginning with law enforcement as the case-finding phase, the courts determine by trial under due process of law what cases shall proceed to the correctional phase. The correctional system or phase attempts to rehabilitate and neutralize the deviant behavior of adult criminals and juvenile delinquents. This is done through probation, imprisonment, parole, or other procedures such as community-based programs.

The development of our modern system of criminal justice was difficult and took a long time to develop. Social control of some sort has existed since humans organized into a society. Social control first began to be enforced by social disapproval and vengeance against the offender by the victim or the victim's family quite early in history. It was not until recent centuries that the punitive reaction to crime in accordance with definite regulations—purposely inflicting pain on the offender because of some assumed value of pain—became popular.

It is impossible to fix an exact date for the beginning of imprisonment as punishment for crime. The only statement in this regard that can be made with accuracy is that punitive imprisonment was not used to any great extent until the middle of the sixteenth century in England and the beginning of the seventeenth century in Continental Europe. Not until the beginning of the nineteenth century did it succeed in displacing the capital and corporal penalties for serious crimes.[82] The eighteenth century may be considered as a period of transition from corporal punishment to imprisonment, although the process of change did not reach its greatest rate until the last quarter of that century.[83]

Throughout history four principal methods of implementing punishment have been used, but there is no distinct "evolution" of any one system from the other. Removal from the group by death, exile, or imprisonment, physical torture, social degradation, and financial loss have all been used differentially in various historical periods, and they are used differentially today. In the United States today imprisonment and fines seem to be the most popular.

In light of the above remarks, this section will focus on the development of correctional institutions in the United States, including life in prison, rehabilitation in the correctional system, and other correctional developments. Attention will also be given to the development of correctional recreation service.

HISTORICAL ORIGINS

The historical development of correctional institutions in the United States followed a pattern of development similar to that which initially developed in England. The colonies inherited the Old World's sanguinary methods of punishment. Eventually, all of them put into effect in varying degrees the English code, which in general prescribed some form of corporal punishment less than death for crimes that were not classified as capital.

When the Revolutionary War came to a close, America had no penal institutions similar to the present state prisons. However, the Quakers provided the keystone around which modern penal reform or state prisons developed in America. In fact, before and after the Revolution the Quakers were quite instrumental in criminal code and institution reform.

Jails

Jails and houses of correction were established in the American colonies soon after settlement. Both were designed after their counterpart in England, and both eventually came to be used as places of punishment after conviction. The difference between the two was in name only. The offenders spent their time together and had no work to do, depending upon charity for their maintenance. There was no attempt to rehabilitate; even religious services were absent.

Prisons and the Prison System

No institutions belonging to the state were established during the colonial period until Connecticut purchased land in 1773 and constructed buildings over an old abandoned mine near Simsburg and turned it into a prison. Offenders were simply dropped down the shaft and lived in three parallel tunnels, supplied by a single pool of fresh water. They were restrained during the night by heavy chains attached to their necks at one end and to the heavy beams above them at the other; in addition, heavy irons were fixed to their feet. Not surprisingly, the first prison riot was there in 1774.[84] This so-called prison was closed in 1776.

After the adoption of the Constitution in 1780, the first state prison was established in the Commonwealth of Massachusetts on Castle Island in Boston harbor in 1784–85. The courts sentenced men to hard labor for a term of years or life in this fortress-prison. Because of security problems a new state prison was begun around 1800. In December 1805 the commonwealth's maximum security "penitentiary prison" at Charlestown received its first prisoner.[85]

The state prison movement spread rapidly during the last part of the eighteenth century and into the nineteenth century. Immediately following the Revolution, the forces of reform in Pennsylvania, including such prominent persons as Benjamin Franklin, Benjamin Rush, and William Bradford, began a savage attack upon the criminal codes of the colonial days. As a result, the criminal codes of Pennsylvania (and subsequently of other states) were changed. In 1794 the list of capital crimes was reduced to death for murder in the first degree and imprisonment for other serious offenses. The concept behind this reform was that imprisonment was in itself a sufficiently severe penalty, and that prisoners should be assisted in their efforts to become rehabilitated.[86]

Meanwhile, two new methods in the treatment of inmates began to emerge as a result of a concern about the twin evils of congregrated confinement and idleness in jails and prisons. Reformers were also concerned with fulfilling the concept of imprisonment as the principal method of punishment. These newer methods took their name from their location: New York State Prison at Auburn (Auburn system), which opened in 1819, and Eastern Penitentiary in Philadelphia (Pennsylvania system), which opened in 1829. The basic difference between them was that Pennsylvania inmates lived and worked in separate cells, which afforded the inmate a means of learning a trade. Each cell also had its own exercise yard. In the Auburn system, prisoners lived in separate cells but worked together in shops. In both systems strict silence rules were enforced in the cells and in work to make discipline easier and to prevent contamination of one prisoner by another. The Auburn system also incorporated the *striped suit* and the *lock step*.[87] In the polemical battle between the advocates of the two systems the Auburn system eventually became the one that persisted in America with some modifications until the early twentieth century.[88]

These prisons, regardless of system, were referred to as penitentiaries. The word *penitentiary* had a significance at the time that the systems were initiated but is no longer applicable. At that early period the prison was not for retribution but for producing "penitence" or penitentiary reformation. The first so-called penitentiary, which was originally a jail (Walnut Street jail), was established in Philadelphia in 1794.

In 1877 another new concept of a correctional institution was implemented outside Elmira, New York. The institution was called a *reformatory*, with emphasis placed on education, productive work, and grading privileges to produce reformation for first-felony offenders between the ages of sixteen to thirty-one years. However, by 1910 the reformatory concept was on the decline resulting from too few and too overworked instructors, poor selection of offenders, and "old guard" prison employees conditioned to the punitive ideology.[89]

Sandwiched between the development of these various systems was the first meeting of the National Congress of Penitentiary and Reformatory Discipline (now called the American Correctional Association) in 1870. At this meeting the members considered the problems and reactions to punitive discipline. They also passed a resolution that established the goal of corrections as the rehabilitation of the offender.[90] Over one hundred years have gone by since that conference, and the field is still coping with the definition of rehabilitation and how to achieve it.

Two other notes of historical value include the first separate women's prison, which opened in Indianapolis in 1872.[91] Since that time separate women's prisons have opened in each state. The other is the establishment of the United States Bureau of Prisons by Congress in 1930. The bureau today operates an integrated system of forty-five facilities. That system is considered to have the best overall treatment program through the use of treatment teams.[92]

Since the early 1900s our prison system

has followed a trend toward treatment or rehabilitation (sometimes referred to as resocialization). However, while rehabilitation or resocialization may be the goal, the type of treatment or rehabilitation may vary widely in definition and implementation. Public and political attitudes, as well as the personality and competence of the administrators, influence institutional programs. Today prison programs can be classified into five broad, overlapping categories of approach to rehabilitation:

1. *The punishment approach*, which satisfies that part of the public interested in vengeance.

2. *The treatment approach*, which puts emphasis on resocialization (education, vocational training, counseling, recreation, library) and medical and dental services.

3. *The combination approach*, which incorporates elements of treatment and punishment.

4. *The custody approach*, which has little regard for either treatment or punishment. This approach has frequently been called *warehousing*; the idea is to keep the offender out of the public's sight.

5. *The work approach*, which uses offenders as a labor force for public works.[93]

As we noted earlier, institutionalization and the use of any of the above approaches to rehabilitation have not as yet provided many examples of successful rehabilitation (or resocialization) in prisons.

Imprisonment

Since the early twentieth century the horrors of prison life have been reduced. Improvements have been made in diet, cleanliness, ventilation, lighting, and methods of discipline. Solitary confinement, except as punishment for serious infraction of regulations, has been generally abandoned, and marks of degradation have been eliminated. Entertainment, programs of athletics, and

recreation have been made available, as well as libraries and educational classes. Also, visiting and correspondence privileges have been introduced, and self-government has been established to a degree in many institutions. While these changes have occurred for the better, a prison, according to some criminologists, is still characterized by deprivation and is as close to a society without culture as can be found in Western civilization.[94]

> The prison is similar to a city, but there ends the similarity because most prisons are unisexual communities housing people whose legal status is either felon or misdemeanant. The social formation and interaction within institutions differs considerably from that in free society. Although the city has a nucleus of permanent population with many transients that give a quality of dynamic movement, the prison has a permanent population, or the feeling of one, only. Nobody is "just passing through" in the same overnight sense as that outside. The prison is a closed community.[95]

> The culture of a prison is characterized by deprivation. Methods of protecting one's self become a real part of the culture. In a culture of deprivation, simple things become important. The day's menu, identifying the movie that is to be shown in the auditorium Saturday or Sunday afternoon, a letter, a visit, and a tour by a college class, all become important. . . .[96]

OTHER CORRECTIONAL DEVELOPMENTS

Juvenile Corrections

Juvenile corrections began to emerge in the nineteenth century between 1847, when state juvenile institutions were initiated in several states, and 1899, when the juvenile court in Chicago separated children from adult offenders through legislative action. The first American institution specifically for juvenile delinquents was opened in New York City in 1825 after more than a generation of discussion. It was under the control of a private association. The first institutions of this type under state control were started in Massachusetts and New York in 1847. Both public and private institutions exist today; some private institutions have changed to public management, though none has changed from public to private management.[97]

The approaches to rehabilitation used in training schools that are built around a cottage system of architecture vary. To a great extent, training schools have incorporated much of what was found in the Elmira system: self-government, religious teaching, academic teaching, industrial training, and release on good behavior, which is similar to parole. In addition, various psychological theories to change behavior are also used. The education, hard work, and discipline approach is the most frequent, although operant conditioning and orthopsychiatric approaches are frequently found. The success of any specific rehabilitation program is not good. There is high recidivism, with many theories as to why. In 1972 the Massachusetts Division of Youth Services abolished the training schools on grounds that they were doing more harm than good.[98]

Juvenile Detention Centers

These centers are a recent development. In lieu of putting the juvenile in a municipal jail or lockup, children of juvenile court age are generally permitted to remain at home. It is frequently necessary, on the other hand, to detain children because of the serious nature of the offense, the condition of the home, or the possibility that the child will try to escape the jurisdiction of the court. The concept of detention centers is to supplement detention with treatment, since such centers are usually the first correctional institution to which a child is exposed.

Juvenile detention centers are found in middle-sized and large urban centers. Regional centers also have been established.

Programs vary widely depending upon the philosophy and resources of the jurisdiction. In general, most centers function with minimal programs. However, testing and other diagnostic procedures are rather frequent in the larger detention centers, sometimes in cooperation with neighborhood child guidance or mental health clinics. Educational programs are usually provided so that the child who is already behind academically will not be further delayed. Likewise, recreation services are an important part of the care and treatment program. The beginning of long-term treatment and the completion of some short-term treatment can be accomplished in the detention facility.[99]

Probation

Probation is the suspension of a sentence with supervision of the convicted offender by an officer of the court in the community. It is used more frequently than any other disposition, both for juveniles and adults. Credit for the development of probation is generally given to John Augustus, a Boston shoemaker who in 1843 voluntarily embarked on a career of visiting the courts and paying the fines and accepting the supervision of many offenders to give them a second chance.[100] By 1925 probation for juveniles was available in every state, and by 1956 all states granted probation to adults, although probation laws differed from state to state.[101]

Parole

Parole is the act of releasing or the status of being released from a penal institution in which one has served a part of one's maximum sentence on condition of maintaining good behavior and remaining in custody under supervision in the community until final discharge. It was initiated by New York State in 1869, although it was not until 1944 that all states had enacted a parole law.[102] Today some states make extensive use of parole, while others make little use of it.

Community-Based Corrections

Community-based corrections is a term used to refer to community-oriented programs and services other than probation and parole that promote the ex-offender's adjustment to the community. The program of services is of recent origin, having begun in the early 1950s. It incorporates halfway houses, guidance centers, work-release and study-release programs, furlough and pass programs, vocational training, job placement and referrals, and other services that help to maintain effective ties between the community and correctional programs.[103]

Organizations and Agencies

Since the Philadelphia Society for Alleviating the Miseries of the Public Prisons was organized in 1787, many organizations have been concerned for the social welfare of juvenile and adult offenders whether in or out of the institution.[104] The International Association of Chiefs of Police, the American Bar Association, the American Correctional Association, the National Prisoners Alliance, and the National Council on Crime and Delinquency, to name a few, have been most helpful in improving conditions by providing service or by communicating to the political leadership the real problems of the correctional system. Likewise, many governmental agencies have contributed to research grants to improve the system: most directly, the Law Enforcement Assistance Administration, the Youth Development and Delinquency Prevention Administration, the United States Department of Labor through its Manpower Development and Training Act and Office of Economic Opportunity, the United States Department of Education, and the National Institute of Mental Health.

CORRECTIONAL RECREATION

None of the early prisons provided recreation for offenders. In fact, the idea of recreation appears to have been completely for-eign to imprisonment. Only since the turn of the century has it been common to find time allotted for informal, unsupervised recreational pursuits in prisons regardless of type. And it is even more recent that recreational activities have been considered a rehabilitation tool in some juvenile and adult institutions.

The first hint of correctional recreation in the New World (1600s) is given to us by Hormachea:

> The House of Burgesses of Virginia passed a series of laws establishing prisons which were the forerunners of the county jail in Virginia. These institutions were to be fashioned after the ordinary Virginia house, and each facility was to have an unfenced yard which would allow the inmate to walk around outside the jail. Inmates were on their honor to make no escape attempt. Later this practice was abandoned. . . . [105]

For many years after imprisonment became the standard punishment, recreation was thought to have no place in prison life. The concept of imprisonment emphasized, as we have noted, the belief that the lot of the offender should be harsh, uncomfortable, and repellent. In prisons that practiced solitary confinement, recreation was limited to solitary exercise in a high-walled yard and to reading the Bible and other religious publications. Yet there appears to be some evidence that offenders made little articles out of whatever material was available. A visitor to Eastern State Penitentiary in Philadelphia in 1830 relates the following concerning one of the offenders he visited:

> He wore a paper hat of his own making. . . . He had very ingeniously manufactured a sort of Dutch clock from some discarded odds and ends; and his vinegar bottle served for the pendulum. He had extracted some colours from the yarn which he worked, and painted a few poor figures on the wall. One, a female, over the door, he called "The Lady of the Lake."[106]

The overcrowding of prisons that necessitated placing two or more adult offenders in one cell and the establishment of dormitories in juvenile institutions brought further relaxation of the rules. As it became apparent that nothing disastrous happened when offenders mixed informally, a few wardens began to grant freedom of the yard and permitted conversation while eating. Such steps were noted as early as the 1850s.[107]

The next step in the development of recreation programs was the introduction of organized sports. As in the case of education, the reformatories led the way. Zebulon Brockway at Elmira, New York, in 1877 brought organized games to a high point during his tenure as superintendent. He believed that such activities would develop self-control and team spirit. Military drills and calisthenics also became a definite part of the Elmira regime.[108]

During the same period as the Elmira Reformatory was developing, the reformatory at Concord, Massachusetts, organized sports and clubs to which all offenders were assigned. The clubs included a YMCA, Reformatory Prayer Meeting, a Catholic Debating Society, a Saturday Scientific and Literary Club, a Baseball and Literary Society, and a Chautauqua Club.[109] If some of these clubs seem uninteresting in terms of present-day organizations for young people, it must be remembered that such activities were very popular immediately after the Civil War.

Gradually more organized recreation was introduced into juvenile and adult prisons as more freedom of speech and action was allowed. The degree of freedom of speech and organized activities depended on the attitude of the individual warden, the directives of state political and administrative groups, and public reaction. Sports, clubs, and lectures that brought offenders together in groups often were avoided because they aroused fear of riots. Gradually, however, occasional privileges became established customs.

By 1910–15 organized recreation programs became a regular part of prison life, especially in the North. Music was introduced; prison bands began to provide concerts as part of Sunday recreation programs. In 1912 the first rationale for the encouragement of recreational activities had been formulated, primarily as a result of a decline in prison industries and an attempt to reduce prolonged idleness.[110] Hence, recreation became a form of discipline and was valued by the wardens as such.[111]

The following two decades witnessed a continuing interest in the rehabilitative functions of recreation activity but not to the extent found in hospitals/institutions. By 1930 the American Correctional Association, in a revision of its Declaration of Principles, noted that "it has come to be recognized that recreation is an indispensable factor of normal life. This principle is now heartily endorsed by prison administrators."[112] In 1939 the American Prison Association pointed out the growing effectiveness of recreation as a rehabilitation tool.[113] A few years later this same association again stated that recreation was conceived of as an integral part of the treatment program—not just to fill a gap in the day—and should loom large in the daily life of any offender.[114]

In subsequent years there was increased interest in the organizational and administrative aspects of organized recreation programs in correctional institutions. In the 1950s, in particular, a number of recreation publications gave attention to the value of recreation.[115] Barnes and Teeters in their 1955 edition of *New Horizons in Criminology* devoted half a chapter to recreation and its importance in treatment and also made suggestions for planning and designing space for recreation activities that would include trees and high bushes for shade purposes.[116]

The 1950s also saw the first scientific surveys of recreational practices in correctional institutions. Principal findings indicated that approximately half of all prisons for adult males employed a full-time director of recreation, that recreational programs in federal institutions were far more advanced than those in state institutions, that baseball was the main outdoor activity while hobby activities were the main indoor activity, and that the failure to implement recreational programs could be attributed to custody problems, lack of funds, and lack of space due to the age of the institution and not to the resistance of prison administrators.[117]

The following decade witnessed a continuing trend. The American Correctional Association (ACA) developed a substantial elaboration of its recreation standards in 1960.[118] The Task Force on Corrections of the President's Commission on Law Enforcement and Administration of Justice gave the weight of its support to these standards when in 1967 it included the ACA recreation standards in its own listing of standards.[119] In 1970 the International Commission of Jurists to the United Nations submitted recommendations regarding standards for treatment of offenders, including four standards concerned with the rights of offenders to recreation and recreation services.[120] More recently the National Advisory Commission on Standards and Goals for Criminal Justice have recognized the value of recreation through standards.

The interest within the correctional community in the rehabilitative value of recreational programs is matched by the support of such programs by many offenders. The *Proceedings of the Annual Congress of the American Correctional Association* are marked by frequent testimony to this effect. Inmate autobiographies and scientific observation provide additional confirmation, although there are dissenting voices.

During the 1970s the National Therapeutic Recreation Society, in association with the National Recreation and Park Association, became involved in the correctional process by establishing task forces, initiating workshops, and scheduling correctional recreation sessions at various Congresses for Recreation and Parks. Also during this period, specifically 1977 and 1978, there were fifteen litigations involving the question of

the offenders' rights to recreation and exercise. In addition, there were more than thirty suits centering on recreation rights, time allotted for recreation, access to recreation while segregated, and pretrial access to recreation by detainees.[121]

Although recreation services appeared to continue to grow in various types of correctional institutions and to have the general support of administrators through the 1970s and into the 1980s, such services never gained the recognition they had in health and health-related facilities. Further, it became apparent that although recreation services had an immediate value in releasing energy not dissipated in work, in relieving tension created by confinement, and in speeding the passage of time, their value as a rehabilitation tool was not being recognized. According to Krug: "Recreation is not an established rehabilitation tool within the prison environment, and it is not a felt necessity to many correctional administrators."[122] Many studies present strong evidence that prison has damaged the offenders and made them less capable of adaption to society than they were when they went to prison.[123]

In the early 1980s a number of publications devoted entire issues to the broad nature of the concerns, problems, and needs of correctional recreation services.[124] Qualitatively, these issues offered strong evidence for the improvement of recreation services regardless of institutional setting. On the other hand, the material presented incorporated only a limited dimension of recreation services for offenders in community-based corrections. One of the greatest challenges of correctional recreation, according to Krug, is the offender's leisure pursuits outside the prison.[125] He comments further:

> The delivery of resource services and counseling to the community resource centers and half-way houses is a strong part of that challenge. . . . The municipal recreation director needs to recognize his or her role as a member of the community service team. . . .

By working together, the municipal recreation director and the local correctional personnel can aid the individual in better construction of his or her leisure lifestyle.[126]

Many criminologists and penologists agree there are problems in the criminal justice system. The question of what must be changed in order that behavior may change is at the core of the controversy. Past and present evidence has yet to provide answers for policy-making decisions.[127] It is obvious that the old ways do not work. The philosophical determinants in the treatment of offenders have changed rapidly throughout history. Today we respect the offender as an individual with rights who is deserving of good treatment, but does this treatment include recreation?

In conclusion, provision of recreation service is considered by many investigators, civic leaders, and individuals associated with the criminal justice system to be one of the most important parts of the correctional process. It is their opinion that recreation services within the correctional process can reduce not only youth crime but adult crime.[128] However, most recreational activities in prison, according to Williams and Ortom, are limited to sedentary, diversional, singular types of pursuits.[129] Consequently, according to Reynolds, "current recreational services in corrections appear to have little effect on the development of alternate leisure life-styles of inmates and therefore exert minimal impact on their rehabilitation."[130] Such a statement may very well support the evidence mentioned by Keve about how prison life damages the offender's ability to adapt to society after prison.

To overcome the problem of recreation services traditionally being directed toward alleviating boredom and filling unobligated time, as opposed to assisting in rehabilitation, Reynolds suggests six principles for "the implementation of a comprehensive program of leisure services, designed to aid in the total rehabilitation of the offender."[131] However, as he further points out, these principles will require a change in philosophy, content, and operation of correctional recreation services:

1. Leisure services must be recognized and acknowledged as an essential and viable component of the total rehabilitative effort of community and institutional correctional programs.

2. Leisure services must become an integral component of the offender's treatment process.

3. The purpose and content of recreational programs in correctional settings must be redefined.

4. The use of community leisure resources must be emphasized.

5. Changes in staff and offender roles and responsibility for leisure must be initiated.

6. The efficacy of the leisure service intervention in corrections must be documented through empirical investigation.[132]

In support of Reynolds's principles are the recent correctional mission statement and national policy statement and standards relative to personnel and facilities developed by the National Correctional Recreation Association (NCRA) and the American Association for Leisure and Recreation (AALR).[133]

This mission statement speaks to the importance and benefits of recreation and leisure in the life of everyone, including the social offender. It further outlines the purposes of the NCRA/AALR regarding leisure services in correctional institutions; namely, relieve daily tension and develop leisure skills through leisure education which can be carried over into the community. The policy statement regards recreation programming as an integral part of the total correction process as well as being a part of therapy and habilitation of the offender. In order to implement the policy statement, guidelines concerned with program leadership, characteristics, and procedures are provided. The personnel standards are concerned with the number of personnel per size of the institution, and the facility standards address the various types of indoor and outdoor facilities that should be available within the institution.[134]

It is hoped that the mission statement and standards for correctional recreation service will provide the impetus to improve the quality of recreation service in correctional institutions so that in the future recreation service will contribute to total rehabilitation of the incarcerated.

SUMMARY

The extensive progress of twentieth-century science, we noted, revolutionized the practice of medicine. Hospitals today are using various methods and procedures to help patients return to a healthy daily environment. In some ways a humanization of hospital ideas and a survival of the Greek temple philosophy that provided music, theater, and recreational activities for patients as a matter of course appears to be returning. Experts in medical care generally agree that modern medicine treats persons as a whole rather than as depersonalized examples of a specific disease. Further, we can say that changes have occurred for the good in ideology, law, technology, and services. This tells us that disabled persons are making the transition from the state of discarded deviants to fully participating members of society. It heralds a brighter tomorrow.

The second section of this chapter focused on the historical development of the correctional system; more specifically, on a historical perspective of reactions to deviant behavior from primitive to modern times. Corrections emerged in the last part of the eighteenth century and throughout the nineteenth century. Jails and workhouses came earlier than the eighteenth century. Twentieth-century refinements have brought corrections to its present state. The section concluded with consideration of the development of organized recreation service within the correctional system. Both positive and negative references were made to its development with recommendations concerning its further growth and development.

NOTES

1. Richard Solecki, *Shanider* (New York: Knopf, 1971), pp. 195–96.

2. Henry E. Sigerist, *A History of Medicine*, vol. 1 (New York: Oxford University Press, 1951), pp. 154–55.

3. Quoted in Elliott M. Avedon, "The Public and Therapeutic Recreation," *Recreation in Treatment Centers* 2 (1963), 42.

4. Virginia Frye, "Historical Sketch of Recreation in the Medical Setting," *Recreation in Treatment Centers* 1 (1962), 40.

5. Felix Marti-Ibanez, ed., *The Epic of Medicine* (New York: Clarkson N. Potter, 1962), pp. 51–52.

6. Elliott M. Avedon, *Therapeutic Recreation Service: An Applied Behavioral Science Approach* (Englewood Cliffs, N.J.: Prentice-Hall, 1974), p. 8.

7. William Henry, "Mental Hospitals," in *A History of Medical Psychology*, ed. Gregory Zilboorg (New York: W. W. Norton, 1941), pp. 558–89.

8. Richard Kraus, *Therapeutic Recreation Service: Principles and Practices*, 2nd ed. (Philadelphia: W. B. Saunders Co., 1978), p. 16.

9. Avedon, *Therapeutic Recreation Service*, p. 8.

10. Exod. 21:23–24.

11. Marti-Ibanez, *Epic of Medicine*, p. 34.

12. George Rosen, *A History of Public Health* (New York: MD Publications, 1958), p. 47.

13. Sigerist, *History of Medicine*, p. 431.

14. Marti-Ibanez, *Epic of Medicine*, p. 63.

15. Ibid., p. 64.

16. Mary Risley, *House of Healing* (New York: Doubleday & Co. 1961), p. 56.

17. Kenneth M. Walker, *The Story of Medicine* (New York: Oxford University Press, 1955), p. 60.

18. N. D. C., *A Short History of Psychiatric Achievement* (New York: W. W. Norton, 1941), p. 37.

19. Risley, *House of Healing*, p. 74.

20. William Durant, *Caesar and Christ* (New York: Simon & Schuster, 1944), p. 334.

21. Ibid., p. 336.

22. Patricia T. Cegelka and Herbert J. Prehm, *Mental Retardation: From Categories to People* (Columbus, Ohio: Charles E. Merrill Publishing Co., 1982), p. 46.

23. Nathaniel W. Faxon, "A History of Hospitals," in *The Hospital in Modern Society*, ed. Arthur C. Bachmeyer and Gerhard Hartman (New York: Commonwealth Fund, 1943), p. 5.

24. Charles M. Frank, *The Historical Development of Nursing* (Philadelphia: W. B. Saunders Co., 1953), pp. 47–53, 68–69, 71.

25. Avedon, "Public and Therapeutic Recreation," p. 43.

26. Risley, *House of Healing*, p. 75.

27. Ibid., p. 145.

28. Marti-Ibanez, *Epic of Medicine*, p. 130; and Avedon, *Therapeutic Recreation Service*, p. 9.

29. Marti-Ibanez, *Epic of Medicine*, p. 130.

30. Risley, *House of Healing*, pp. 157–69.

31. Gladys Sellew and M. E. Ebel, *A History of Nursing*, 3rd ed. (St. Louis: C. V. Mosby Co., 1965), p. 132.

32. Sigerist, *History of Medicine*, p. 223.

33. Cegelka and Prehm, *Mental Retardation*, p. 48.

34. Ibid., p. 49.

35. Edgar A. Doll, "A Historical Survey of Research and Management of Mental Retardation in the United States," in *Readings On The Exceptional Child: Research and Theory*, ed. E. P. Trapp and P. Himmelstein (New York: Appleton-Century-Crofts, 1962), p. 384.

36. Donald A. Read and Walter H. Greene, *Health and Modern Man* (New York: MacMillan, 1973), p. 484.

37. Risley, *House of Healing*, pp. 176–77.

38. Henry, "Mental Hospitals," pp. 323–24.

39. Ibid.

40. Risley, *House of Healing*, p. 216.

41. James O. Hepner and Donna M. Hepner, *The Health Strategy Game* (St. Louis: C. V. Mosby Co., 1973), p. 9.

42. Hyman Pleasure, "The Mental Hospital," in *Rehabilitation Medicine and Psychiatry*, ed. Jack Meislin (Springfield, Ill.: Charles C Thomas Publishers, 1976), p. 234.

43. Risley, *House of Healing*, p. 206.

44. National Council on the Aging, *Senior Centers: Report of Senior Group Programs in America* (Washington, D.C.: the council, 1975), p. 3.

45. Thomas G. Morton, *History of Pennsylvania Hospitals, 1751–1895* (New York: Arno Press, 1973), p. 149.

46. Frye, "Historical Sketch of Recreation," p. 41.

47. J. Sanbourne Bockovern, "Moral Treatment in American Psychiatry," *Journal of Nervous and Mental Diseases* 123, no. 8 (1956), 167–94; and Zilboorg, *History of Medical Psychology*, p. 149.

48. Norma Dain, *Concept of Insanity in the United States 1789–1865* (New Brunswick, N.J.: Rutgers University Press, 1964), pp. 117–19.

49. Cited in Williams R. Dunton, Jr., *Occupational Therapy* (Philadelphia: W. B. Saunders Co., 1915), p. 14.

50. Cited in William R. Dunton, Jr., "History of Occupational Therapy," in *Occupational Therapy*, 2nd ed., ed. William R. Dunton, Jr. and Sidney Light (Springfield, Ill.: Charles C Thomas Publishers, 1957), p. 8.

51. Ibid.

52. Florence Nightingale, *Notes on Nursing: What It Is and What It Is Not* (New York: D. Appleton & Co., 1873), pp. 95–104.

53. Risley, *House of Healing*, p. 203.

54. Sellew and Ebel, *History of Nursing*, p. 247.

55. D. Zietz, *Child Welfare* (New York: John Wiley & Sons, 1959), p. 125; and H. Lende, *What of the Blind?* (Chicago: American Foundation for the Blind, 1938), p. 17.

56. President's Committee on Mental Retardation, *Mental Retardation: Past and Present* (Washington, D.C.: U.S. Government Printing Office, 1977), p. 23.

57. Cegelka and Prehm, *Mental Retardation*, p. 53.

58. L. Kanner, "Emotionally Disturbed Children: A Historical Review," *Child Development* 33, no. 9 (1962), 97–102.

59. Lillian Summers, "The American Red Cross Program in Recreation in Military Hospitals: A Retrospective View," *Recreation in Treatment Centers* 1 (1962), 18.

60. Ibid.

61. R. F. L. Ridgway, "Recreation for Mental Cases," *American Journal of Psychiatry* 78, no. 7 (1921), 87–95.

62. William Menninger and Isabelle McCall, cited in Lee E. Meyer, "Recreation and the Mentally Ill," in *Recreation and Special Populations*, 2nd ed., ed. Thomas A. Stein and H. Douglas Sessoms (Boston: Holbrook Press, 1973), p. 147.

63. Bertha E. Schlotter and Margaret Svendsen, *An Experiment in Recreation with the Mentally Retarded*, rev. ed. (New York: National Mental Health, 1951).

64. Peter A. Witt, "A History of Recreation for the Mentally Retarded," unpublished, personal copy.

65. Arthur Williams, "Notes on History and Theory," in *Recreation: Pertinent Readings—Guideposts to the*

Future, ed. Jay B. Nash (Dubuque, Iowa: William C. Brown Co., 1965), p. 19.

66. Ira J. Hutchison, Jr., "Recreation and Racial Minorities," in *Recreation and Special Populations,* p. 330.

67. Frye and Peters, *Therapeutic Recreation,* p. 23.

68. Ibid., p. 25.

69. C. C. Bream, Jr., "Rehabilitative Recreation in the Veterans Administration," *Recreation in Treatment Centers* 1 (1962), 36.

70. Lee E. Meyer, "Recreation and the Mentally Ill," in *Recreation and Special Populations,* p. 152.

71. Risley, *House of Healing,* p. 176.

72. National Center on the Aging, *Senior Centers,* p. 2.

73. Ibid., p. 10.

74. George D. Butler, *Introduction to Community Recreation* (New York: McGraw-Hill Book Co., 1940), p. 223.

75. James F. Murphy, "Recreation and the Economically Deprived," in *Recreation and Special Populations,* pp. 300–302.

76. Richard Kraus, "Providing for Recreation and Aesthetic Enjoyment," in *Governing the City,* ed. Robert H. Connery and Demetrios Caraley (New York: Praeger Publishers, 1969).

77. Murphy, "Recreation," p. 302.

78. National Park Service, Division of Special Programs and Populations, Department of Interior, brochure, n.d.

79. David C. Park, "Therapeutic Recreation: A Community Responsibility," *Parks and Recreation* 5, no. 7 (1970), 25.

80. P. Roos, B. McCann, and M. Addison, *Shaping the Future: A National Forum on Community-Based Services and Facilities for Mentally Retarded People* (Baltimore: University Park Press, 1980).

81. Richard C. Scheerenberger, *Public Residential Services for the Mentally Retarded, 1979* (Madison, Wis.: National Association of Superintendents of Public Residential Facilities for Mental Retardation, 1980).

82. Thorsten Sellen, "Imprisonment," in *Encyclopedia of the Social Sciences* 8 (London: Oxford University Press, 1948), p. 617; and Max Griinhut, *Penal Reform* (London: Oxford University Press, 1948), pp. 11–13.

83. Harry Elmer Barnes, *The Evolution of Penology in Pennsylvania* (Indianapolis: Bobbs-Merril Co., 1927), p. 54.

84. Neil C. Chamelin, Vernon B. Fox, and Paul M. Whisenand, *Introduction to Criminal Justice* (Englewood Cliffs, N.J.: Prentice-Hall, 1975), p. 296.

85. Robert M. Carter, Daniel Glaser, and Leslie T. Wilkins, *Correctional Institutions* (Philadelphia: J. B. Lippincott Co., 1972), p. 19.

86. Robert G. Caldwell, *Criminology,* 2nd ed. (New York: Ronald Press Company, 1965), p. 503.

87. Elmer H. Johnson, *Crime, Correction, and Society,*

rev. ed. (Homewood, Ill.: Dorsey Press, 1968), pp. 480–81; and Richard R. Korn and Lloyd W. McCorkle, *Criminology and Penology* (New York: Holt, Rinehart & Winston, 1967), pp. 383–84.

88. Edwin H. Sutherland and Donald R. Cressey, *Criminology,* 9th ed. (Philadelphia: J. B. Lippincott Co., 1944), pp. 484–85.

89. Blake McKelvey, *American Prisons* (Chicago: University of Chicago Press, 1936), pp. 109–13.

90. Donald Clemmer, *The Prison Community* (New York: Rinehart & Co., 1958), p. 138.

91. Joy S. Egman, *Prisons for Women* (Springfield, Ill.: Charles C Thomas, Publishers, 1971), p. 135.

92. Carter, Glaser, and Wilkins, *Correctional Institutions,* 2nd ed., Chap. 7.

93. James A. Inciardi, *Criminal Justice* (San Francisco: West Publishing, 1984), pp. 621–26.

94. Chamelin, Fox, and Whisenand, *Criminal Justice,* p. 392.

95. Ibid., pp. 377–78.

96. Ibid., p. 386.

97. Ibid., p. 298.

98. Ibid., p. 375.

99. Ibid., p. 325–27.

100. Johnson, *Crime, Correction, and Society,* pp. 666–67.

101. Ibid.

102. Sutherland and Cressey, *Criminology,* pp. 584–86.

103. Chamelin, Fox, and Whisenand, *Criminal Justice,* Chap. 16.

104. Caldwell, *Criminology,* p. 503.

105. Quoted in Carroll Hormachea, "New Slants on Old Correctional Recreation Ideas," *Parks and Recreation* 16, no. 2 (1981), 31.

106. Quoted in Harry E. Barnes and Negley K. Teeters, *New Horizons in Criminology,* 2nd ed. (Englewood Cliffs, N.J.: Prentice-Hall, 1955), p. 678.

107. McKelvey, *American Prisons,* p. 41.

108. Zebulon Brockway, *Fifty Years of Prison Service* (New York: Charities Publications, 1912), pp. 420–22.

109. McKelvey, *American Prisons,* pp. 114–17.

110. *Proceedings of the Annual Congress of the American Prison Association* (Washington, D.C.: the association, 1912).

111. Clemmer, *Prison Community,* Chap. 9.

112. American Correctional Association, *Manual of Correctional Standards* (Washington, D.C.: the association, 1959), pp. 603–4.

113. John Law, L. W. Doves, and Gerald Curtain, "Physical Education and Recreation," in *Correctional Education Today,* ed. American Correctional Association (Washington, D.C.: the association, 1939), pp. 222–40.

114. Darwin E. Clay, "Physical Education and Recrea-

tion in Correctional Treatment," *Proceedings of American Correctional Association* (Washington, D.C.: the association, 1946), pp. 137–44.

115. Garrett Heyne, "Penal Institutions," *Annals of the American Academy of Political Science* 313 (1957), 71–75; and Harold D. Myer and Charles K. Brightbill, *Recreation Administration: A Guide to Its Practice* (Englewood Cliffs, N.J.: Prentice-Hall, 1956).

116. Barnes and Teeters, *New Horizons in Criminology*.

117. Margaret J. Staples, "A Survey of Recreation in Prisons" (unpublished manuscript, Temple University, 1950), cited in Harry E. Barnes and Negley K. Teeters, *New Horizons in Criminology* (Englewood, N.J.: Prentice-Hall, 1951), pp. 676–77; and material digested from a master's thesis by Richard Haley, University of Colorado, 1949, cited in Barnes and Teeters, *New Horizons in Criminology*, p. 686.

118. American Correctional Standards, *Manual of Correctional Standards* (1966), pp. 519–40.

119. President's Committee on Law Enforcement and Administration of Justice, *Task Force Report: Corrections* (Washington, D.C.: U. S. Government Printing Office, 1967), pp. 209–10.

120. International Commission of Jurists to United Nations, "Standard Minimum Rules for the Treatment of Prisoners." Report submitted by the Commission to the Fourth United Nations Congress on the Prevention of Crime and Treatment of Offenders, Kyoto, Japan (1970).

121. Cited by James L. Krug, "Correctional Recreation: A Statement on Progress," *Parks and Recreation* 14, no. 11 (1979), 36–39.

122. Krug, "Correctional Recreation," p. 36.

123. Paul W. Keve, "Reintegration of the Offender into the Community," in *Holistic Approaches to Offender Rehabilitation*, ed. Leonard J. Hippchen (Springfield, Ill.: Charles C Thomas, Publisher, 1982), pp. 415–35.

124. "Special Issue: Recreation in Corrections," *Parks and Recreation* 16:2 (1981); and "Correctional Recreation," *Journal of Physical Education and Recreation* 52, no. 4 (1981).

125. Krug, "Correctional Recreation," p. 38.

126. Ibid.

127. Thomas G. Eymon, "Research Needs in Correctional Classification," in *Holistic Approaches*, pp. 466–82.

128. Chamelin, Fox, and Whisenand, *Criminal Justice*, p. 372.

129. Larry R. Williams, "An Analysis of the Recreational Pursuits of Selected Parolees from a State Correctional Institution in Pennsylvania," *Therapeutic Recreation Journal* 6, no. 3 (1972), 134–40; and Dianne J. Orton, "An Investigation of the Past, Present and Future Recreation Pursuits of Adult Inmates in Two Iowa Correctional Institutions," *Therapeutic Recreation Journal* 11, no. 2 (1977), 66–69.

130. Ronald P. Reynolds, "Leisure Services: An Essential Aspect of Offender Rehabilitation," in *Holistic Approaches*, p. 325.

131. Ibid., p. 327.

132. Ibid., pp. 327–38.

133. National Correctional Recreation Association/ American Association for Leisure and Recreation, "National Mission Statement, Policy Statement, Personnel Standards, Facility Standards for Correctional Recreation."

134. Ibid.

SUGGESTED READINGS

BARNES, HARRY E. *The Story of Punishment* (2nd ed.). Montclair, N.J.: Patterson Smith, 1972.

CARTER, JEAN M., GLEN E. VAN ANDEL, and GARY M. ROBB. *Therapeutic Recreation: A Practical Approach.* St. Louis: Times Mirror/Mosby College Publishing, 1985, pp. 35–49.

CLEMMER, DONALD. *The Prison Community.* New York: Rinehart & Company, 1958.

"Correctional Recreation." *Journal of Physical Education and Recreation* 52, no. 4 (1981).

DOLAN, JOSEPHINE A. *The History of Nursing.* Philadelphia: W. B. Saunders Co., 1969.

ELKIN, E. "Historical Perspectives." In *A National Forum on Residential Services*, ed. *National Association for Retarded Citizens.* Arlington, Texas: the association, 1977, pp. 5–12.

ERIKSON, JOAN M. *Activity, Recovery and Growth: The Community Role of Planned Activities.* New York: W. W. Norton, 1976.

HAYNES, FRED E. *The American Prison System.* New York: McGraw-Hill Book Co., 1939.

HENRY, WILLIAM. "Mental Hospitals." In *A History of Medical Psychology*, ed. *Gregory Zilboorg.* New York: W. W. Norton, 1941, pp. 558–89.

IRWIN, JOHN. *The Felon.* Englewood Cliffs, N.J.: Prentice-Hall, 1970.

KRANNER, L. *A History of the Care and Study of the Mentally Retarded.* Springfield, Ill.: Charles C Thomas, Publishers, 1964.

KRAUS, RICHARD. *Therapeutic Recreation Service: Principles and Practices* (3rd ed.). Philadelphia: Saunders College Publishing, 1983, pp. 18–27.

LEWIS, OLIVER F. *The Development of American Prisons and Prison Customs, 1776–1845.* Albany, N.Y.: Prison Association of New York, 1922.

NORRIS, ALBERT S., ANTHONY E. RAYNES, and ROBERT L. KELLEY. "Mental Hospitals." In *Handbook of Psychiatry* (2nd ed.), ed. *Philip Solomon* and *Vernon D. Patch.* Los Altos, Calif.: Lange Medical Publications, 1969.

RISLEY, MARY. *House of Healing.* New York: Doubleday & Co. 1961.

ROWTHORN, ANNIE W., "A History of the Evolution and Development of Therapeutic Recreation Services for Special Populations in the United States from 1918 to 1977." Ph.D dissertation, New York University, 1978.

SENNA, JOSEPH A., and LARRY J. SIEGEL. *Introduction to Criminal Justice* (3rd ed.). St. Paul: West Publishing Co., 1984.

"Special Issues—Recreation in Corrections." *Parks and Recreation* 16, no. 2 (1981).

TEETES, NEGLEY K. *The Cradle of the Penitentiary: The Walnut Street Jail at Philadelphia, 1773–1835.* Philadelphia: Pennsylvania Prison Society, 1955.

WARD, DAVID A., and GENE G. KASSEBAUM. *Women's Prison.* Chicago: Aldine Publishing Co., 1965.

5

Professional Development

The preceding chapter considered the historical evolution of therapeutic recreation in health and health-related facilities and correctional institutions. During this historical evolution a variety of matters normally associated with the process of professionalization developed. Today the professional status of therapeutic recreation has become a pressing issue.

In retrospect, patterns can be identified in the process of professionalization. Historically, specializations have arisen in response to the identified needs of society. From this response fundamental skills and knowledge bases are identified by trained personnel and are handed down using the apprenticeship method. In an apprenticeship information is transmitted in an informal setting such as a home by someone considered knowledgeable in the field to those less knowledgeable. Eventually, educational programs are developed that teach theory and skill. Payment for services is provided, and formal rules of practice (codes) are devised and enforced. The methods for enforcement of these codes are established by the professional group, and a profession thus develops group consciousness.[1]

The historical development of therapeu-

tic recreation reflects a similar pattern of professionalization. As we have noted, in the late nineteenth century and the early years of this century recreation service in hospitals/institutions was provided by volunteers with varied backgrounds. The early training of such individuals was accomplished through apprentice education, with knowledge passed on by word of mouth. From this base therapeutic recreation broadened and expanded its components and the related skills and techniques. Gradually recreation services of a therapeutic nature became a formalized service in various hospitals and institutions; likewise, community recreation services developed for the ill and disabled, with the training of personnel provided through in-service training programs, workshops, and conferences. It was through the general acceptance of recreation services in agencies following World War II that the education process for therapeutic recreation became formalized, and the beginning of a theoretical base was established. As group consciousness arose, therapeutic recreation specialists began to organize into professional organizations.

A brief historical evolution of therapeutic recreation raises the question of whether therapeutic recreation really is a profession. Has it emerged, or is it maturing? What are the characteristics of a profession? These and related questions are considered in this chapter.

THE NATURE OF THERAPEUTIC RECREATION

A number of therapeutic recreation specialists have attempted to define therapeutic recreation. Some have defined a *concept* of therapeutic recreation; others have stated *beliefs* about therapeutic recreation; and still others have defined a *philosophy* of therapeutic recreation. But the question is still frequently asked: What is therapeutic recreation? Perhaps the answer is so obvious that a precise definition is unnecessary, or the many variables operating make a precise definition impossible. Any discussion of what therapeutic recreation is can be approached from a number of avenues. For example, therapeutic recreation can be defined according to the actions used in performing the service, the roles of the individuals who do therapeutic recreation, the functions of the therapeutic recreator, the consumer's image of therapeutic recreation, the image of therapeutic recreation that therapeutic recreation peers have, the philosophy of therapeutic recreation as perceived by practitioners, the settings in which therapeutic recreation is performed, and the value placed on the individual who needs therapeutic recreation. These avenues (and others) certainly emphasize the complex nature of therapeutic recreation.

DEFINITIONS AND CONCEPTS

Over the years a variety of terms have been used to express in some philosophical fashion (including practice and service) the nature of therapeutic recreation. The term initially used to describe recreation services to the ill and disabled was *hospital recreation*, with emphasis on the recreation experience within hospitals or institutional settings. Another term used for a brief period was *medical recreation*, which suggested that rec-

reation service was under medical approval. Still another term, which overlapped the previous two and was extensively used into the mid-1960s, was *recreation therapy*. This perspective considered recreative experiences or activities as treatment tools that were prescribed as part of therapy; the concern was with illness and treatment of disease. In community settings the terms *recreation to the ill and handicapped* and later *recreation for special populations* have been used to describe recreation services to individuals with limited impairments or disabilities. More recently the terms *community-based programs for special populations* and *special recreation* have been applied. In 1966 the term *therapeutic recreation* replaced the older terms except for those terms related to the community setting. The rationale at that time for a change in terminology was the unification of the various perspectives.[2]

Only recently has therapeutic recreation clarified its purpose, although controversial and analytic discussion of this focal issue has been going on for some years and will undoubtedly continue into the future. Earlier terms, definitions, concepts, and theories regarding therapeutic recreation reflected not only the influence of the individual's own philosophy of recreation, education, and experience but that of the agencies, the therapeutic value of recreation to special population members, and the impairment or limitation of the special population member. (See the various journal and text publications mentioned in this chapter that discuss these early definitions, concepts, and theories of recreation services to the ill and disabled.) These efforts suggest a deliberate approach to a thorough analysis of therapeutic recreation. Such constructive efforts provide the therapeutic recreation profession with the structural framework within which the process and knowledge of therapeutic recreation can be examined, critically analyzed, revised, and improved continually in a sound scientific manner.

The first attempt to create a philosophical base for recreation services to the ill and disabled is found in the publication *Basic Concepts of Hospital Recreation.*[3] In 1953 a committee of the Hospital Recreation Section—American Recreation Society (HRS-ARS) was appointed to conduct a study on recreation concepts in hospitals. A part of the Statement of Tenets of this publication reads as follows:

WE BELIEVE,

That wholesome recreation is an essential ingredient of mental, emotional, and physical well-being.

That in keeping with the modern medical concept of treating the whole man, recreation, under medical guidance, has a vital and an important role in the treatment, care, and rehabilitation of ill and disabled people.

That recreation assists the physician in his work of helping the patient get well by:

1. Facilitating favorable adjustment of the patient to treatment and hospital environment.

2. Contributing to the development, restoration, or maintenance of sound mental, emotional, and physical health.

3. Providing the physician with opportunities to observe patient response to medically approved recreation activities.[4]

A few years later during the 1956 annual conference of the American Association for Health, Physical Education and Recreation, Bernie E. Phillips, author of the "Recreational Therapy" column in the *Journal of Health, Physical Education and Recreation,* raised the philosophical issue during a presentation of what to call recreation leaders who provide recreation services in hospitals.

Can we agree . . . that a person needs recreation whether or not he is in the hospital . . . that he needs recreation as he needs food, exercise, rest, faith, and shelter . . . that those deficient in recreation, whether in amount or kind, must be prescribed recreation just as those deficient in certain foods must be prescribed diets . . . that, further, there are many in the hospital with no recreation deficiency who, nevertheless, need recreation just as there are those with no diet deficiency who must eat?

If we can agree on this simple reasoning, it is not, then a case of whether or not recreation in the hospital is more Recreational Therapy than it is Therapeutic Recreation . . . or just plain Recreation. It is, in instances, all of these.

Can we agree further to use the term Recreational Therapist to identify the professional recreation leader who is engaged in "hospital recreation," "recreation rehabilitation," or "recreation therapy" . . . the leader who, in varying circumstances, finds himself playing the role of the *educator* or *therapist,* as well as the *recreator?*[5]

During the 1958 annual conference of the National Association of Recreational Therapists (NART) the following concept of the use of recreation as a therapeutic tool was offered:

Recreation Therapy, or Therapeutic Recreation, is the constructive use of recreational activities as tools to give the patient a group of experiences that would provide a positive meaning for him in relation to the medical problem he has.[6]

As recreation service to the ill and disabled expanded, attention was focused on the appropriate use of the term *professional* and the concept of *professionalism.* In an attempt to resolve issues associated with the concept of professionalism and develop an ideology, a position statement on therapeutic recreation was drafted and initiated during the Ninth Southern Regional Institute on Therapeutic Recreation at the University of North Carolina in 1969.[7] During the annual conference of the National Therapeutic Recreation Society (NTRS) in the same year, the statement was discussed further, and in 1970 at Indiana State University the statement was the topic of a work-study conference.

At the same time and into the late 1970s various authors expressed their views with suggested models regarding the purpose, function, and role of therapeutic recreation. Some of these models tended to be specific, but others were broader and more encompassing of the scope and practice of therapeutic recreation. The models made reference to a continuum approach that incorporated a range of recreative experiences based upon the functioning or limitation of the individual. The role of the therapeutic recreation specialist was determined by the function of the individual and the type of services offered by the agency—therapy (rehabilitation), therapeutic, or recreation.

As a result of continued dissatisfaction about various therapeutic recreation concepts among prominent leaders in the field, a Philosophical Statement Task Force was established in 1977 by Gary Robb, then president of NTRS, to study and make recommendations concerning a definition and philosophical statement of therapeutic recreation. Between 1977 and 1981 various committees appointed by succeeding presidents of NTRS continued the work of the initial committee. Eventually four alternative positions or purposes of therapeutic recreation were developed.[8] These positions were further developed and interpreted so that in 1981 the NTRS board of directors, after a vote by the membership regarding each position, endorsed with modification the "leisurability" purpose of therapeutic recreation as follows:

> The purpose of therapeutic recreation is to facilitate the development, maintenance, and expression of an appropriate leisure lifestyle for individuals with physical, mental, emotional, or social limitations. Accordingly, this purpose is accomplished through the provision of professional programs and services which assist the client in eliminating barriers

to leisure, developing leisure skills and attitudes, and optimizing leisure involvement. Therapeutic recreation professionals use these principles to enhance clients' leisure ability in recognition of the importance and value of leisure in the human experience.

> Three specific areas of professional services are employed to provide this comprehensive leisure ability approach toward enabling appropriate leisure lifestyles: therapy, leisure education, and recreation participation. While these three areas of service have unique purposes in relation to client need, they each employ similar delivery processes using assessment or identification of client need, development of a related program strategy, and monitoring and evaluating client outcomes. The decision as to where and when each of the three service areas would be provided is based on the assessment of client needs and the service mandate of the sponsoring agency. The selection of appropriate service areas is contingent on a recognition that different clients have differing needs related to leisure involvement in view of their personal life situation....

> These three service areas of therapeutic recreation represent a continuum of care, including therapy, leisure education, and the provision of special recreation participation opportunities. This comprehensive leisure ability approach uses the need of the client to give direction to program service selection. In some situations, the client may need programs from all three service areas. In other situations, the client may require only one or two of the service areas....[9]

Although the official statement on therapeutic recreation may serve the purpose for which it was intended, there is evidence that it has not satisfied everyone. Most recently new philosophical concepts and service models have appeared. In 1984 the newly formed American Therapeutic Recreation Association (ATRA) viewed therapeutic recreation services as contributing "to the rehabilitation, habilitation, education, and medical treatment of clients in health care and human service settings."[10] ATRA defines therapeutic recreation as follows:

Therapeutic Recreation is the application, by qualified professionals, of appropriate intervention strategies using recreation services to promote independent functioning and to enhance optimal health and well being of individuals with illnesses and/or disabling conditions. Therapeutic Recreation places a special emphasis on the development of an appropriate leisure lifestyle as an integral part of that independent functioning.

The underlying philosophy of Therapeutic Recreation is that all human beings have the right to and need for leisure involvement as a necessary aspect of optimal health and, as such, Therapeutic Recreation can be used as an important tool for these individuals in becoming and remaining well.[11]

Carter, Van Andel, and Robb in 1985 suggested a model of professional service that they refer to as "A Helping Model." In this model the emphasis is on the interpersonal aspects of actions that are therapeutic recreation and on identifying the behavioral stimulus for the person in need so as to designate the action to take.[12] Carter comments as follows regarding the development of this model:

Our thoughts were that the role of the helper is dependent upon the functioning abilities and needs of the participant. A second thought is the wholistic concept recognizing the influence of the community-agency-participant on one another during the therapeutic recreation process of assessment, plan, implement, and evaluate as being interactive and also as influencing the intended outcomes. The model attempted to tie together the purpose of therapeutic recreation with the process of programming and the roles of the therapeutic recreator. We also hoped to recognize the concomitant values on the total (whole) wellness of the participant. Finally, we hoped to present a model that would encourage the profession to keep "questioning" rather than remain tied to one viewpoint.[13]

In that same year Mobily suggested an existential approach to therapeutic recreation in both practice and education,[14] while

Sylvester challenged the therapy component of the NTRS Leisure Ability model by proposing that the "elements of freedom, responsibility, power and intrinsic value" found within the definition and concept of leisure be incorporated into the therapy or treatment concept; while therapy may be required it does not preclude leisure.[15] Halberg and Howe-Murphy called for a therapeutic recreation philosophy that does not involve settings but rather involves a philosophy that addresses "our unique professional capabilities and will enhance our ability to be responsive to changing societal conditions" and, in addition, a philosophy that will "contribute to both a better understanding of and a decreased reliance on the models of allied fields, thus further strengthening the identity of our own field."[16]

Most recently two additional perspectives have emerged. In fact, one may be a reemergence of the early term and concept of "recreation for special populations," which Kennedy, Austin, and Smith refer to as "special recreation."[17] Special recreation takes a nonclinical approach to providing recreation service to the disabled with emphasis on freely chosen recreation participation. Although these authors recognize that a difference exists between therapeutic recreation and special recreation, they also recognize that an overlap exists. They explain the overlap as follows:

... a therapeutic recreation program (directed primarily toward a specific therapeutic outcome through a planned intervention) offers the client an accompanying benefit of a recreative experience, or ... a special recreation program (aimed primarily toward the provision of a recreative experience) serves as an intervention, bringing about a desired therapeutic benefit.[18]

In a more recent publication Howe-Murphy and Charboneau take an "ecological perspective" on therapeutic recreation.[19] This perspective incorporates some ideas from Rusalem's earlier "ecological model."[20] Howe-Murphy and Charboneau write that therapeutic recreation

is based on a recognition of the many elements necessary for play, and on a realization that functional impairments (disabling conditions) can be possessed by both the individual and the environment. Therefore, the term will refer to a planned process of intervention directed toward specific environmental and/or individual change. The goals of the change process are to maximize the quality of life, enhance the leisure functioning of the individual, and promote acceptance of persons with disabilities within the community. The processes by which purposeful change occurs are variable, encompassing both the promotion of individuals (individual, community, environment) and the elimination of individual and environmental barriers.[21]

It is worthwhile to note that few authors addressed the issue of therapeutic recreation failure on the part of the client. Unless the therapeutic recreation specialist is realistic about the possible negative outcome of the therapeutic recreation experience, the specialist may very well be prone to disappointment and frustration. It is important for the specialist to recognize that efforts to return the client to a state of wellness and ability to participate in recreative experience are not always successful. Although it was developed in conjunction with the provisions of services to mentally retarded persons, as the authors have indicated elsewhere, the principle of dignity of risk associated with Wolfensberger's concept of normalization has wide potential applicability to a variety of disabling conditions and therapeutic recreation.[22] In fact, the concept speaks directly to the point that clients have the "right to fail."[23]

The unique function of therapeutic recreation is to assist the client, sick or well, in the performance of those leisure activities or experiences contributing to health or its recovery, including general recreative participation. The fulfillment of this function involves essentially three major phases of ther-

apeutic recreation practice: (1) identification of the client's need for help; (2) assistance in, or ministration of, help needed; and (3) validation that the help given was indeed the help needed. For our purpose here, a *need* is thought of as anything individuals require to maintain or sustain themselves in their situation; *help* is thought of as any measure or action that enables individuals to overcome whatever interferes with their ability to function capably in relation to their situation. A need for help, then, is any measure or action required and desired by the individuals (recreative experience) that has the potential for restoring or extending their ability to cope with the demands implicit in their situation.

Functional ability, or ability to cope, is an intrinsic quality of individuals. It is something they must develop within themselves; no one can give it to them or develop it in them or for them. By the same token, to be helpful, help must be used by individuals and must succeed in enhancing or extending their capabilities.

Certainly the continued advancement of therapeutic recreation in recent years has compounded the difficulty in defining, theorizing, and conceptualizing therapeutic recreation. Therapeutic recreation is multifaceted and multidimensional. We cannot help but feel that maybe there is no one definition or purpose of therapeutic recreation because of the many variables operating: persons, needs, settings. As long as available definitions and purposes of therapeutic recreation are unsatisfying to therapeutic recreation students and specialists, such individuals should continue to strive to assemble definitions that represent their ideas and reflect the service of therapeutic recreation as they see it. This would seem to be more important than continuing to look for one definition of therapeutic recreation that will be universally accepted. A variety of resources should be used, including the potential of each concerned specialist to describe therapeutic recreation. The definition of therapeutic recreation should be a foundation for functioning; then the specialist is ready to move on to the essential actions of therapeutic recreation for which the definition is the springboard or beginning.

The need for sound theories and concepts to guide the practice of therapeutic recreation has been expressed in the literature. In practice, basic scientific theories can be accepted initially, and then tested and evaluated as the specialist deliberately programs for clients. Theories that guide the specialist can be retested and reexplored to assess their value and the extent to which they help to improve the practice of therapeutic recreation. "Hunches" can be defined and new ideas used to pursue further theories and actions, thereby setting up a continual cycle of activity—selecting a theory, using that theory to prescribe and plan therapeutic recreation, testing the effectiveness of the action in terms of benefit to the patient, revising, redefining, perhaps determining a new theory or selecting a different one to use, testing and reevaluating for future actions. Hence, the deliberate use of theories assists in the sound planning and implementation of therapeutic recreation action and results in effective therapeutic recreation practice. Eventually, from sound therapeutic recreation practice a body of theory will emerge that can be labeled the theory of therapeutic recreation.

CRITERIA OF A PROFESSION

There are no absolute, inclusive, and exclusive criteria to specifically define a profession. Professional status is a dynamic social concept that is relative to ever-changing and evolving social values, expectations, and ideals of service. It may help to clarify our thinking and be a provocative experience to first consider some generally accepted criteria of all professions and then, specifically, therapeutic recreation.

Around the turn of the century professionalism was a topic of emphasis and priority in occupational circles. Abraham Flexner identified areas needing attention in the medical profession and developed criteria for a profession. These criteria were to be applicable to many different professional areas, such as social work, nursing, and others. The following are seven characteristics of professional activity listed by Flexner:

1. Essentially involves intellectual operations accompanied by a large degree of individual responsibility.
2. Is learned in nature, and its members constantly resort to the laboratory and seminar for a fresh supply of facts.
3. Is not entirely academic and theoretical; however, it is definitely practical in its aims.
4. Possesses a technique capable of communication through orderly and highly specialized education discipline.
5. Is a brotherhood of individuals whose activities, duties, and responsibilities tend to completely engage them. It is well organized.
6. Is concerned with the public interest, and its motives are altruistic.
7. Has a definite status—social and professional.[24]

William Wickenden, while president of Case School of Applied Science, gave an address before the Engineering Institute of Canada in which he described the characteristics of the professional person. He mentioned four distinctive marks. The first is a *"type of activity,* which carries high individual responsibility and which applies special skills to problems on a distinctly intellectual plane." The second is a *"motive of service,* associated with limited rewards as distinct from profit." The third is the *"motive of self-expression,* which implies joy and pride in one's work and a self-imposed standard of excellence." And the fourth is a "conscious *recognition of social duty* to be fulfilled among other means by guarding the ideals and standards of one's profession, by advancing it in public understanding and esteem, by sharing advances in technical knowledge, and by rendering gratuitous public service, in addition to that for ordinary compensation, as a return to society for special advantages of education and status."[25]

Wickenden went on to describe the attributes that mark the life of a group of persons as professional in character:

> We may place first a *body of knowledge* (science) and of *art* (skill) held as a common possession and to be extended by united effort. Next is *an educational process* based on this body of knowledge and art, in ordering which the professional group has a recognized responsibility. Third is a *standard* of personal qualifications for admission to the professional group, based on character, training, and proved competence. Next follows *a standard of conduct* based on courtesy, honor, and ethics, which guides the practitioner in his relations with clients, colleagues, and the public. Fifth, we may place a more or less formal *recognition of status*, either by one's colleagues or by the state, as a basis for good standing. And finally, there is usually *an organization* of the professional group, devoted to its common advancement and its social duty, rather than to the maintenance of an economic monopoly.[26]

Wilbert E. Moore in 1970 suggested that we should view occupations as distributed along a continuum, with professionalism regarded as a scale and with professions differing from nonprofessional occupations quantitatively rather than qualitatively.[27]

Since 1977 therapeutic recreation specialists as well as the National Therapeutic Recreation Society and more recently the American Therapeutic Recreation Association have more consciously addressed the issues relating to professionalism. They are examining therapeutic recreation according to professional criteria to determine its standing as a profession.

Some characteristics of a profession frequently cited in the literature today include the following:

Provides services vital to human and social welfare.

Develops a body of knowledge on which skills and services are based and expands this body of knowledge through investigation, analysis, and research.

Involves essentially intellectual operations, accompanied by individual responsibility.

Educates its practitioners in institutions of higher education.

Establishes and controls policies and activities; that is, in most instances its practitioners have relative independence in performance of their functions and activities.

Attracts individuals whose primary motivation lies in service as opposed to personal and financial gain.

Develops a code of ethics that guides the conduct of its practitioners.

Provides one association that fosters and ensures quality of practice.[28]

The compulsion to achieve personal identity impels maturing individuals to prove their worth, find their place in the sun, establish status positions, and gain the symbolic prestige of social recognition and acceptance as independent, responsible people. Likewise, in its evolutionary development therapeutic recreation has experienced its adolescent growing pains and has sought to establish its unique identity. It has struggled to be freed from its identity association with other organizations and to fulfill its function as an equal partner with other helping professions. In this maturing process, professional status has symbolized for therapeutic recreation an intrinsic personal as well as professional sense of attainment.

In the following pages we consider some of those criteria or attributes that make up the profession of therapeutic recreation. There is no particular order or hierarchy in the presentation of these attributes.

ORGANIZATIONS

For a discipline to be considered a profession, it is imperative that a professional organization be established. This has happened in therapeutic recreation. In fact, there are two organizations today involved in the therapeutic recreation movement; at one time, however, there were three, then one, and now two.

A professional group exercises its prerogative to function autonomously. Its membership formulates policies and standards. They use independent methods for the self-determination and control of professional activities. A true profession is committed to maintain and improve its services and the welfare of its practitioners through organized endeavor.

It was not until shortly after World War II that individuals employed as recreation therapists or hospital recreation workers in military and Veterans Administration hospitals and in state institutions for the mentally ill and mentally retarded began to organize themselves. The first of these organizations, established in 1948, was the Hospital Recreation Section of the American Recreation Society. (A listing of the leadership of the HRS-ARS can be found in Appendix C.) The section issued its first quarterly newsletter in 1950. It was later incorporated into the American Recreation Society's *Bulletin*, which eventually became the *American Recreational Journal*. As noted above, the section published the well-received document, *Basic Concepts of Hospital Recreation*.

Two other organizations, the Recreation Therapy Section of the American Association for Health, Physical Education, and Recreation (now called the American Alliance for Health, Physical Education, Recreation and Dance), formed in 1952, and the

National Association of Recreation Therapists (NART), established in 1953, furthered the early movement of therapeutic recreation. Membership in the former organization consisted primarily of those employed in special schools with an educational background in recreation, physical education, and adapted physical education. For a number of years the section produced a monthly column titled "Recreational Therapy," which appeared in the AAHPER's *Journal of Health, Physical Education, and Recreation*.

The NART membership consisted primarily of recreation workers employed in public and private institutions and schools for the mentally ill and mentally retarded in the southern and midwestern states. (A listing of the leadership of the RTS-AAHPER and NART can be found in Appendix C.) This organization published a quarterly publication, *Recreation for the Ill and Handicapped*.

As might be expected, philosophies, interests, programs, and opinions differed among the three organizations; thus, a desire arose for some form of organization through which ideas could be exchanged and concerted action be taken. In 1953 representatives from each organization met, which resulted in the formation of the Council for the Advancement of Hospital Recreation (CAHR). The council not only provided a framework wherein communication was established to further the concepts and interests of hospital recreation but also eventually established standards of qualifications for hospital recreation workers in 1956.

Within a few short years it became apparent that while the CAHR did provide a channel for communication among the three organizations, a single strong organization was also needed that would speak for all recreation specialists working in various settings that provided care and treatment to the ill and disabled, as well as those providing special services in the community. Between 1958 and 1962 representatives from the three organizations met for the purpose of resolving differences of philosophies so as to unite in one organization that could speak for the needs of this profession in its own right. Differences could not be resolved, however, and the Committee on Merger was disbanded.

During the early 1960s an interesting phenomenon occurred, namely a concern for unity within the total park and recreation movement. As a result of this concern, five national organizations representing various park and recreation interest areas merged in 1965, forming the National Recreation and Park Association (NRPA). To represent the various interests of those organizations that had merged, branches were established. Sensing the urgent need to maintain unity, representatives from NART and the former HRS-ARS (now part of NRPA) again met in 1965 to attempt to resolve previous differences. By mid-1966 both organizations had received favorable responses from their membership for the movement to develop a branch within the NRPA. During the National Park and Recreation Congress in October 1966 the National Therapeutic Recreation Society (NTRS) was born. (A listing of the leadership of the NTRS since its inception can be found in Appendix C.)

According to its charter and bylaws, the purpose of the NTRS is as follows:

> The purpose of this society shall include and conform to the purposes of the National Recreation and Park Association, Inc. These shall include, but not be limited to: gathering and disseminating facts and information with reference to therapeutic recreation; furthering the rehabilitation of participants through recreation; engendering a spirit of cooperation between all professions and agencies related to our common cause; and developing standards for personnel, programs and facilities that will result in improved services for the participant.[29]

Since the initial establishment of NTRS there has been a growing concern among members employed primarily in health-care settings about the society's inability to meet the needs of clinical practitioners.[30] As a result of this concern, whether directly or indirectly motivated, another organization was established. The American Therapeutic Recreation Association (ATRA) was founded in 1984. (A listing of the leadership of the ATRA can be found in Appendix C.) According to its first president, Peg Connolly, it differs from other professional organizations concerned with therapeutic recreation in that ATRA "is not a special interest group of some larger public or lay organization but an independent, professional association devoted solely to the advancement of Therapeutic Recreation." It was founded "in recognition of the increased accountability demands and dramatic changes and challenges facing health care and human services today."[31]

In addition to the national organizations, nearly every state has an organized constituent group of therapeutic recreation specialists within its NRPA affiliate state society or as a separate group. This allows for local control of therapeutic recreation policies and statewide support for therapeutic recreation practice.[32]

PUBLICATIONS

One of the most valuable services of any organization and one that reflects professionalization is to provide publications that contribute to the advancement of its membership educationally and in service. To a great extent, the advancement and acceptance of therapeutic recreation can be attributed to the publications of all three early organizations, as noted above, and the NTRS in more recent years. Since the formation of ATRA, it has published only newsletters, which is not unusual for a newly formed organization.

The official quarterly publication of the NTRS, the *Therapeutic Recreation Journal*, has been widely accepted by recreation professionals as well as by other professionals in other disciplines. An earlier publication was the *Therapeutic Recreation Annual,* which evolved from *Recreation in Treatment Centers,* a publication initially produced by the HRS-ARS. Other publications have included *Impact, Communiqué* (a joint branch publication of NRPA), *NTRS Yearbook,* and various society newsletters. In association with NRPA, a number of specific publications and special magazine issues concerned with a variety of topics as they relate to special populations have appeared; examples include *Recreation in Nursing Homes, Community Recreation Programming for Handicapped Children,* "Trends for the Handicapped," "Leisure and Handicapped People," and *Therapeutic Recreation—State of the Art,* prepared for the Thirteenth World Congress of Rehabilitation International in Israel.[33]

In recent years more textbooks and special publications concerned with therapeutic recreation have appeared, and many articles written by therapeutic recreation specialists have been published in the above journals and other professional and scientific journals. The first so-called textbook appeared in 1952, written by John E. Davis, Sr. and titled *Clinical Applications of Recreational Therapy.*[34] (According to a reference by B. E. Phillips in the December 1955 issue of the *Journal of Health, Physical Education and Recreation* 26, no. 9, p. 46, a recreation therapy text was coauthored by Davis and William R. Dunton as early as 1933. Unfortunately, no title or publisher was given, and additional research on the subject produced no results.) Initial textbook editions with author(s) and year of first edition include Hunt (1955); Rathbone and Lucas (1959); Pomeroy (1964); Frye and Peters (1972); Kraus (1973); Stein and Sessoms (1973); Avedon (1974); Shivers and Fait (1975); O'Morrow (1976); Gunn and Peterson (1978); Austin (1982); Reynolds and O'Morrow (1985); Carter, Van Andel, and Robb (1985); Kennedy, Austin, and Smith (1987); Crawford and Mendell (1987); and Howe-Murphy and Charboneau (1987).[35]

EDUCATION

Professional education deals with practice in a particular field. Students are informed of the current practices of their profession, and under teacher guidance and observation they participate in those practices as part of a planned curriculum. However, professional preparation extends beyond practice. Future practitioners are also given a theoretical basis so that they may act with intelligence and good judgment. This comprehensive background of knowledge and principles is provided so that the practitioners will be qualified to evaluate and improve practice. Professional study prepares people to act with maximum competence in the conduct of their occupation.

The growth of university curricula in therapeutic recreation has been varied and extensive in recent years. With the initiation of more recreation programs in hospitals/institutions and the demand for trained leaders and administrators in the late 1940s, educational institutions began to offer concentrations or options in hospital recreation or recreation therapy. The first institutions to offer a concentration in this specialization at the graduate level were the University of Minnesota and the University of West Virginia in 1951.[36] Kraus, in his review of professional education, indicated that by 1953 six colleges and universities were offering undergraduate and graduate degrees in hospital recreation.[37] In 1969 Stein reported that 35 of 114 institutions were offering a major in therapeutic recreation.[38] According to the 1984 Society of Park and Recreation Educators' curriculum study, 98 undergraduate and 55 graduate programs (master's and above) in therapeutic recreation existed among 260 institutions of higher education that responded to the survey.[39] This finding supports an earlier study of Anderson and Stewart, who found that there was a considerable expansion of therapeutic recreation programs during the 1970s and projected a continued growth in the 1980s.[40]

Curricula in the early 1950s incorporated

courses that reflected the function, duties, and/or responsibilities a therapeutic recreation specialist might encounter in the performance of a specific job.[41] In 1961 the National Recreation Association sponsored a Therapeutic Recreation Curriculum Development Conference to identify general competencies needed by recreation specialists working with the ill and disabled.[42] As a result, educational institutions began to implement suggestions from the conference.

Since the early 1970s a shift has occurred wherein attention has been focused on specific undergraduate competencies the student needs to attain by the time of graduation. (The list of competencies can be found on p. 318.) These competencies have been developed by a NTRS Committee on Curriculum Development and Standards, approved by the NTRS Board of Directors, and incorporated into the educational standards of the Council on Accreditation, which is sponsored by the NRPA in cooperation with the American Association for Leisure and Recreation and recognized by the Council on Postsecondary Accreditation. As of October 1987 there were sixty-two therapeutic recreation programs of study or options within the seventy-three recreation, leisure services, and resources education curricula so accredited.[43]

The baccalaureate program has both theoretical content and field experience. Typically, there is an emphasis on scholarship, with students expected to develop their abilities in organizing, extending, testing, communicating, and applying knowledge of the field of therapeutic recreation. Generally speaking, programs of study in institutions of higher learning provide students with an opportunity to acquire the following information:

1. A knowledge of developing theories and practice of therapeutic recreation and the basic skills and techniques of the therapeutic recreation field

2. A knowledge of the broad function the profession is expected to perform in society

3. Competency in selecting, synthesizing, and applying relevant information from various disciplines

4. Competency in collaborating with members of other disciplines and with the general public

5. The ability to assess therapeutic recreation needs and provide for therapeutic recreation intervention

6. The ability and motivation to evaluate current practices and try new approaches

7. A foundation for graduate study in therapeutic recreation

As a result of acquiring the above knowledge in a baccalaureate program, students should have the following skills:

1. Assess, plan, implement, and evaluate services with special populations, families, and communities

2. Utilize theoretical and empirical knowledge from the physical and behavioral sciences and the humanities as a source of making therapeutic recreation practice decisions

3. Utilize decision-making theories in determining therapy/therapeutic plans, designs, or interventions for achieving comprehensive therapeutic recreation goals

4. Treat therapeutic recreation interventions as hypotheses to be tested; anticipate a variety of consequences and make decisions; select and evaluate the effectiveness of alternative approaches

5. Accept individual responsibility and accountability for therapeutic recreation interventions and their results

6. Use therapeutic recreation practice as a means of gathering data for refining and extending therapeutic recreation service

7. Share in the responsibility for the health and welfare of all people with colleagues on the interdisciplinary health team and

in the community by collaborating, coordinating, and consulting with them

8. Assist in restructuring the therapeutic recreation delivery system through an understanding of the present and emerging roles of the therapeutic recreation specialist

As the demand for better recreation service to ill and disabled individuals as well as for better trained leaders increased, many universities initiated institutes, workshops, and seminars to discuss a broad range of therapeutic recreation topics. During the 1950s and 1960s, for example, the University of North Carolina and the University of Minnesota conducted institutes in alternating years. In recent years the following universities have been among those that sponsored therapeutic recreation conferences: Maryland, Temple, George Washington, Texas Women's, Pennsylvania State, Indiana, New York, Oregon, Iowa, and Missouri. In 1971 the University of Illinois initiated the first Midwest Symposium on Therapeutic Recreation. Subsequently, regional symposiums have been conducted on an annual basis throughout the United States. Another educational experience directed toward those already in practice is the Therapeutic Recreation Management School established in 1978 at Ogelbay Park, Wheeling, West Virginia. This school, co-sponsored by the Wheeling Park Commission and the Department of Recreation, University of Maryland, offers an annual one-week session of classroom study.

The NTRS has also been concerned with continuing education and training. Educational sessions and mini institutes on therapeutic recreation topics have been a part of the annual NRPA Congress since the formation of NTRS. In addition, NTRS has sponsored or cosponsored in association with NRPA regional conferences, symposiums, and institutes to further the knowledge and professional growth of therapeutic recreation specialists in the field and those about to enter it.

STANDARDS

Equally as important as therapeutic recreation education or curricula are standards—personnel, education, and practice standards respectively. Standards in general are minimal competency guidelines or criteria developed by professional organizations to ensure, upgrade, or improve the quality of education and service being provided. For our discussion here, standards may be divided into two major types. One is *credentialing*, which refers both to practitioners and educational programs to prepare practitioners. (The latter form of credentialing is generally referred to as *accreditation*, which was briefly considered in an earlier chapter.) Personnel credentialing recognizes the competency of individuals and includes the practice of licensure, certification, and registration. The second major type is *program or practice standards*, which address the quality of practice or service being delivered to the public in health or community facilities.

As you can imagine, there is a relationship between accreditation and certification as well as between credentialing and standards of practice. In fact, there is a very close relationship among the various standards. The goal of promoting professional competency is an extremely worthy one. Benefits achieved from that goal are realized by members of the profession itself as well as by members of the public who interact with the profession. The hallmark provides prestige, recognition, and earning power for the individual and enrollment power for the institution/department. Equally important, credentialing enables the public (as well as government and private third-party payers for professional services) to distinguish those who have attained some qualifying level of competency from those who have not.

The various types of credentialing are defined as follows:

Accreditation: the process by which an agency or organization evaluates and recognizes an institution as meeting predetermined qualifications or standards

Licensure: the process by which an agency of government grants permission to an individual to engage in a given occupation upon finding that the applicant has attained the minimal degree of competency required to ensure that the public health, safety, and welfare will be reasonably well protected

Certification: the process by which a governmental or nongovernmental agency grants recognition to an individual who has met certain predetermined qualifications set by a credentialing agency or association

Registration: the process by which qualified individuals are listed on an official roster maintained by a governmental or nongovernmental agency[44]

The voluntary registration program initially established through CAHR has continued throughout the years with various revisions. Today the field has a two-level certification program—professional and paraprofessional—which is administered through the National Council for Therapeutic Recreation Certification and is fiscally, legally, politically, and managerially independent of both the NTRS and NRPA. (The NCTRC standards are found in Appendix D.) In addition, the council is in the process of developing a national written therapeutic recreation examination. The council and the certification program provide for a better and stronger relationship with regulatory groups like the Joint Commission on Accreditation of Hospitals and the Commission on Accreditation of Rehabilitation Facilities. Moreover, various agencies and departments in government in addition to the private sector are requiring certification as a requirement for employment.

Although certification is the process level of choice within the therapeutic recreation field at present, considerable attention is being given to licensure. In fact, the NTRS

Board of Directors has approved a Therapeutic Recreation Model Practice Act and is currently developing the political process of how to introduce the act into various state legislatures. Utah and Georgia at present have therapeutic recreation licensure laws. Licensure, as noted, is the legal indication that an individual has at least the minimum knowledge and skills for safe and effective practice. Licensing is part of the policing power of each individual state and guaranteed by the United States Constitution. There are two kinds of licensure laws, *mandatory* (compulsory) or *permissive* (voluntary). Mandatory licensure usually requires everyone who practices a specific specialty for compensation to be licensed. Permissive licensure permits an individual in a particular specialty to practice without a license as long as the individual does not claim to be licensed or use the initials that signify a specific licensure (for example, R.N. for professional nurse). Obviously, mandatory licensure assures the public of greater protection and is therefore much stronger than permissive licensure. Both Utah and Georgia have mandatory licensure.

Therapeutic recreation accreditation has been a stimulant to the improvement of therapeutic recreation education since its addition to the National Council on Accreditation standards in 1976. Therapeutic recreation accreditation is voluntary. The institution requests this service for its program of study when applying for overall park and recreation accreditation and pays for the evaluation. There is no guarantee that the end result will be accreditation. The common denominator is quality. Increasingly, accreditation is sought because of the significance of this accreditation to the prospective student, the faculty member, and the community.

The NTRS works continually and in many ways to improve the quality of therapeutic recreation service to the public, assuming responsibility for the competency of its members and defining and interpreting its principles and standards of practice. As early as 1965 a committee within NTRS began the process of developing standards, and by 1979 general standards associated with major health settings had been developed.[45] In 1978 the NTRS Board of Directors approved community therapeutic recreation standards—*Guidelines for Community-Based Recreation Programs for Special Populations.*[46] In subsequent years, 1980 and 1982 respectively, two additional publications were published—*Standards of Practice for Therapeutic Recreation Service* and *Guidelines for Administration of Therapeutic Recreation Service in Clinical and Residential Facilities.*[47] These publications are intended to serve both as a guide to the development of efficient therapeutic recreation service and as a yardstick against which these services can be measured.

RESEARCH

Research is regarded as a vital and basic component in the process of professionalization. It has often been stated that the primary task of any profession is the development and refinement of theories and concepts into an organized body of knowledge that can serve as a guide to practice. In reality, research is an enabling process to extend, correct, or verify knowledge, whether that knowledge aids in the construction of a theory or in the delivery of services. The need to develop a better knowledge base for therapeutic recreation through research has been repeatedly emphasized. In 1955, for example, the Recreation Therapy column in the *Journal of Health, Physical Education and Recreation* commented about the need for more and better research regarding basic practice knowledge and skills.[48] More recently Compton stated: "Building a body of knowledge in recreation service to special populations or in therapeutic recreation is not only desirable but mandatory. . . . The systematic investigation of selected leisure behavior phenomena as they relate to special populations is essential to research efforts in our

profession."[49] In a like manner Bullock, McGuire, and Barch have commented: "The validity and credibility of therapeutic recreation as an allied health profession can only be established through research. In addition, systematic investigation is needed to assist in developing and evaluating programs, understanding human behavior and its relationship to leisure involvement, and providing data relevant to the practice of the profession."[50]

It is difficult to pinpoint when therapeutic recreation research efforts started. Formal therapeutic recreation research may have had its beginnings in the efforts of Bertha Schlotter and Margaret Svendsen in working with the mentally retarded in 1932 at the Lincoln State School and Colony in Illinois.[51] We have been led to believe that the *Basic Concepts of Hospital Recreation* was the result of research;[52] likewise, early contributors to our field documented the importance of recreative experiences with the ill and disabled and pointed out significant data, which resulted in education, practice, and organizational reform.

The growth of therapeutic recreation curricula also had a great effect on therapeutic recreation education and practice as faculty and students gradually became more interested in, and sophisticated about, research. As a result, educators and students became involved in establishing more objective methods of obtaining reliable knowledge about therapeutic recreation subjects and practices. In addition to curriculum advancement, the *Therapeutic Recreation Journal* published reports, articles on research methods, and news about research activities. Likewise, the *Journal of Leisurability*, the *Journal of Leisure Research*, special publications of the NRPA and AAHPERD, and some university departments have published research studies and carried abstracts of studies in therapeutic recreation. Lastly, the sponsorship of research studies, institutes, and seminars by public and private agencies, especially federal governmental agencies, through grants of various kinds has helped to further the importance of research.

While research is currently recognized as an important process in therapeutic recreation education and practice, the growing pains, problems, and weaknesses common to other professions in the early days of their development relative to research have also plagued therapeutic recreation research. A major effort in the early decades of the so-called therapeutic recreation scientific movement, for example, was arousing interest in initiating investigations. Even today, according to some individuals in our field, there is a definite need to improve the quality of research, and rightly so. Much of the research in the past, and to some extent the present, in their opinion, has been localized, trivial, biased, fragmentary, and defective in design and methodology; it made little if any contribution to a body of organized knowledge and practice. However, we must also recognize that well-trained investigators do not spring up overnight.

The limited training and experience of therapeutic recreation investigators has hampered the development of the therapeutic recreation research movement. At an earlier period of time therapeutic recreators lacked the necessary foundation in basic sciences, mathematics, psychology, and logic. Some were not thoroughly familiar with the literature in the field and the various research techniques and procedures. Since the late 1970s and early 1980s a more positive and critical attitude has developed toward research, so that today more programs of study have developed instructional materials to prepare students for research. At the same time those in the field have started to recognize that merely collecting data and describing phenomena does not advance knowledge appreciably. Hence, they have endeavored to explain phenomena, and in doing so they have begun to develop theories and concepts. Moreover, the therapeutic recreation research movement has progressed to the point where therapeutic recreators are beginning to survey and

analyze the weaknesses in the overall production of studies. They are finding that the development of research has been uneven, and that there is a need to strive for a greater balance and comprehensiveness in investigative efforts not only in the quality of research but in its focus. The active, expanding therapeutic recreation research movement is passing from its infancy to a more sophisticated stage of development. To aid in this continued development, a Therapeutic Recreation Research Colloquium was initiated at Indiana University (Bloomington) in 1984 and is now in its fifth year as it travels to different universities each year.

CODE OF ETHICS

A code of ethics is considered an essential characteristic of a profession. It expresses the ideals of the profession and establishes standards of conduct for its members to follow in their day-to-day activities. Professions recognize the need for codes of ethics that will guide the members in their practice, and they realize that the procedures and methods by which members seek to further their professional positions must be governed by standards of conduct and good taste. Standards are designed not only to protect the members but also to bring better service to the public.

Ethics is not an easy word to define; essentially it refers to standards of conduct based on moral judgments and values. *Moral*, in turn, is defined as "relating to the distinction between right and wrong." Individuals, of course, may have their own specific ideas of what is right or wrong; these will derive from their background, their religion, their philosophy of life. Generally speaking, though, there are certain standards of "right" behavior accepted by almost everyone: one should not lie, steal, harm others, and so on.

These principles of conduct have developed over the centuries, not just from the teachings of organized religion but also from the effects of any act or behavior upon the well-being of society in general. In general, most moral concepts revolve around the good of the whole. None of us can do just what we please for very long, much as we might like to. We must be concerned with the welfare of the group or community to which we belong as well as with our own happiness.

It has been said that modern codes of professional ethics as well as older ones derive from an admixture of ethics and etiquette.[53] Ethics deals basically with the rightness or wrongness of an individual's actions in the light of principles arising out of the nature of human beings. They establish guides that govern specific situations in such a way that the rights and dignity of the individual are the basic criteria of behavior.

Medicine was the first profession in the United States to adopt a code of ethics; law was the second; pharmacy followed; veterinary medicine was next. In 1929 the National Education Association adopted a code for teachers. Interest in a code of ethics for therapeutic recreation can be traced to NTRS committee actions that began in 1973. Since NTRS is a branch of the NRPA, its Statement of Professional Ethics adopted in 1976 is found in the "Suggested Principles of the Code of Ethics of the Recreation and Park Profession."[54]

Various themes may be identified in the statement. The importance of special recreation for those with limitations is one theme. The responsibility of providing quality service and the dignity of the client are others. Confidentiality and privacy as well as the role of the therapeutic recreator as an advocate are still other themes. The last theme is concerned with consultation services and fees for services. Generally speaking, the statement is designed to create a sensitivity to ethical standards and is concerned with the therapeutic recreation specialist's relation to therapeutic recreation, to the client, to therapeutic recreation as a profession, and to allied professions. The statement in its entirety is reproduced here:

I. The therapeutic recreation professional believes in the value and importance of special recreation services for persons who are limited in their opportunities because of physical, social or mental disabilities. He/she is committed to the continuous task of learning and self-improvement to increase his/her competency and effectiveness as a professional.

II. Above all else, the therapeutic recreation professional is guided by the accepted responsibility of encouraging and providing quality service to the client/consumer as an individual human being. He/she makes an honest effort to meet the habilitative, rehabilitative and leisure needs of the client/consumer and takes care that the client/consumer is not exploited or otherwise abused. This includes but is not limited to the guarantee of basic human rights under law.

III. The therapeutic recreation professional engages only in those activities which bring credit to himself/herself and to the profession. He/she shows respect for fellow colleagues in word and deed. When he/she becomes aware of unethical conduct by a colleague or fellow professional, appropriate and prescribed professional channels will be followed in reporting said conduct.

IV. The therapeutic recreation professional observes the principle of confidentiality in all written and verbal communications concerning clients/consumers, fellow colleagues and/or matters of professional privilege.

V. The therapeutic recreation professional serves as an advocate for therapeutic recreation by interpreting the purposes and values of the profession to client/consumers, other professionals, and the community at large. He/she accepts responsibility for improving communications and cooperative effort among the many professional fields serving special populations. He/she encourages and participates in demonstration and investigative projects aimed at upgrading professional services and communicates the results of his/her efforts.

VI. The therapeutic recreation professional obligates himself/herself to providing consultation service to consumers, other professionals, community agencies and institutions. Fees for service, where appropriate, are made known to client/consumers prior to entering into any contractual relationships.[55]

In addition to standards or guidelines set by the profession, individual facilities or agencies may provide ethical guidelines for various professionals. An example of this is a human subject committee that reviews proposed research studies to determine if there are risks to clients and their rights.

PROVIDES NEEDED SERVICE

There is a philosophical concept that affirms that awareness of a need constitutes an implicit moral obligation to do something to meet that need. This is indeed a hard ideal, and because of its implications we tend to liken it to other demanding philosophies—impractical ideals impossible of application. However, a review of the historical development of therapeutic recreation service indicates that as a discipline we met a need and are meeting a need now. It is enough to say that historically the status of therapeutic recreation has been closely related to the prevailing philosophies of its contemporary society, and its progress, like that of all fields of human endeavor, arose out of consciousness of need and a demand for appropriate action to meet that need. The value system of a society ultimately determines the action taken. Thus, therapeutic recreation service expresses an organized response to a consciousness of social need and demand for a particular service.

From a more practical perspective, it is evident that society in general approves of therapeutic recreation and respects it—as indicated by the number of programs of study found in institutions of higher learning and the number of therapeutic recreators who are hired for positions in public and private agencies. In addition, as people have been helped with their personal and family problems through therapeutic recreation, they have usually become exponents of therapeutic recreation and its services. Equally important has been the general support by the public of those attributes associated with professionalization, especially credentialing standards—accreditation, certification, and licensure.

Regardless of the philosophical and practical aspects relating to providing a needed service, therapeutic recreation must continue to change, adapt, and enlarge its scope in response to the needs, expectations, demands, and opportunities of society. Although therapeutic recreation has been motivated from its beginnings by a concern for those with physical, mental, emotional, and social limitations, it must also play an ever more significant role in promoting the health and well-being of the larger society and its individual members.

PROFESSIONAL STATUS

Professional status can be earned only by the quality of practice; it cannot be acquired by self-seeking. It bears repeating that professional status is a social recognition granted to a particular group of people who are united by an allegiance to a common socially approved objective, in the attainment of which specific acquired knowledge and learned specialized skills are utilized.

Collective professional status is increasingly being accorded to therapeutic recreation specialists and to therapeutic recreation as a discipline. But it is well to remember that when professional status is attained by a representative group, this does not automatically confer professional status upon each individual member of that group. If the specialist is to gain and maintain the right to the privileges associated with professional status, each specialist as an individual must accept and conform to the professional ideals and achieve the competence in the practice of those duties that is in accordance with professional standards of excellence. It is also true that it is the collective achievement of individual specialists that alone determines the status of therapeutic recreation in contemporary society.

Professional status when won is maintained only by continued vigilance and adherence to the ethical principles, the competence in practice, the quality of service given, and the growth in the knowledge and skills of the profession. The heights reached and won by the therapeutic recreation specialists of the past and present were not attained by any single flight of accomplishment but have been attained and can be maintained only by consistent toiling upward by all specialists toward the goals of the calling of the therapeutic recreation specialist. Ultimately, status and accomplishments are determined by the preparation and qualities that are reflected in the excellence of the service performed by therapeutic recreation specialists.

SUMMARY

Although there is concern about the professional development of therapeutic recreation, progress is being made; the body of therapeutic recreation knowledge is evolving, and pertinent research is beginning to take place. New emphasis is being put on the intellectual, on judgmental aspects of therapeutic recreation, and on the assumption of individual responsibility. The therapeutic recreation organizations have, through the years, established policies and standards of practice, and personnel standards have been developed, approved, and established. Although therapeutic recreation specialists have little control over their function in many agencies, some changes for the good are occurring. Finally, more and more individuals are being attracted to therapeutic recreation service as a result of a service motive. At what point therapeutic recreation achieves complete professionalism will depend to a large extent on the goals and action of its educators and especially its practitioners.

Therapeutic recreation cannot expect the field to gain public and professional recognition as a full-fledged profession without building a body of competent research and knowledge. But before this can be accomplished, the therapeutic recreator as well as the researcher must become acquainted with pertinent studies, learn to make some judgment as to which research is valid, begin to test theories in various settings, and add his or her own contributions. It is important to appeal to facts for answers to problems rather than becoming involved in endless emotional arguments with associates, other professionals, and the public concerning who is right.

NOTES

1. William J. Goode, "Encroachment, Charlatanism, and the Emerging Professions: Psychology, Sociology, and Medicine," *American Sociological Review* 25, no. 12 (1960), 902–14; and Harold L. Wilensky, "The Professionalization of Everyone?" *American Journal of Sociology* 120, no. 2 (1964), 141–46.

2. Janet R. MacLean, "Therapeutic Recreation Curriculum," *Recreation in Treatment Centers* 12 (1963), 23–29.

3. Hospital Recreation Section, *Basic Concepts of Hospital Recreation* (Washington, D.C.: American Recreation Society, 1953).

4. Ibid., p. 2.

5. B. E. Phillips, "Recreation Therapy," *Journal of Health, Physical Education and Recreation* 27, no. 5 (May-June 1956), 52.

6. Charlotte Cox and Virginia Dobbs, "Before the Merger: The National Association of Recreation Therapists," *Therapeutic Recreation Journal* 4, no. 1 (1970), 7.

7. "Therapeutic Recreation Position Paper." Developed at the ninth Southern Regional Institute on Therapeutic Recreation, University of North Carolina, Chapel Hill, 1969.

8. National Therapeutic Recreation Society, *Alternative Positions and Their Implications to Professionalization* (Alexandria, Va.: National Recreation and Park Association, 1981).

9. National Therapeutic Recreation Society, "Philosophical Position Statement of the National Therapeutic Recreation Society," May 1982.

10. *American Therapeutic Recreation Association Newsletter*, 1984, p. 2.

11. Ibid.

12. Marcia Jean Carter, Glen E. VanAndel, and Gary M. Robb, *Therapeutic Recreation: A Practical Approach* (St. Louis: Times Mirror/Mosby College Publishing, 1985), pp. 65–66.

13. Marcia Jean Carter, personal correspondence, Feb. 4, 1986.

14. Kenneth E. Mobily, "A Philosophical Analysis of Therapeutic Recreation: What Does It Mean to Say 'We Can Be Therapeutic'?" part 1, *Therapeutic Recreation Journal* 19, no. 1 (1985), 14–26.

15. Charles D. Sylvester, "Freedom, Leisure and Therapeutic Recreation: A Philosophical View," *Therapeutic Recreation Journal* 19, no. 1 (1985), 6–13.

16. Kathleen J. Halberg and Roxanne Howe-Murphy, "The Dilemma of an Unresolved Philosophy in Therapeutic Recreation," *Therapeutic Recreation Journal* 19, no. 3 (1985), 7, 15.

17. Dan W. Kennedy, David R. Austin, and Ralph W. Smith, *Special Recreation: Opportunities for Persons with Disabilities* (Philadelphia: Saunders College Publishing, 1987).

18. Ibid., p. 14.

19. Roxanne Howe-Murphy and Becky G. Charboneau, *Therapeutic Recreation: An Ecological Approach* (Englewood Cliffs, N.J.: Prentice-Hall, 1987).

20. Herbert Rusalem, "An Alternative to the Therapeutic Model in Therapeutic Recreation," *Therapeutic Recreation Journal* 7, no. 1 (1973), 8–15.

21. Howe-Murphy and Charboneau, *Therapeutic Recreation*, 9–10.

22. Wolf Wolfensberger, *The Principle of Normalization in Human Services* (Toronto: National Institute on Mental Retardation, 1972), pp. 196–98.

23. Ronald P. Reynolds and Gerald S. O'Morrow, *Problems, Issues and Concepts in Therapeutic Recreation* (Englewood Cliffs, N.J.: Prentice-Hall, 1985), p. 156.

24. Abraham Flexner, "Is Social Work a Profession?" (New York: New York School of Philanthropy, 1915).

25. William E. Wickenden, "The Second Mile." Address delivered before the Engineering Institute of Canada, 1941.

26. Ibid.

27. Wilbert E. Moore, *The Professions: Roles and Rules* (New York: Russell Sage Foundation, 1970), p. 4.

28. Goode, "Encroachment, Charlatanism, and the Emerging Professions"; Wilensky, "Professionalization of Everyone?" and Everett C. Hughes, "Professions," in *The Professions in America*, ed. Kenneth S. Lynn (Boston: Houghton Mifflin Co., 1965), pp. 1–14.

29. National Therapeutic Recreation Society, charter and bylaws, n.d., p. 1.

30. See Carol Ann Peterson, "A Matter of Priorities and Loyalties," *Therapeutic Recreation Journal* 18, no. 3 (1984), 11–16, for a discussion regarding the organization structure of NTRS/NRPA and the concerns of clinical therapeutic recreation specialists.

31. Both statements are from Peg Connolly, "A Message from the President," *American Therapeutic Recreation Association Newsletter*, 1984, p. 1.

32. See *National Therapeutic Recreation Society: The First Twenty Years 1946–1986* (Alexandria, Va.: NTRS, 1986) for a historical account of NTRS as an organization.

33. Dorothy A. Mullen, *Recreation in Nursing Homes*, National Recreation and Park Association Management Aids, series no. 88 (Washington, D.C.: the association, 1970); George T. Wilson, *Community Recreation Programming for Handicapped Children*, National Recreation and Park Association Management Aids, series no. 96 (Arlington, Va.: the association, 1974); "Trends for the Handicapped," *Trends*, Park Practice Programs, 3rd qtr. (Arlington, Va.: National Recreation and Park Association, 1974); "Leisure and Handicapped People," *Parks and Recreation* 12, no. 11 (1977); and Gerald S. Fain and Gerald L. Hitzhusen, eds., *Therapeutic Recreation—A State of the Art* (Arlington, Va.: National Recreation and Park Association, 1977).

34. John E. Davis, *Clinical Applications of Recreational Therapy* (Springfield, Ill.: Charles C Thomas, Publisher, 1952).

35. Valerie V. Hunt, *Recreation for the Handicapped* (Englewood Cliffs, N.J.: Prentice-Hall, 1955); Josephine L. Rathbone and Carol Lucas, *Recreation in Total Rehabilitation* (Springfield, Ill.: Charles C Thomas, Publishers, 1959); Janet Pomeroy, *Recreation for the Physically Handicapped* (New York: Macmillan, 1964); Virginia Frye and Martha Peters, *Therapeutic Recreation: Its Theory, Philosophy and Practice* (Harrisburg, Pa.: Stackpole Co., 1972); Richard Kraus, *Therapeutic Recreation Service: Principles and Practices* (Philadelphia: W. B. Saunders Co., 1973); Thomas A. Stein and H. Douglas Sessoms, eds., *Recreation and Special Populations* (Boston: Holbrook Press, 1973); Elliott M. Avedon, *Therapeutic Recreation Service: An Applied Behavioral Science Approach* (Englewood Cliffs, N.J.: Prentice-Hall, 1974); Jay S. Shivers and Hollis F. Fait, *Therapeutic and Adapted Recreational Services* (Philadelphia: Lea and Febiger, 1975); Gerald S. O'Morrow, *Therapeutic Recreation: A Helping Profession* (Reston, Va.: Reston Publishing Co., 1976); Scout Lee Gunn and Carol Peterson, *Therapeutic Recreation Program Design: Principles and Procedures* (Englewood Cliffs, N.J.: Prentice-Hall, 1978); David Austin, *Therapeutic Recreation: Processes and Techniques* (New York: John Wiley & Sons, 1982); Ronald P. Reynolds and Gerald S. O'Morrow, *Problems, Issues and Concepts in Therapeutic Recreation* (Englewood Cliffs, N.J.: Prentice-Hall, 1985); Carter, Van

Andel, and Robb, *Therapeutic Recreation*; Kennedy, Austin, and Smith, *Special Recreation*; Michael E. Crawford and Ron Mendell, *Therapeutic Recreation and Adapted Physical Activities for Mentally Retarded Individuals* (Englewood Cliffs, N.J.: Prentice-Hall, 1987); and Howe-Murphy and Charboneau, *Therapeutic Recreation.*

36. American Recreation Society, *The Hospital Recreation Section: Its History, 1948-1964* (Washington, D.C.: the society, 1965), p. 3.

37. Kraus, *Therapeutic Recreation Service*, 2nd ed. (1978), p. 75.

38. Thomas A. Stein, "Therapeutic Recreation Education: 1969 Survey," *Therapeutic Recreation Journal* 4, no. 2 (1971), 4–7, 25.

39. Richard Gitelson, "The 1984 SPRE Survey: Park and Recreation Enrollment Stabilizes," *Parks and Recreation* 20, no. 4 (1985), 65.

40. Stephen C. Anderson and Morris W. Stewart, "Therapeutic Recreation Education: 1979 Survey," *Therapeutic Recreation Journal* 14, no. 3 (1980), 4–10.

41. Kraus, *Therapeutic Recreation Service*, 2nd ed. (1978), 65–69.

42. Comeback, *Therapeutic Recreation Curriculum Development Conference* (New York: Comeback, Feb. 1961).

43. Donald Hinkel, personal communication, November 4, 1987.

44. U.S. Department of Health, Education and Welfare, *Health Resource Statistics 1976-1977*, DHEW publication no. (PHS) 79-1509 (Washington, D.C.: U.S. Government Printing Office, 1977), pp. 6–7.

45. Glen E. Van Andel, "Professional Standards: Improving the Quality of Services," *Therapeutic Recreation Journal* 15, no. 2 (1981), 25–30.

46. Jacquelyn Vaughan and Robert Winshow, eds. *Guidelines for Community-Based Recreation Programs for Special Populations* (Alexandria, Va.: National Recreation and Park Association, 1979).

47. *Standards of Practice for Therapeutic Recreation* (Alexandria, Va.: National Recreation and Park Association, 1980); and National Therapeutic Recreation Society Standards Committee, *Guidelines for Administration of Therapeutic Recreation in Clinical and Residential Facilities* (Alexandria, Va.: National Recreation and Park Association, 1982).

48. B. E. Phillips, "Recreation Therapy," *Journal of Health, Physical Education and Recreation* 26, no. 2 (1955), 52.

49. David M. Compton, "Research Priorities in Recreation for Special Populations," *Therapeutic Recreation Journal* 18, no. 1 (1984), 9–17.

50. Charles C. Bullock, Frances M. McGuire, and Elizabeth M. Barch, "Perceived Research Needs of Therapeutic Recreators," *Therapeutic Recreation Journal* 18, no. 3 (1984), 17–24.

51. Bertha Schlotter and Margaret Svendsen, *An Experience in Recreation with the Mentally Retarded*, rev. ed. (New York: National Mental Health, 1951).

52. Hospital Recreation Society, *Basic Concepts.*

53. Edmund Pellegrino, "Ethical Implications in Changing Practice," *American Journal of Nursing* 64, no. 9 (1964), 110–11.

54. "Suggested Principles of the Code of Ethics of the Recreation and Park Profession," (Arlington, Va.: National Recreation and Park Association, 1977).

55. "Code of Ethics—National Therapeutic Recreation Society," *Therapeutic Recreation Journal* 18, no. 1 (1984), 62–63.

SUGGESTED READINGS

"A Report on the NTRS President's Commission for the Assessment of Critical Issues." *Therapeutic Recreation Journal* 12, no. 2 (1978), 38–41.

AUSTIN, DAVID, and BENJAMIN K. HUNNICUTT. "National Therapeutic Recreation Society: The First Twelve Years." *Therapeutic Recreation Journal* 12, no. 3 (1978), 4–14.

BULLOCK, CHARLES C., FRANCIS M. MCGUIRE, and ELIZABETH M. BARCH. "Perceived Research Needs of Therapeutic Recreators." *Therapeutic Recreation Journal* 18, no. 3 (1984), 17–24.

CARTER, MARCIA J. "Registration of Therapeutic Recreators: Standards from 1956 to Present." *Therapeutic Recreation Journal* 15, no. 2 (1981), 17–22.

COMPTON, DAVID M. "Research Priorities in Recreation for Special Populations." *Therapeutic Recreation Journal* 18, no. 1 (1984), 9–17.

GOODE, WILLIAM J. "Community within a Community: The Professions." *American Sociological Review* 22, no. 7 (1957), 194–200.

HALBERG, KATHLEEN J., and ROXANNE HOWE-MURPHY. "The Dilemma of an Unresolved Philosophy in Therapeutic Recreation." *Therapeutic Recreation Journal* 19, no. 3 (1985), 7–16.

HOSPITAL RECREATION SOCIETY. *Basic Concepts of Hospital Recreation.* Washington, D.C.: American Recreation Society, 1953.

HUGHES, EVERETT C. "Profession." In *The Professions in America*, ed. Kenneth S. Lynn. Boston: Houghton Mifflin Co., 1965.

HUNNICUTT, BENJAMIN K. "A Rejoinder to the Twelve-Year History of the National Therapeutic Recreation Society." *Therapeutic Recreation Journal* 13, no. 3 (1978), 15–19.

MEYER, LEE E. *Philosophical Alternatives and the Professionalization of Therapeutic Recreation.* Arlington, Va.: National Recreation and Park Association, 1980.

MOBILY, KENNETH E. "A Philosophical Analysis of Therapeutic Recreation: What Does It Mean to Say 'We Can Be Therapeutic'?" Part I. *Therapeutic Recreation Journal* 19, no. 1 (1985), 14–26.

———. "Quality Analysis in Therapeutic Recreation Curricula." *Therapeutic Recreation Journal* 17, no. 1 (1983), 18–25.

MOORE, WILBERT E. *The Professions: Roles and Rules.* New York: Russell Sage Foundation, 1970.

NATIONAL THERAPEUTIC RECREATION SOCIETY. *Alternative Positions and Their Implications to Professionalization.* Alexandria, Va.: National Recreation and Park Association, 1981.

NATIONAL THERAPEUTIC RECREATION SOCIETY. "Philosophical Position Statement of the National Therapeutic Recreation Society," May 1982.

O'MORROW, GERALD S. "Therapeutic Recreation Accreditation: Its Problems and Future." *Therapeutic Recreation Journal* 15, no. 2 (1981), 31–38.

PETERSON, CAROL ANN. "A Matter of Priorities and Loyalties." *Therapeutic Recreation Journal* 18, no. 3 (1984), 11–16.

———. "Pride and Progress in Professionalism." In *Expanding Horizons in Therapeutic Recreation,* ed. Gerald Hitzhusen, pp. 1–9. Columbia, Mo.: Department of Recreation and Park Administration, University of Missouri, 1981.

SHAPIRO, IRA G. "The Path to Accreditation." *Parks and Recreation* 12, no. 1 (1977), 29–31, 68.

SYLVESTER, CHARLES D. "Freedom, Leisure and Therapeutic Recreation." *Therapeutic Recreation Journal* 19, no. 1 (1985), 6–13.

SYLVESTER, CHARLES, ET AL. *Philosophy of Therapeutic Recreation: Ideas and Issues.* Arlington, Va.: National Recreation and Park Association, 1987.

VAN ANDEL, GLEN E. "Professional Standards: Improving the Quality of Service." *Therapeutic Recreation Journal* 15, no. 2 (1981), 25–30.

6

Therapeutic Recreation:
Process and Models

The previous chapters have discussed therapeutic recreation as an area of service by describing our clientele, the settings in which we practice, and the historical and professional development of the field. This chapter describes the *process* of therapeutic recreation and briefly discusses its application in the medical-clinical, custodial, therapeutic milieu, education and training, and community models of human service.

PROCESS

The term *therapeutic recreation process* will be used herein to describe the series of steps the therapeutic recreation specialist takes to meet the needs and problems of special population members through recreative experiences. This view implies that the therapeutic recreation process is concerned with moving members from a particular point in the environment, where they are involved in activity as a result of unconscious needs or interests or are unable to participate because of a variety of circumstances, to a point where they are able to fulfill their responsibility for meeting their own recreation needs and interests at a conscious level—or short of this, participating in recreative experiences to the extent possible within the limitations imposed by the circumstances. The latter, in most instances, refers to those members who are impaired severely by developmental deficits, physical injury or illness, or psychological and social disabilities.

PROCESS MODELS

Since the late 1960s several authors have expressed thoughts similar to the above, and it is appropriate that we briefly review some of them. Of particular interest are those process or continuum models suggested by Berryman, Ball, Frye and Peters, and Gunn and Peterson.

Berryman contributes a model wherein recreational activities become "experiential bonds," joining the member with the environment.[1] Initially, the specialist presents activities that are expected to have a positive effect on the special population member, thereby establishing the first bond between the member and the environment. As new recreative experiences are introduced by the specialist, new bonds are created. Eventually, members no longer need the assistance of the specialist and pursue recreative experiences on their own, establishing new bonds between themselves and the environment. Moreover, according to Berryman:

> The self-actualization process continues ad infinitum with recreative experiences creating ever new bonds between the self and his environment and Self and Environment continue to establish new relationships and additional expansions.[2]

Ball, in her continuum model, outlines a series of four progressive stages that a member may move through to reach a "true recreative experience" (Table 6.1).[3]

Ball assumes that the member may also function simultaneously in all four stages:

> An individual might have a work experience (typing copy for the newspaper), a recreation education experience (learning the skills and knowledge about volley ball, and developing attitudes towards participating), a therapeutic recreation experience (participating in a party) and a recreation experience (listening to music). No one of these experiences negates the other and in fact, they probably complement each other and help the individual to gain or regain a balance in living.[4]

A clinical model that appeared in Frye and Peters' *Therapeutic Recreation* has also precipitated thought and discussion among therapeutic recreation specialists. This model identified five stages:

1. Recreator administers highly structured program under medical orders.
2. Recreator "sells" program to patient, motivates patient to participate.
3. Recreator and patient construct program together.
4. Recreator advises patient and community.
5. Patient is free to participate in any activity available to him.[5]

The model proposed by Gunn and Peterson is not that much different from what has been discussed by the previous writers and the authors. Generally speaking, it promotes independent leisure functioning in special population members through the use of various activities, facilitation techniques, and programs in various settings. Their approach, however, is a systems approach. It incorporates determining purposes, goals, and objectives; designing a program based on purposes; determining a delivery system; implementing the program; monitoring, evaluating, and revising the program, if needed, with appropriate feedback at each step in the sequence. They further suggest that the systems approach not only has value in individual and group program planning but can be used to develop a total therapeutic recreation service within a specific setting.[6]

TABLE 6.1. Recreative Progression

	EXPERIENCE	TYPE OF TIME	MAJOR MOTIVATION
1	Activity for sake of activity	Obligated time	Drive is outer directed.
2	Recreation education	Obligated time	Drive is outer directed.
3	Therapeutic recreation	Unobligated time	Motivation is inner directed but choice of experiences is limited.
4	Recreation	Unobligated time	Motivation is inner directed.

SOURCE: Edith L. Ball, "The Meaning of Therapeutic Recreation," *Therapeutic Recreation Journal* 4, no. 1 (1970), 18.

In developing a personal concept of the therapeutic recreation process, you must be aware of your own personal philosophy and views of human values, ethics, and beliefs. The authors propose the following thoughts concerning the nature of the therapeutic recreation process, based on their own philosophical views.

Therapeutic recreation can be considered a process wherein recreative experiences are used to bring about a change in the behavior of individuals with special needs. There is no stereotyped, only one way to proceed through the phases of the therapeutic recreation process, nor is there a definite pattern to follow in moving back and forth among the different phases. These are factors that are determined according to the needs of the patient in each situation and the abilities of the individual therapeutic recreation specialist. Some situations deal with several facets of patient care and treatment; others deal with a limited number of problem areas. The focus of the process is on the use of recreative experiences to (1) enhance growth and development of the individual, and (2) enable the individual to meet the responsibility of fulfilling his or her own leisure needs.[7]

PROCESS RATIONALE

Before we proceed with a discussion of the therapeutic recreation process, it is well for us to consider briefly the rationale for such a process. In the past, therapeutic (hospital) recreators often provided recreation service without determining how these services would affect the behavior of special population members. Activities, the primary source of service, were designed to appeal to large groups of individuals. Enjoyment was a major concern. Recreators were referred to by terms that did not have a professional connotation. Although their activities were generally accepted, the acceptance was because patients were kept busy, not because activities made a major contribution to treatment or a particular goal. In recent years our approach to programming has become more sophisticated, and our image as recreators has become more therapeutic, more professional. Today we are considered a professional discipline with professional procedures and services. However, if we are to continue to develop as a professional discipline and be accepted by other professionals, especially in health settings, and make contributions in a professional manner, we must continue to improve our procedures in offering recreation services. Other professional disciplines utilize a standardized procedure in providing their services; we cannot do otherwise.

Two factors have had a profound effect upon the development of a standardized procedure in the delivery of recreation services to special population members in health settings. One is the right-to-treatment litigation; the other is the economic recession that occurred during the mid-1970s and led eventually to the concept of accountability.

The right-to-treatment litigation relates to civil commitment procedures and is associated with the mentally ill, the mentally retarded, the aged, and a variety of other individuals who have been committed to hospitals/institutions. Although there were some early precedents in right-to-treatment decisions, the breakthrough came in *Wyatt v. Stickney* (December 1971), in which the U.S. Supreme Court held that involuntarily committed patients "unquestionably have a constitutional right to receive such individual treatment as will give each of them a realistic opportunity to be cured or to improve his or her mental condition." (3345. SUPP, p. 341) The court found that the defendant's treatment program was deficient because it failed to provide a human psychological and physical environment and a qualified staff in sufficient number to administer adequate treatment and individualized treatment plans. The court proposed detailed standards, which it defined as "medical and constitutional minimums."[8]

As a result of this litigation, various state

courts and legislative bodies established standards mandating changes in staffing, physical resources, and treatment process. (Various accrediting bodies also tightened up their standards.) Moreover, these standards affected both voluntarily and involuntarily committed patients. Guidelines were included relative to procedures for planning, implementing, and evaluating the program. Although the standards or guidelines that have been developed tend to reinforce a medical model of treatment (which has used a systematic standardized procedure approach for many years), they have promoted a more effective delivery of recreation services.

The concept of accountability as it relates to recreation services is of more recent origin. Beginning with our growth following World War II and until the economic recession that began about 1974, programs were justified on a philosophy of the importance of recreation. The programs in those days were operational through dollar appropriations. Today conditions have changed.

It is a conservative estimate that more than $100 billion are spent annually on health care. Costs have skyrocketed. Today's emphasis is on cost containment; a cost-benefit evaluation is being placed on all health-care services. Therapeutic recreation service will continue to receive direct appropriations (and probably always will to some degree, particularly in governmental agencies), but more and more funds will be coming from *third-party carriers*—commercial insurance companies and federal programs such as Medicare, Medicaid, and the like. It is anticipated that these programs will not only increase dramatically in the future but will dominate the entire health industry. However, third-party insurance does not help a person forever. Independence must be achieved in some way by most people because premiums or appropriations must at least match the outlay. Therefore, a host of controls are being placed on all health-care services.

One of the controls is that every patient must have an *individual treatment plan* (ITP), and this plan must be written into the medical record of the patient. In the medical record will be a statement of the problem, followed by a treatment plan that includes who provides the services to meet the plan and how long will it take to bring about a change in the behavior of the patient, including projected discharge or release. Generally speaking, the therapeutic recreator will be involved in all aspects of developing and implementing this plan, to the extent deemed necessary by the specific agency.[9]

Another control is that all treatment plans will be monitored. A peer committee verifies that the treatment provided is consistent with the state of the art or with established successful procedures. For years physicians reviewed procedures used by other physicians. Accrediting bodies (JCAH) have used a monitoring procedure for some years to determine whether a hospital or institution should be accredited. Recreation services may eventually be required to establish peer review committees. The federal government has already initiated committees that regularly monitor services provided through Medicare, and Medicare is found in nearly all types of health settings. In short, our profession, like other professions, is now expected to document its plans, procedures, goals, and objectives. Those who are knowledgeable and skillful in working in this type of atmosphere will thrive and the profession will prosper. Those who cannot will experience great difficulties.

As a result of PL 94-142, therapeutic recreators who provide recreation services in special education to special population children in local education agencies are expected to participate in the *individualized education plan* (IEP) for each child. This will occur whether the specialist is employed directly by the educational agency or is a staff member of the local municipal park and recreation department which has been contracted to provide recreation services. The IEP is similar in nature to the ITP; a study is made of leisure needs, a plan is developed, evaluation occurs, and each step is recorded. In addition, therapeutic recreators working in public and voluntary recreation agencies that provide recreation service to special population members are expected to establish programs based on sound principles of program development and use adequate and proper evaluation tools. Such procedures are recorded so as to provide for better accountability.

PROCESS GOALS

From the various models presented, it would appear that there are several steps through which the specialist proceeds to effect change in the special population member. However, all have one aspect in common—helping the special population member respond in a more rewarding manner. It is a form of assistance to bring more happiness to individuals, to permit members to function better, and, in general, to give them a more satisfactory way of life.

Webster's Third International Dictionary defines *process* as an action of moving forward, progressing from one point to another on the way to a goal, or to completion; it is the continuous movement through a succession of developmental stages; it is the method by which something is produced, something is accomplished, or a specific result is attained.[10]

To perceive a process as an action suggests a power behind the action or a mover of the action, hence control and/or systematic movement. Conscious and deliberate effort must be exerted to arrive at a desired goal.

The therapeutic recreation process is oriented toward the future. Both specialist and special population member have come together to help the member function more effectively in the future. The specialist, however, must focus on the past, present, and future. The primary goal of the specialist is to assist the member to achieve those goals that lead to more rewarding behavior. However, in order to attain this long-range goal, it may be necessary to first attain certain more immediate goals. This requires a systematic and complex planning process. Adequate planning involves not only a knowledge of human beings, of their specific problems, and of their adaptive behavior, but also a means of applying that knowledge to the promotion and maintenance of the special population members as they respond in a holistic manner to their environment. Thus, the essential characteristics of the therapeutic recreation process are that it is planned, it is person centered, and it is goal directed.

COMPONENTS OF THE THERAPEUTIC RECREATION PROCESS

Dividing the process into phases is an artificial separation of actions that cannot be separated in actual practice since the basic concept of the process suggests it is a unified whole. The whole process is dynamic since data from one phase can alter or support the other phases. However, to ensure a deliberateness and thoughtfulness in proceeding through the process and to facilitate discussion, the therapeutic recreation process is divided into the following phases or steps:

1. *Assessment* of the special population members' therapeutic recreation needs (including the collection of information about the members)

2. *Development (planning)* of goals for therapeutic recreation action

3. *Implementation* of therapeutic recreation action to meet goals

4. *Evaluation* of the effectiveness of therapeutic recreation action

The therapeutic recreation specialist and the special population member are viewed as partners in the therapeutic recreation process. It is this "complex interaction," according to Collingwood, that provides "the sources of gain for clients."[11] Each member is also viewed as a unique individual in the units of a social system. The specialist draws heavily on perception, communication, and decision making as well as knowledge of activities in the use of the process. The member also utilizes these skills by participating in assessing, planning, implementing, and evaluating. Thus, there is a cyclical nature to the therapeutic recreation process, and the movement is constant among the components (Figure 6.1).

The skills the specialist must have are intellectual, interpersonal, and technical. Intellectual skills entail solving problems, thinking critically, making judgments, and analyzing activities. Interpersonal skills relate to the abilities to communicate; listen; convey interest, knowledge, and information; establish rapport; and obtain needed data in a manner that enhances the individuality of the special population member as a person. These skills foster relationships with members, the family, coworkers, colleagues, and the community in general.

Interpersonal skills cannot be overemphasized regardless of the problem or setting. In dealing with members having physical problems, interpersonal skills are extremely important in supplementing technical knowledge in the treatment of a member as an individual. When dealing with members having emotional problems they become preponderantly so. In fact, it has been suggested by some psychiatrists that a proper relationship may be of greater importance than the activity itself. This concept is offered because some therapeutic recreation specialists are so action oriented that they develop feelings of guilt if they are not providing direct leadership to special population members all the time.

Technical skills relate to methods, procedures, and the ability to direct and conduct activities to bring about the desired results or behavioral responses of the member. However, students are cautioned that lead-

FIGURE 6.1. Cyclic Nature of the Therapeutic Recreation Process

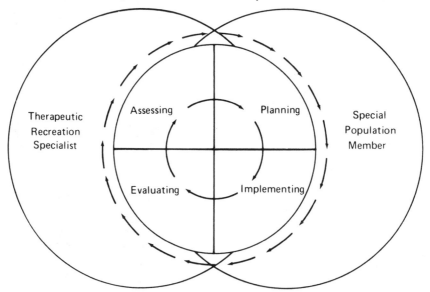

ership behavior changes from setting to setting. These skills are always necessary, but the emphasis may vary with the special population member and the agency involved.

For the therapeutic recreation specialist to engage successfully in the process, it is important to recognize the following premises about the special population member:

1. A special population member is a human being endowed with worth and dignity.

2. An individual has basic human needs.

3. Problems result when needs are only partially met or are unmet.

4. Inability of individuals to fulfill their basic needs may entail the intervention of someone else who can help them meet their needs or fill the needs directly until such time as the members can resume that responsibility for themselves.

5. The therapeutic recreation specialist is interested in rendering high-quality service to special population members, no matter what their problem or disability, lifestyle, economic status, culture, or beliefs might be.

6. To utilize the therapeutic recreation process and to develop goal-directed recreative experiences, the specialist must have knowledge of theories from the biological, emotional, and social and behavioral sciences and must have knowledge of the concepts of therapeutic recreation and recreative activities as well.

7. The heart of the specialist-member interaction is the development of a helping relationship in which the specialist fosters the member's personal growth and development. Thus, the leader is in reality a therapeutic agent.

8. The practice of therapeutic recreation involves the ability to focus on a person's needs and requires the full attention and energy of the specialist when engaged in the practice of therapeutic recreation. Bridges tells us that "we must approach patients as human beings, use our awareness and our perceptiveness; but most important, we must approach patients with an aliveness, with feeling, and with the urge to communicate our whole selves. Only in this manner can we genuinely confront the patients' false solutions constructively and transmit a vision of what life could be."[12]

9. Specialists strive to meet their own self-development through the practice of therapeutic recreation.

10. Every member has the right to enjoy quality leisure and park and recreation programming and to participate in such.

11. Therapeutic recreation specialists need to focus on preventing illness, maintaining wellness, and rendering services to those who have physical, emotional, social, and intellectual problems through leisure and recreative experiences.

ASSESSMENT

Assessment is the first phase in the therapeutic recreation process. It is the act of reviewing a situation for the purpose of determining the member's problem. It consists of identifying and obtaining data about the member from many sources; these data are then classified, analyzed, and summarized to determine problems or needs.

Data Collection

Data collection is time consuming but is an absolutely essential part of problem identification. Data can be collected from many sources. The member's past history, health and social history, and past and present leisure and recreative experiences are all areas that contribute to the assessment.

Past and present practices in play and recreation cannot be considered apart from other influences experienced by the individual. Thus, to understand the influence that play and recreation exert upon the individual, there is a need for some knowledge of the setting within which these influences were experienced. Home influences, parental relationships, presence or absence of brothers and sisters, emotional or physical maladjustments or deficiencies, social problems, housing conditions, opportunity to use varied and extensive play materials, presence or absence of adult leadership, and extent and quality of neighborhood and school resources favorable to the development of recreation habits all have a telling effect upon the character of recreation needs and interests. Environment, whether urban or rural, also contributes to recreation needs and interests. Data collection involves astute observation, purposeful listening, a broad knowledge of human behavior, and an understanding of what needs to be known and where to obtain that information.

Verbal Communication

Communication is an act by means of which one human being conveys (usually verbally) to another his or her ideas, thoughts, needs or feelings. It is not only an activity of daily living like mobility or self-care, but it is also a necessary tool to effect changes in behavior. As Austin comments " . . . the ability to maintain effective interpersonal communication is important and is a basic competency needed by the therapeutic recreation specialist in order to perform as a viable helping professional. If the therapeutic recreation specialist cannot communicate with his or her clients, the therapeutic recreation process is almost certainly doomed to failure."[13]

If a formal interview is used to collect data, the format will vary according to the setting, the services rendered, and the role of the specialist. Although core data about the member will always be needed, specific areas of information will differ if the member, for example, is being admitted into a mental health center or is being interviewed or observed in a long-term health-care facility or correctional institution.

Personal interviews must be carefully used lest they become too formalized. Thus, group interviews are often more successful as the initial application of the interview method. A subsequent interview with the individual appears to be a more logical outcome. Regardless, the well-structured interview can serve to achieve the following purposes, according to Ferguson (who also provides a good overview of interview techniques and questioning strategies in the same article):

Assess client readiness for treatment, both physically and emotionally.

Assess client rationality and appropriateness for specific activity participation.

Identify the client's leisure behavior patterns.

Provide increased insight into the personal leisure values of the client.

Determine the strength of relationships between the client and family.

Note personal strengths and assets of the client.

Determine what lifestyle adjustments may be needed for healthy leisure function.

Assess available leisure support systems or resources in the community.

Examine economic factors influencing the client's leisure.[14]

Special population members should feel that the specialist is interested in them. Specialists must communicate—both verbally and nonverbally—that they view members with respect and dignity. The fact that the specialist calls the member by name, listens with full attention, anticipates questions, and speaks *with* the member rather than *to* the member, conveys respect. The specialist should refrain from using language unfamiliar to the member and guard against responding to questions in a condescending manner. Finally, the specialist should tell the member how the information being requested will be used as well as the plan for continuing the interaction into the planning, implementing, and evaluating phase. Ideally, such an interview begins a relationship based on trust, respect, concern, and interest.

In some instances checklists and questionnaires are used. The specialist, however, will often seek additional information that has not been addressed by these tools. At times it may be appropriate for the member to fill out recreative information sheets. This, of course, is only appropriate if the member can read and write, is oriented and aware, and has the strength to do so. In any case, personal verification should follow.

Frequently the former recreational interests of the individual will give valuable clues as to the therapeutic activities to be utilized; frequently the type of activity chosen may lay a foundation for the development of a future leisure pursuit for the individual.

Observation

Up to this point verbal interaction between specialist and member has been emphasized. Intelligent observation is important to sound therapeutic recreation practice; it should be both systematic and scientific. It is just as important as the interview to the identification of the problem and the subsequent planning and evaluating of therapeutic recreation service. In interacting with some special population members, observation is the only technique available. With other members verbalization may be at such a low level that observation is the only method that will provide cues for behavior change. The specialist's skillful observation also aids other members of the treatment team in determining a total approach to the problem.

Observation is a descriptive, not an interpretive or evaluative, act. It is made by the five senses. Observation is influenced by the specialist's past experience and ability to be thorough, by the ability of the specialist to pick up subtle clues, and the ability of the observer to remain objective.

The specialist can consciously develop skills in observing. It is not possible to note everything that comes within our range of vision; therefore, specialists must learn to be selective in their observations. This entails learning what to look for, and becoming trained to observe significant factors in the member's appearance and behavior. Observations should be as objective as possible and described in terms of a factual record.

Although the specialist's observations may intentionally be made to appear casual in order not to arouse anxiety in the member, in actual fact such observations are always systematic; the specialist is aware of what to look for and differentiates the normal from the abnormal. It is only through a knowledge of normal behavior that digressions from the normal are recognized. The specialist's observations are scientific in that they are objective and are based on knowledge of the sciences.

In general, the personal approach to observation of special population members includes:

1. *General appearance.* The general appearance of members can provide clues to physical and emotional health. The depressed member, for example, may stand with a stooped, defeated posture.

2. *Interpersonal interaction.* Observing the members' interpersonal behavior tells the specialist about their patterns of socialization, anxiety level, acceptance or rejection of the problem, and ability to cope with the present situation.

3. *Motor activity.* Members' agility, range of motion, and ability to manage themselves are all indications of their place on the dependence-independence continuum.

4. *Body language.* By general definition, body language means the behavioral patterns that individuals use to communicate nonverbal messages. According to Tubbs and Moss, nonverbal behaviors can be classified into three categories: visual cues (facial expression, eye contact, body movement, hand gestures, and physical appearance and the use of objects); vocal cues (volume, rate and fluency, pitch, and quality); and spatial and temporal cues (time and space-physical position in relation to others).[15] Stance, distance relationship, facial expression, and posture tell much about how members think and feel. Body language is particularly significant when the member is or becomes mute; even though the member does not communicate verbally, he or she does not stop communicating altogether. The real value of body language, however, remains in its blending with the spoken word to convey thoughts, ideas, and feelings.

Techniques

It is impossible here to discuss in any detail the personal approach and observation techniques to use with special population individuals having specific problems. However, it does seem important that we consider a few in a general way.

Most persons with physical injuries suffer from fears. The most common fear is that of pain and disfigurement. However, the focus of the person's attention on pain changes when he or she becomes absorbed in an activity. The fear of disfigurement is frequent, and many persons are embarrassed because of a disabled part and may try to hide it. Until the individual realizes that this reaction tends to draw more attention to the condition, it is often difficult to gain full cooperation. Fear of permanent disability is also a problem in the satisfactory recovery of an individual. When a condition is permanent, the patient must adjust to it and learn to live with it.

The potential specialist with an active, open mind and a will to learn will be rewarded by acquisition of the ability to adjust and to work effectively with emotionally ill patients. The attitude toward mental illness and the approach to the patient determine to a great extent the quality of the care and treatment that is provided. Persons suffer from emotional problems that are the result of an accumulation of unsuccessful efforts on the part of the individual to adjust to the environment, as we have noted earlier. Whether mental problems are organic, functional, or toxic in origin, individuals are hospitalized because they have been unable to cope with the larger society.

A tactful approach is of importance in working with emotionally disturbed persons. As a result of emotional difficulties, a patient's standard of values may be momentarily submerged beneath the drive of more powerful instinctive tendencies, rendering him or her incapable of temper control. The ability to empathize with the member is important, but at the same time an objective attitude must be maintained. The value of active listening cannot be overemphasized. However, suspicion should not be aroused in individuals that their personal affairs have been discussed. Frequently individuals regard the specialist as they would a member of their family. The importance of keeping this relationship within normal limits cannot be overstressed.

In approaching newly blinded persons, tact and resourcefulness are essential, and there must be knowledge of the special techniques used. It is important to help them to think of themselves as individuals. Being treated differently causes many blind people to feel they are different. The effort must be made to help the blind realize that in spite of the disability, their individuality is not lost and that if they are otherwise physically and mentally capable, they are able to lead normal, active lives. It must be recognized that although the shock of blindness has its emotional effect on the individual, the reaction is not the same in all persons, and the needs of the individual must always be foremost in planning the approach. To most blinded persons, the loss of sight is not so disturbing as the loss of freedom of motion and the resulting dependence upon others.

The first contact with a geriatric resident in a nursing home should be made in the individual's room, if possible, since it is the resident's homeground, and the first step is to gain his or her confidence. Old age may deprive people of confidence; they feel helpless, useless, and unwanted. Other attributes of old age must also be taken into consideration: reduced physical mobility, poor eyesight, diminished hearing, cosmetic changes, lessened ability to concentrate for long periods of time, and lack of finer movements, to name a few. In addition, practitioners have pointed out that unfortunately many recreational programs are designed for the ambulatory resident.

The specialist must recognize that it is difficult to motivate some geriatric residents to participate because of fear of ridicule and failure and lack of confidence.[16] However, once they are involved, their energy and enthusiasm become remarkable. Also, it is extremely important for residents to become involved in activities as soon after entering the nursing home as their medical condition permits. One of the most important aspects of geriatric therapeutic recreation is its potential for prevention. Many of the effects of long-term degenerative diseases of the aged, both physical and mental, can be reduced if the individual remains active.

Instruments

Assessment of an individual is both subjective and objective. It is not uncommon for the specialist to be unable at times to determine the functioning level of a special population member even after observation in an activity. The specialist, therefore, may want to use an instrument to obtain more meaningful data on the functioning of the member. Assessment instruments are frequently used to determine the performance level of the member while eliminating any biases the specialist might have in gathering information. Using such instruments is comparable to the physician's scheduling laboratory tests to obtain additional information prior to the diagnosis or the psychiatrist's ordering a series of psychological tests to better determine the individual's capacity to interact intellectually and emotionally with his environment. Naturally, the usefulness of any test depends to a great extent on the ability of the specialist to administer the test and interpret the results. Some tests are extremely simple to administer and interpret while others are more complex and involved.

Assessment instruments cover a broad range of factors including cognitive, affective, and psychomotor skills; self-help and everyday community-living skills; and leisure or recreational skill preference. Assessing favorite leisure activities of a special population member is an important step in the initial stages of leisure counseling. Identifying fine motor or gross motor ability with the developmentally disabled is another example of the use of an assessment instrument. Assessment instruments are also valuable tools in determining goals and objectives in planning and for evaluative purposes.[17]

A word of caution, however, is needed about the use of assessment and evaluation instruments. No matter how carefully obtained, the results may not do justice to the breadth of a member's behavior. No one person is exactly the same as any other person. Test results are at best a limited description of capabilities and should be used in conjunction with other data available.

While there is a continued need for further development and research of assessment and evaluation instruments, several commonly used instruments presently being employed include, but are not limited to, Leisure Activities Blank (LAB), Self Leisure Interest Profile (SLIP), Mirendia Leisure Finder, Leisure Satisfaction Scale, Mundy

Recreation Inventory, Comprehensive Evaluation in Recreation Therapy Scale (CERT), Goal Attainment Scale (GAS), Linear Model for Individual Treatment (LMIT), Joswiak's Leisure Counseling Assessment and Recreation Therapy Assessment, and the Leisure Skills Curriculum Assessment Inventory. An entire issue of the *Therapeutic Recreation Journal* was devoted to a variety of assessment factors, including assessment instruments and techniques with various disabilities and in various settings.[18]

Problem Identification

For a number of years *diagnosis* was a forbidden word in therapeutic recreation. A literal definition of the word, with no qualifier preceeding it, suggests it is a good term to use when conveying the idea that we are seeking knowledge or information about what needs to be improved, what is causing the difficulty, or what is interfering with normal functioning. With this in mind, therapeutic recreators can use the word *diagnosis* as effectively as the physician can or any person who is trying to discover where efforts must be applied to perform service for the benefit of the member.

After the data are collected and sorted, it is possible to identify the member's problem. Problem identification begins with an identification of the member's needs. The word *need* is used in many ways, sometimes as a noun and sometimes as a verb. It is used to denote a lack of something or to mean a requisite for bodily, psychic, or social functioning. It is used frequently in everyday conversation. A need is not necessarily a problem, but a special population member can develop a problem when a basic human need is not filled or is filled only partially.

By definition, a problem is an interruption in the member's ability to meet a need. According to some investigators, problems exist when there is no straight-line action possible.[19] This means a progression of events toward need gratification has been interrupted, altered, or disturbed; in some way, need gratification is not clearly or discernibly evident.

The therapeutic recreation specialist's function is to assess the problem and the extent of the problem. In contrast to goals of some professions, specialists do involve themselves with basic human needs that affect the total person rather than just one aspect. To focus on one aspect, such as a physical problem, to the exclusion of other areas is to assess the member's problem in a limited manner. This limited perspective could create rather than solve problems for the member.

Other members of the treatment team contribute to the specialist's understanding of the member and his or her problems. Observation and interpretation may be communicated by the physician, social worker, nurse, security officer, and vocational therapist, to name only a few, through written notes on the member's record and through consultation with other specialists.

Specialists will try to satisfy the needs of each member. Their effectiveness in assessing these needs depends upon knowledge of basic needs relative to age and sex—roles, expectations, and behaviors relating to infancy, childhood, adolescence, and adulthood. The specialist may use a variety of models to designate basic human needs. Reference has been made to Maslow's Hierarchy of Needs.[20] Two more such models are Erikson's Eight Ages of Man[21] and Duvall's Family Development.[22] All are popular and useful models in determining basic human needs.

When assessing needs of special population members from different racial groups, the specialist needs to know their customs, rites, rituals, roles, traditions, expectations, and views. Likewise, religion, formal or informal education, and socioeconomic status affect each member's needs. It is also important to assess the member's perception of his or her status.

To assess biological, physical, emotional, and social status, the specialist needs a model of wellness to serve as a base. The model must incorporate such factors as age, sex, socioeconomic status, and culture. Knowing what is expected or normal for bodily and psychosocial functions provides the framework within which the status of each can be assessed for a special population member.

The specialist must have a knowledge of pathological and psychopathological problems important to the member at various age levels, for each sex, for the major racial and cultural groups, and for specific geographic areas of certain environments. The specialist who works with the social offender likewise must have a knowledge of the social problems that result in incarceration.

With a knowledge of normal human function and a working knowledge of major pathophysiological, psychopathological, and sociological problems, the specialist is prepared to begin the assessment phase of the therapeutic recreation process.

Assessment takes place through either verbal communication or observation or both. There is no specific personal approach that can be used with all individuals. Each participant is a unique individual with his or her own needs and interests. The individual must be considered as a human being with a problem, not as a number, a case. As Frye and Peters so well state:

> Human characteristics are so complex that no two individuals are alike. Those qualities of behavior, emotional tendencies, habit patterns, character traits, attitudes, and so on which characterize an individual considered collectively, make up his personality, and each individual has a distinct and different personality.[23]

The selection of techniques and their appropriate use are based upon how well they facilitate obtaining information. A technique is not effective or ineffective by itself. How appropriately it can be used and the outcome will determine its value. Its worth depends upon its potential to influence the outcome of therapeutic recreation service.

PLANNING

The planning phase begins when the specialist determines that a problem exists and terminates with the development of the plan. It involves setting goals, designing methods for implementing the plan, and providing the framework for evaluation. Said in another way, the specialist determines goals and articulates them in plans. Plans are formulated from decisions. Decisions guide action because they are selected choices that actions follow. (In some healthcare settings, program plans may be referred to as *treatment protocols*; however, the term is extremely limited in its use.)

Goal Setting

Judicious, careful, and deliberate goal setting is vital to this phase of the therapeutic recreation process. The specialist considers possible actions and their consequences in order to determine the best actions. The goals should be realistic and attainable in terms of both the potentialities of the member and the ability of the specialist to help the member meet the goals. However, the student should keep in mind that other factors, such as specific physical and/or emotional limitations or incarceration, as well as the function of the agency and its administrative policies and directives, influence goal setting.

When dealing with individuals who have recently acquired a physical disability, for example, it is extremely important to fully understand the problem before activities are selected and initiated. In other words, the choice of activity may be governed by the extent of the injury. In some cases special equipment may be needed to adapt the activity to the individual's need. However, the use of special equipment is justified only when it accommodates a permanent disability or is a necessary temporary expedient. The obvious danger is, of course, fostering too great a dependence on adaptations that may not be practical beyond the period necessary.

Other influencing factors would include the time needed to resolve the behavioral problem, particularly from the member's point of view; the attitude of society and other professionals; the cost to the member as well as the service's own funding; and the availability of resources.

Objectives are stated in terms of the special population member's goals, rather than the specialist's goals or activities; then the specialist's action is planned to help the member achieve these goals. Without goals or objectives the plan loses its therapeutic value. Also, depending upon the setting, goals and objectives usually are complementary to the facility's treatment goals.

Experienced therapeutic recreation specialists realize that if activities are offered for activities' sake, they lose their value and may detract from rather than contribute to the optimal growth and development of special population individuals. For this reason specialists must exercise great care in the proper selection of activities. The specialist is not so much concerned with what the individual accomplishes in the activity as with what the activity does to the individual; not so much with how the individual plays the game as with how the game affects the emotional, physical, and social state of the individual.

The goals describe the behavior the member is expected to attain. Behavioral objectives are usually written in sentence form and include the subject (special population member), an action verb that describes the desired behavior, the conditions under which the activity is to take place, and a standard for judging the action.[24] The advantages of the behavioral approach, according to Musgrove and others, are as follows:

1. Instead of using a "hit or miss" method, the problem of programming is solved by a comprehensive view of the entire program and recognition of all the subelements and their relationships to the overall program.

2. By stating the objectives in terms of behavioral performances to be accomplished by the client, the emphasis is taken off the person leading the activities and put on the person for whom the program is designed.

3. The statement of objectives in behavioral terms forces the provider of the activities to take a critical look at the program to determine if individual needs are being met.

4. The systematic process of behavioral objectives is an efficient method for programming and should eliminate waste of time and effort.

5. The designer of the objectives should continually evaluate and revise the objectives. This should keep the objectives relevant in addition to avoiding inflexible and highly structured programming.[25]

Another method of goal setting is the utilization of standards. The profession of therapeutic recreation is directing its efforts toward developing standards of service; these standards as they relate to programs are broadly stated at present. Most standards are stated in terms of a general systematic, goal-directed, problem-solving approach. For the most part they do not differ that much from the behavioral-objective approach discussed above.[26]

Another approach used quite frequently in larger hospitals/institutions places the member in activities that have their own goals and objectives. In other words, goals and objectives have been developed for a specific activity, and the member is referred to that activity. Even when goals and objectives have been established for the member, they are usually very general, and ongoing evaluation is limited. Only after a considerable period of time in the activity can any sort of evaluation be made. The specialist is never quite sure whether goals are being reached. Evaluation is unfortunately sketchy and based strictly on subjective impressions.

Activities

Once goals have been identified by the member and the specialist, an ordering or priority is established. The specialist should designate possible activities for each behavioral problem; however, activities offered by the member should also be considered. The possible success of each activity in solving a behavioral problem is estimated, based on scientific principles and/or sound research. Variables such as age, sex, lifestyle, education, socioeconomic status, and cultural background of members and their physiologic and emotional status, as they relate to and affect suggested solutions, should be considered. To do this the specialist must know a member well enough to know the usual effect a given activity has on that member and what this specific activity is likely to mean to the member. The specialist must also know the level of participation and involvement and the meaning of participation and involvement. The specialist predicts as accurately as possible the consequences of each activity. This requires that the specialist know which activities are appropriate for a dependent, a semidependent, or an independent member; which are appropriate for an acutely ill, chronically ill, convalescent, or aged member; and lastly, which are appropriate for those with a disability who might be living in the community. Then the activities most likely to be successful in resolving or diminishing the behavioral problem are selected.

Resolving the behavioral problem may be a multifaceted process with immediate, intermediate, and long-range implications. An immediate goal is one that can be accomplished in a short span of time. An intermediate goal can be attained over a period of time, while a long-range goal is oriented toward the future. The most urgent goal, or the one that should be achieved first, is determined before long-range or more distant goals are set. Goals for the member will include preventive and rehabilitative as well as the immediate aspects.

Behavioral problems that can be resolved by the intervention of the therapeutic recreation specialist must be differentiated from those that require assistance from other members of the health or correctional team or from members in the community. A well-designed and well-developed referral system should be established so that appropriate persons can be involved. In some settings, methods and forms are available for referral use.

When the appropriate activities or services most likely to be successful are selected, specific action on the part of the specialist to achieve the immediate, intermediate, and long-range goals must be delineated. Such action must be clear, purposeful, capable of being accomplished, and adapted to the particular lifestyle, beliefs, and expectations of the special population member. Since therapeutic recreation action is designed to solve a behavior problem, the outcomes expected as a result of that action should be stated in terms of the member's behavior. Only by recording the member's behaviors can therapeutic recreation specialists judge the impact of their actions.

The Plan

During the entire planning phase activity is directed toward quality and quantity of therapeutic recreation actions that will be needed to resolve or minimize problems. This activity culminates in the formulation of the therapeutic recreation plan.

The format for this plan should flow from the goals set. A well-devised plan provides a description of the member and his or her problems and a plan of action to solve them. The development of a therapeutic recreation plan is a creative, intellectual activity. It is an expression of a specialist's knowledge and ability. A clearly stated plan is the most effective means of assuring that the member's problems will be solved and his or her basic human needs fulfilled.

Sharing the plan with appropriate health, correctional, and community team members fosters a better understanding of the member, and the efforts of all are more likely to complement each other. Team members will find that they can function in their specific role more effectively and successfully when the roles of associates are clarified. Other team members should be encouraged to utilize the therapeutic recreation plan as a resource.

Evaluation Criteria

As the specialist plans for the delivery of services, it becomes evident that some means of evaluating these services is also necessary. If the therapeutic recreation actions are designed to help the member meet a need or solve a problem, then an evaluation plan to determine if the expected outcomes of the actions are forthcoming must be developed.

When planning evaluation criteria for therapeutic recreation action, it is important to include a precise idea or description of the expected outcomes. The terminal expectations should be described in unambiguous terms so that all those concerned will know what to expect. Again, they should be written in behavioral terms.

The therapeutic recreation plan details the member's problems and needs, the goals or priorities that have been set, the activity approaches that have been selected, and the evaluative criteria that will measure the actions. It reflects the objectives or goals and is not merely a listing of therapeutic recreation activities. In reality, the therapeutic recreation plan has many purposes. It provides for:

1. *Individualization.* A plan that meets the member's needs, problems, and priorities.
2. *Continuity.* A plan that provides for short-term and long-term goals; information about the member's desires, preferences, and expectations; and information about the member's problems and the proposed activity approaches.
3. *Communication.* A plan that provides

data about the past and present problems and becomes a resource to refer to at any one time.

4. *Evaluation.* If the specialist or other members of the team consistently keep the total plan current, it provides a means of evaluating the process. Evaluation is an ongoing process that occurs each time a goal is reached, and there is a response to a specific approach.
5. *Comprehensive treatment.* A plan that involves the whole person. The member's psychic, social, physical, emotional, and intellectual needs are considered.
6. *Team spirit.* The member is usually the recipient of the cooperative effort of several persons. Working together, the health, correctional, or community team shares its ideas, observations, and suggestions about the member and participates in selecting therapeutic recreation approaches. This participation creates a sense of responsibility in the team, for they all share in the process of planning. The essence of effective and successful activities is a planned, well-organized program carried out in close coordination with the team's findings.

In sum, taking the time to collect data, to develop objectives, and to devise a plan with evaluative criteria is time well spent. Failure to undertake these endeavors before implementation contributes to the misuse of time and the wasted efforts and talents of therapeutic recreation specialists and other personnel. The cost in economic, physical, and emotional terms can hardly be estimated. Economically and ethically, the profession of therapeutic recreation cannot permit this misuse of human and material resources.

IMPLEMENTATION

Once the therapeutic recreation plan has been developed, the implementation phase begins. Depending upon the nature of the behavioral problem and the condition, ability, and resources of the special population member, as well as the nature of the therapeutic recreation action planned, the member, the member and specialist, the specialist alone, or the therapeutic recreation team members who might function under the primary specialist's supervision may implement the plan.

The Specialist's Role

The implementation phase draws heavily upon the intellectual, interpersonal, and technical skills of the specialist. Decision making, observation, and communication are significant skills that enhance the success of action.

Just as the specialist's philosophy, education, and experience influenced the character of the plan, so will these factors significantly affect implementing the plan. The emphasis, focus, and creativity will be affected by the specialist's strengths, limitations, prejudices, stereotypes, knowledge of human behavior, strength of convictions, ability to handle human closeness, and ability to use himself or herself therapeutically.

In order to be successful in implementing the plan, the specialist must command respect and confidence. If the specialist's thinking is muddled and confused relative to the task ahead, these traits are reflected in individual contact; if dislike, jealousy, and self-pity are harbored, similar feelings are aroused in the member by their projection. The specialist's personal inhibitions should be understood and an effort made to correct them if effective assistance is to be given in meeting the individual member's needs.

With the therapeutic recreation plan as the blueprint and the immediate, intermediate, and long-range goals in focus, the plan is put into practice. The plan is not carried out blindly with all thinking and decision making accomplished during the previous two phases. The specialist continues to collect data about the member's problems, reactions, and feelings. Additional informa-

tion is obtained from other team members and the community. At the same time the specialist records the reaction of the member to the plan. While brevity and clarity are desirable in recording progress, the record's use will be diminished considerably if brevity becomes the exclusive goal.

The success or failure of the plan depends upon the specialist's intellectual, interpersonal, and technical ability. This includes the ability to judge the value of new information that becomes available during implementation and the innovative and creative ability to make adaptations. The specialist must also have the ability to react to verbal and nonverbal cues, validating inferences based on observation. Paramount during the interaction is the specialist's confidence in his or her ability to perform the independent functions inherent in the therapeutic recreation plan.

The amount of time spent with the individual or group varies significantly, ranging from short to prolonged interaction. This encounter could range from minutes to hours or from days to weeks or could last a year, either continuing or intermittent. Interaction should be planned precisely, with allowances made for the unexpected.

It is essential that each interaction be goal directed and purposeful. Interaction demands alert, observant, attentive behavior by the specialist. Likewise, the specialist must be fully aware of the need to communicate with the member who does not respond in the usual and expected manner.

The specialist must be aware that some special population members may resist change even after they have participated in therapeutic recreation service. This may be the result of emotional dependence on the specialist, general opposition to any kind of change, clinging to existing satisfactions, financial cost of change, and the like. When such a situation occurs, the specialist must reevaluate the approach taken. Many resistance forces can be converted into change. Resistance comes into being originally in response to certain needs. If the person is saying, in effect, that the status quo must be maintained because it is the best way to meet leisure needs, the specialist might be able to show that the same need would be met even more satisfactorily in a different set of circumstances. The very energy that the member once used to maintain the status quo may then shift direction and give impetus to change.

Continuing Evaluation

In each contact with the member the specialist not only focuses on the purpose or goal of the interaction, but also utilizes his or her perceptual ability to obtain data about the member that would indicate that the planned action is correct. The specialist also seeks data that would indicate other problems due to unmet or poorly met basic human needs.

As the specialist implements the therapeutic recreation plan, he or she learns more about the member's reactions, feelings, strengths, limitations, coping ability, preferences, satisfactions, and dissatisfactions. The specialist learns the member's response to planned therapeutic recreation action, additional ways available to the member and to the specialist to perform actions, the need for additional actions, and any untoward response to the planned action. These data are synthesized and utilized to further develop the therapeutic recreation plan and are the basis for recording data about the member on appropriate progress note forms.

As a result of the member's response during the implementation, priorities may have to be reassigned, and replanning may be required. Judgment is needed to know what to do with the information obtained, what information is needed, whether a new plan is needed, and what the plan of action should be.

Thus, the implementation process includes assessing, planning, and evaluating. Implementation is an action-oriented phase of the therapeutic recreation process in

which the specialist is responsible for implementing the therapeutic recreation plan that was developed. The intellectual, interpersonal, and technical actions employed during this phase are based on the plan designed for the member according to the member's assessed problems.

EVALUATION

Criteria

Evaluation, the fourth and last component of the therapeutic recreation process, follows the implementation of actions. It implies measurement against predetermined criteria that are stated in terms of how the member is expected to respond to the planned action. Further, if the specialist has used the logical, goal-directed problem solving approach, evaluation should have a high level of success. Evaluating the effect of actions during and after the implementation phase determines the member's response and the extent to which immediate, intermediate, and long-range goals are achieved. The evaluation must continue in a purposeful, goal-directed manner.

Evaluation is the natural intellectual activity completing the process phase because it indicates the degree to which the therapeutic recreation diagnosis and actions have been correct. Evaluation will also pinpoint omissions in the assessment, planning, and implementation phases. Since evaluation deals with immediate, intermediate, and long-range goals, the evaluation process is continued until all these goals are realized. Both the specialist and special population member are the immediate agents of evaluation. Other persons, such as the member's family and other facility or community personnel, may also be involved. Based upon the behavioral expectations of the member relative to the immediate, intermediate, and long-range goals, measurement data are collected so that value judgments can be made.

At present there is a paucity of tools whereby the specialist can evaluate actions with a high degree of objectivity. However, various tools are beginning to appear more frequently.[27] For the immediate future, subjectivity will enter into many of our evaluation procedures. Thus, specialists use their senses to collect data, employ communication techniques to elicit subjective responses, utilize those objective tests available, and then make a decision about the member's behavioral response. Data collected from the member about what has occurred and how it was interpreted tell the specialist whether behavior change has taken place.

The use of measurable criteria for evaluation of therapeutic recreation action gives predictability to the action and reliability to the evaluation. When the performance criteria are stated in behavioral terms, evaluation is relatively simple. Criteria stated in behavioral terms describe the desired outcome of the action, the conditions under which the desired outcome will occur, and the acceptable performance. A number of persons can recognize the desired behavior, thereby providing objectivity to the evaluation when it is stated in behavioral terms. The more measurable and objective the criteria, the more reliable the evaluation will be; and the more clearly the criteria are stated in behavioral terms, the more probable it is that the specialist will be able to evaluate the therapeutic recreation action.

Results

The outcome of evaluation may be any one or a combination of the following:

1. The member responded as had been expected and the problem is resolved.

2. Behavioral manifestations indicate the problem has not been resolved; evidence demonstrates that immediate (but not intermediate and long-range) goals have not been achieved. Reevaluation will continue.

3. Behavioral manifestations are similar to those evidenced during the assessment phase. There is little or no evidence that the problem has been resolved. Reassessment with replanning is needed.

4. Behavioral manifestations indicate new problems. Assessment, planning, and implementation of a plan of action to resolve these problems are in order.

Reasons for Failure

Sources for explanations of why predicted behavior outcomes were not realized include the member, the specialist, other persons of importance to the member, and other team members.

Concerning the member, possible causes for failure to realize goals can include an increase in pathophysiology, psychopathology, or social problems, loss of self-esteem, loss of job, lack of interest in and attention to problems, and withholding important data about self and situation.

If the specialist is the source, reasons the member's problem has not been resolved may include overlooked data, failure to validate information, lack of knowledge about the member's situation, failure to recognize the member's strengths and need for independence within the limits of his or her problems, inappropriate activity program, failure to consider the value of input from others, and failure to recognize one's own intellectual, interpersonal, and technical limitations.

Concerning the others significant to the member, goals may not be achieved because these others are not available or not interested in the member; the member's problem, the solution, and expected behavioral change are not understood; fears and anxieties exist between the member and others; transportation is lacking; and moral, cultural, and religious influences may interfere.

Reasons for the failure to achieve the goals planned for the member in relation to other team members include conflict of goals for the member, failure to see the impact of the focus upon the whole member, inability to function as a team member, failure to see value in the therapeutic recreation plan, and acts that depersonalize the member.

The fourth component of the therapeutic recreation process, evaluation, the framework for which has been prescribed, stems from the process itself. Evaluation is always expressed in terms of achieving expected behavior change. The entire focus of the process is goal directed. It is systematically geared to solving the special population member's diagnosed problems by prescribing specific therapeutic recreation actions that would successfully induce a specific behavioral effect denoting that the member's problem has been resolved.

Evaluation aids the specialist to determine problems that have been resolved, those that need to be reprocessed, and new problems that have arisen.

Reports and Record Keeping

Before bringing this chapter to a close, a few brief comments are needed about reports and records since documentation is now a priority. Progress reports keep the treatment team informed about the progress of the patient. How detailed these reports should be depends upon the type of care and the circumstances. The type of record kept would differ greatly from that for a research project. There may also be a marked difference between the type of record made for a patient whose disability is neither serious nor permanently disabling and that made for a more severely disabled individual. In all reports the materials should be factual and not an expression of opinion.

The quality of the recording about the member and what the specialist chooses to document give direct evidence of the status of goal achievement and individual member reactions, and designates the direction for continued problem solving. Placing a low value on recording or making insufficient or inappropriate recordings is an affront to the member and demonstrates the specialist's limitations. Automatic notations or general statements give little or no indication of the member's individuality, problem, and reaction to the planned action. Recordings should be related to the problem; they describe the specialist's actions and the results and include additional data. The written report of therapeutic recreation service given serves to direct continuing action.

Recordings should reflect the member's unique situation and should be identified easily by the quality of their content. The recording should contain the information needed to give a profile of the member. Rules that set limits on what and how much should be recorded—supposedly to save time—can be a waste of time. The specialist must decide what to write, how much to write, when to write, and what is important. Such writing is a professional and not a clerical activity.

Recordings become more frequent when the member's behavior changes rapidly. If changes occur slowly and are infrequent, there will be less to record, but the information will not lose its significance. When recordings become copious or their use is minimized because the specialist does not have the time to review them, the information should be summarized periodically in coordination and in conjunction with the therapeutic recreation plan.

To assist students in writing reports and progress notes, a progress note terminology guide is provided in Appendix A.

RELATIONSHIP: PROCESS AND HUMAN SERVICE MODELS

The previously described therapeutic recreation process is not limited to any particular environment—clinic, hospital, institution, community, or other agency. The process, in fact, may be used in any setting where there are special population members. It is flexible, adaptable, and adjustable to a number of variables, yet sufficiently structured so as to provide a base from which many therapeutic recreation actions can proceed. At this point it will be helpful to briefly overview the human service models where the process of therapeutic recreation is currently employed. Subsequent chapters will provide a detailed description of the application of the process in each of these models.

In Chapter 3 we considered those agencies and institutions that offer health, social, and correctional rehabilitation service. We also noted that therapeutic recreation as a service usually does not operate independently outside an agency or organization. It is found most often within a system that provides a specific kind of care or service. These *human service models* differ in historical development, orientation, mode of intervention, and the professional groups that are most commonly found in the various service models. While there is specialization of function in these models, there is also overlapping. For the most part, these models provide treatment (therapy), rehabilitation, counseling, training and/or reeducation, and a social service. Since there are a number of different models with many variations, we shall limit the discussion to the more prominent ones and the provisions of therapeutic recreation within them. It is anticipated that further exploration of these models, including the provision of therapeutic recreation, will occur in a therapeutic recreation programming course.

It is important to note that the emphasis placed on therapeutic recreation service varies greatly among the agencies and organizations that provide human services. Although the goals of any care system are to provide human services to its clients and to use the resources, knowledge, and technologies available to prevent and alleviate disability and social disobedience, the efforts of the agency are influenced by economics, administration and organizational structure, and the value context that society places upon particular services. Therefore, therapeutic recreation specialists must continue to strive for a certain level of autonomy in relationship to other care workers as well as to seek recognition for our unique role in care and treatment.

MEDICAL-CLINICAL MODEL

This traditional model, for the most part, is found today in general medical and surgical hospitals and medically oriented physical rehabilitation institutes and centers. However, it was not too many years ago that this model was the only one found in psychiatric institutions and other kinds of health facilities. In this model it is important to recognize that medicine dominates the other health professionals. To a large extent, this dominance is supported by political and legal factors.

The model is characterized by a doctor-centered, illness-oriented approach to patient care and treatment. Treatment is directed at the disease rather than the whole person. Professional disciplines involved in the treatment process carry out the physician's orders to meet medical goals and objectives.

In the past few therapeutic recreators were found working in this specific model. If they were, they usually were assigned to the occupational therapy department in the physical medicine and rehabilitation service. In more recent years there has been an increase not only in the number of therapeutic recreators found in the model but also in the number of therapeutic recreation or recreation therapy departments established in hospitals and responsible for services throughout the hospital. Today therapeutic recreators are found working in physical medicine and rehabilitation, in inpatient and outpatient psychiatric services, and in pediatric, orthopedic, cancer, cardiac, renal, and burn units. Their responsibilities include providing diversional recreation services as well as treatment or remedial recreation services per referral or prescription from the physician.

The recreation treatment program in this model may be directed toward any disease aspect—physical, emotional, social, or intellectual. It is more likely, however, to be directed toward the physical since this model is characterized by individuals having short-term physical problems, although in centers of a physical rehabilitational nature the length of stay is usually longer.

Taking into consideration the services available in a general medical and surgical hospital, the recreation treatment program for a recent unilateral below-knee amputee might involve the development of as nearly normal a range of motion as possible in the affected extremity. One specific prescribed activity might be shuffleboard. As the individual progresses, additional activities can be used to assist in the development of strength in the stump and security in movement. Thereafter, the program includes utilization of community resources to increase skill confidence and enhance acceptance of the prosthesis. Incorporated within the use of community resources might be a program of leisure education or counseling.

Diversional programs in this model are many and varied. Some may consist of audiovisual programs in a pediatrics ward, closed-circuit bingo, arts and crafts projects brought to the bedside, and even a babysitting service so parents can leave their children during an examination. In the latter example, the program may be staffed by volunteers.

West suggests that therapeutic recreation services in this model should be structured around the following objectives:

1. To provide through recreation an outlet for the stress and emotional frustration created by illness, disability, and the inability to participate in normal activities

2. To overcome social isolation, boredom, and loneliness while away from family and friends

3. To provide functional activities that will aid the patient's social and psychological adjustment and physical independence

4. To provide activities, diversional in nature, that will offer the opportunity for the constructive use of hospital leisure time

5. To educate and counsel the patient in the use of activities that can be used after discharge as a continuation of the therapeutic regimen or to support health maintenance

6. To assist all health-care professionals in the planning and administering of optimal and comprehensive health care for the entire community[28]

CUSTODIAL AND LONG-TERM CARE MODEL

Since the first edition of this publication there have been significant developments in the care and treatment of special populations in long-term residential institutions, whether hospital/institutions, prisons, or nursing homes. In fact, the custodial model has been replaced by the long-term care model, although shades of the former model still exist in some settings, most notably in correctional institutions. At present there is no generally accepted definition of the long-term care model nor is there a specific title that encompasses the model relative to the health-care setting. Generally speaking, in a health context the model refers to one or more services provided on a sustained basis to enable individuals whose functional capacities are chronically impaired to be maintained at the maximum levels of health and well-being. While this so-called definition contains elements of the custodial model (characterized by conformity, order, subordination of individual needs to the institutional routine, and even punishment for deviation from routines), it does incorporate a health-oriented care and treatment component, which was extremely limited in the early model.

The model is the result of a rising social consciousness on the part of professionals, the public, and government regarding people who are ill and cannot meet their needs through their own resources. The underlying concept here is that all people share certain basic human needs, that they have a right to services designed to maximize their own and their families' capacities to meet those needs, and that they should be furnished services when their needs cannot be met through their own social, emotional, physical, and financial resources. This constellation of needs—referred to as "quality of life" or social needs—include needs for interpersonal contacts and relationships, recreational and occupational experiences and activities, maintenance of roles, and a sense of mastery, autonomy, and some degree of self-determination or control over one's own life.

Although facilities for long-term care (homes for aged, hospitals for chronically ill, nursing homes, geriatric centers, county homes, veterans' homes, hospitals or institutions for the mentally ill and developmentally disabled), have undergone major changes in the positive sense, problems still exist. Distinctions between facilities are blurred, and different facility names mean different things to different people in different places at different times. The professional literature and the popular press are replete with documentation of the sad plight of many of the institutionalized. Undeniably, in some facilities the provision of care and treatment is at a level that should not be tolerated, to say nothing about profiteering, fire hazards, unsanitary conditions, inadequate food, and even cruel treatment. Government legislation and regulations vary widely from region to region, state to state, and in some instances even from county to county and community to community. The population is also changing. New groups of people are entering the long-term care model, and these individuals have better education and better standards of living, are more sophisticated and articulate in their demands, and have higher expectations of care and treatment. Much remains to be done if facilities of a long-term care nature are to reach that positive goal of maximizing

the functioning level and well-being of the long-term patient.

At this time there appears to be no general consensus about what the philosophy of care should be, but there is a consensus that one of the broadest areas of neglect in the long-term care model has been the psychosocial needs of the patients. It is recognized by professionals that the frontiers of care must be pushed beyond subsistence and survival to dignity and enjoyment. While a good deal has been written about the devastating impact of lack of attention to the social and psychological needs of the institutionalized, implementation of this understanding through appropriate programs and services has lagged. Similarly, though there is widespread recognition of the need for therapeutic recreation services as an integral part of the programming in long-term care facilities, their full development has not taken place.

In the past recreation service in the custodial model was limited (if any at all): an evening of games, an occasional dance, and motion pictures for those who were ambulatory and somewhat active. Social interaction was possible only for the more oriented patient. For the most part, activities were of diversional nature to keep the patient busy, quiet, and out of trouble.

Unfortunately, some nursing home programs still provide only the type of recreation service just mentioned. Because people have a tendency to stereotype the elderly, programs are based upon these stereotypes, and those who conform are considered typical. The main purposes of the program are keeping the resident occupied and having pleasant experiences. Further, only those residents who are ambulatory are encouraged to come to the activity room. This kind of situation exists in far too many nursing homes. But according to Halberg, residents should be helped to utilize their ability, no matter how limited, for meaning and satisfaction as well as for fun. This suggests an activity program that has as its purpose as many kinds of opportunities as possible with as few limitations as possible.[29] As Teaff states regarding recreative experiences for the elderly in institutions: "The opportunity to exercise abilities and continue life tasks must be provided . . . , maximizing and reinforcing independence, dignity, and respect."[30]

In many correctional institutions that still abide by the concept of punishment rather than rehabilitation, recreation programs consist of sports and athletic events to reduce tension and boredom. It is not unusual to find that recreation activities are used as a reward for good behavior. The findings reported by Decker in a recreation study completed for the Oregon State Division of Corrections in 1969 can still be applied today to many correctional institutions in the United States.

1. The role and values of recreation are not emphasized.

2. There is no professional staff member trained in recreation.

3. The emphasis is on custodial care and security.

4. Professional guidance and assistance in recreational services are not readily available to the staff.

5. Where recreation programs do exist, they often are instituted with little planning and few long-range objectives in mind.

6. The administrative climate is not conducive to evaluation and change.

7. The professional recreator's efforts have not been directed toward explaining and increasing the role of recreation in the institutional setting.[31]

THERAPEUTIC COMMUNITY OR THERAPEUTIC MILIEU MODEL

This model is the result of the shift away from a custodial to a humanitarian orientation in psychiatric care and treatment. This shift was one of a number of significant developments that took place in the 1950s. These other developments, which contrib-

uted to this model and will be considered later, included psychopharmacology, institutional decentralization, and community-based programs and services. In this model, which incorporated two other models—milieu therapy and therapeutic community—institutionalization is viewed not as a means of removing individuals from society, but rather as an opportunity to give them a sheltered milieu in which specific therapeutic experiences could be provided. In some respects it is a return to moral treatment. Generally speaking, the model suggests that individuals are affected and even changed by their relationship with others and their environment.[32] Treatment is focused on as many aspects of the patient as possible—physical, emotional, social, vocational, recreational—and on a wide range of patients' relationships, and no longer exclusively on physiological disease or psychological conflict.[33]

Variations of the model have been applied in nearly all, if not all, settings that offer health or social service to people. From one perspective, the model may no longer be a model in name because it has been so well integrated into some settings that it seems as if it has always existed. In the main, however, it dominates psychiatric hospital/institution practice in the large state psychiatric institutions, the Veterans Administration psychiatric hospitals, the small private psychiatric institutions, the inpatient and outpatient psychiatric units of general hospitals, and the community mental health clinics or centers. Although the model remains the same, the application of the model will vary and be unique to the type of setting in which one implements it—whether it has many or few patients, whether the staff-patient ratio is high or low, by what kinds of patients are admitted, whether the institution has a long history of a custodial orientation or is a new one with a reformist base.

In brief, the therapeutic milieu model can be defined as the means of organizing a community treatment environment so that every human interaction and every treatment technique can be systematically utilized to further the patient's aims of controlling symptomatic behaviors and learning approaches to psychosocial skills. Moreover, the therapeutic milieu involves the *entire* setting—utilizing both staff and patients in the treatment process. Everyone taking part in the activities of the therapeutic community shares in the commitment to the institution's effectiveness as a therapeutic agent. It is the responsibility of all individuals who make up the therapeutic community to make sure that the hospital/institution functions as closely as possible in accordance with its goals and to see that the social structure is organized to facilitate optimal participation, interaction, and involvement.[34]

The role of the therapeutic recreation department or service in this model is to focus on every aspect of the patient's life. The therapeutic milieu model provides a climate most favorable to the use of recreative experiences as a socializing therapy. These experiences may range from basic socializing activities to reality-oriented social functions that are a part of everyday living. As Edelson points out, "an individual's approach to playtime accurately reflects the organization of his drives and controls."[35] Thus, therapeutic recreative experiences can serve as a means of helping the individual regain social competence, confidence, and acceptance. An example of a change in psychosocial skills that the authors recall follows:

A middle-aged farmer's wife entered with a retarded depression. After a favorable response to drug therapy, she indicated some disappointment with the lonely, grim quality of her life. She was on beck-and-call to feed the men whenever they came in from work, and she never went into town except with her family. In fact, she had forgotten how to drive. The remainder of her hospitalization was used to teach her to drive, to play cards, and to bowl, to schedule these activities into her life, and to enlist the family's cooperation in her regular involvement in church social functions, card clubs, and family group activities.

The therapeutic environment consists of the patient, the therapeutic recreation specialist, the activity (or service), and the physical environment. All of these elements combined in accordance with the treatment plan constitute a milieu therapy approach for therapeutic recreation.

In the medical model, the responsibility for the treatment plan rests with the physician. But in milieu-oriented settings this responsibility often rests with all personnel concerned with a given patient who meet together and arrive at a consensus about the treatment for the patient. The goal is open and easy communication. The traditional hierarchical and authoritarian professional roles and relationships are minimized. The therapeutic recreation specialist is a member of this treatment team. As such, the specialist not only is responsible for bringing into focus the importance and use of recreative experiences as a therapeutic tool and the use of such experiences for diagnostic and evaluative purposes, but also becomes involved with other professional workers in determining the total therapeutic plan. Further, treatment team meetings allow the specialist to educate and consult with others about therapeutic recreation. Thus, the base of the specialist's therapeutic relevancy is broader.

EDUCATION AND TRAINING MODEL

This model cuts across all kinds of settings, residential and nonresidential. It is found within the models just discussed. It is found in special schools and training centers for the mentally retarded, in settings that provide health services to those with specific sensory and nonsensory disabilities, and in prisons and training schools for juvenile and young adult offenders. The model is also applied in sheltered workshop settings and can be utilized on a temporary basis, if not on a permanent basis in some situations, with the homebound.

The model focuses on (1) formal or informal academic educational programs; (2) prevocational or vocational preparation programs or workstudy programs; and (3) socialization training. The importance of these areas is justified by the belief that special population members will view themselves and will be viewed by others in a more positive way if they have developed some academic and vocational skills and are capable of socializing. If, on the other hand, people lack skills in these areas, they will probably be relatively less happy and less adjusted, have little or no social status in their family or community, be an economic burden to others, and be susceptible to patterns of social and personal misbehavior. Moreover, the economic consequences of a member's being unable to work and requiring care in some kind of setting are substantial in our present-day society.

The role of the therapeutic recreation department or service in this model is dependent to a large degree on the setting wherein the model is found. But regardless of setting, emphasis will be placed on the use of recreative experiences to develop a positive self-concept, social skills and activity skills that can be used in leisure pursuits following release or discharge, and leisure counseling to include the importance of developing a personal philosophy about leisure.

The concept of self develops, to a large extent, on the basis of direct comparison of one's performance with the performance of others. Self-concept is formed according to how the members believe others view them. Thus, if activities are either too difficult to realize or improper, and if modifications in them do not occur, members will perpetually fail and will lose faith in themselves and in their ability to perform in a reasonably satisfactory way.

It seems important to mention that the majority of special population members have not experienced social situations that offer opportunities to practice appropriate responses or what constitutes a proper man-

ner of behavior. Indeed, for many, attempting to behave in socially proper ways has not always been a rewarding experience because of imperfect performances. It is especially important, therefore, that activities focus on social skill competencies that are reasonable to achieve and are consistent with the character, needs, situation, and prognosis of each person.

There are few publications today that concern themselves with special populations that do not mention the importance of leisure activities for these individuals *following release or discharge*. It has been said that one of the major problems in the area of health, social, and correctional service is not the person who *is* institutionalized but the person who *has been* institutionalized—the former patient or offender. The period immediately following release or discharge appears to be extremely crucial with respect to whether a person remains in the community or returns to the institution.

Some administrators of rehabilitation programs in the early 1960s noted that successful vocational training was often followed by failure to keep a job because an individual either lacked the social skills necessary to get along well with others on the job or did not have the activity skills necessary to participate in leisure activities after a full day of work.[36] As a result, according to Haun, individuals often engaged in seemingly delinquent acts, or in self-created games of a bizarre nature or returned to play patterns found in an early development period while losing interest in more highly developed activities.[37]

Therapeutic recreation specialists must be exceedingly sensitive to the environment to which the patient returns. Services must be directed toward greater conformity to the normative demands of the larger community. Therapeutic recreation specialists, therefore, must offer activities that develop activity skills and provide a leisure counseling service to meet the post-discharge needs of the special population member.

COMMUNITY MODEL

The community, as the term is used here, means those people as a whole found in a specific geographic area—town or city—who share common needs and interests or are linked together as a group and individually by those needs and interests. This does not mean a community in which all norms, beliefs, values, drives, motives, and ways of life are standardized. But it does suggest that community means that there is a common life of some kind and that there is value in identifying with, and sharing in, this common life. Implicit in this definition is that individuals whom we have identified as special population members are members of this community. As indicated, the vast majority of these members are found in the community, not in an institution or special school or rehabilitation center. They have as much right to be associated with and feel part of this common life as the individual with no physical, emotional, and/or social problems. But according to one source, the "disabled have a significantly higher proportion of idle/leisure time but they have a significantly lower quality of life than the general population."[38] This conclusion is based on the statistic that 80 percent of all disabled are underserved or unserved in recreation.[39]

As noted earlier, recreation service to special population members has been provided since the early 1900s. Such services, however, were found primarily in larger communities; in addition, the services were limited and restricted to special disabilities—cerebral palsy, mental retardation, and the like. Since the early 1950s we have witnessed a gradual movement toward integrated programming, which has met with varying degrees of success depending upon the attitude of the community and sponsoring agency toward special population members as well as the type of services being provided. In more recent years municipal recreation programming settled into a threefold

approach: sheltered, semisheltered, and nonsheltered (integrated). In some instances voluntary service organizations and public park and recreation departments combined to provide the recreation services; in other instances each provided separate services, often in duplication.

Since 1970 several major legislative acts (for example, Rehabilitation Act of 1973 and Education for All Handicapped Children Act of 1975) have had positive effects on community recreation services for special population members. Likewise, in recent years advocacy groups at national, state, and local levels are requesting more recreation services. The President's Committee on Employment of the Handicapped has had for several years a subcommittee on recreation and leisure. This same President's Committee and the NRPA cosponsored in 1974 a National Forum on Park and Recreation Needs of the Handicapped. In 1975 the National Institute of New Models for Community and Leisure for Handicapped Children and Youth was established at the University of Iowa under the direction of Dr. John Nesbitt through a grant from the U.S. Bureau of Education for the Handicapped.

The role of the therapeutic recreator in the community now and for the foreseeable future will be, as Humphrey has indicated, that of a "catalytic and resource leader."[40] In this leadership role the specialist will function as a consultant, public relations expert, advocate, community planner, educator-teacher, supervisor, and leader. The specialist might also serve as coordinator of a recreation service referral or on a coordinating council responsible for offering assistance and advice to recently discharged or released patients and offenders in locating recreative resources in the community.

As noted, leisure service agencies are giving more attention to offering recreation opportunities to special populations. Likewise, other community agencies are initiating leisure services. Therapeutic recreation specialists by virtue of their specialized knowledge and experience can add, when requested, to the competence of the central administration by assisting and participating in leisure service program development and in production and direction of inservice workshops, by serving on committees, by working on experimental or pilot projects, and by providing fieldwork supervision to students in schools offering course work in therapeutic recreation.

In these days of rapid social change the specialist might very well work with an anti-poverty program in helping local community representatives determine what kind of recreative services are wanted, what they think about current services, what really is available, and why so many people are not making use of the services they obviously need. The specialist will help communities involved in such programs do something for themselves, not do it for them, creating the ability to move toward independence rather than dependence.

Increasingly we are observing that therapeutic recreation specialists are employed in various youth-serving agencies, either helping juvenile delinquents find their way into positive recreation opportunities through referrals to public recreation agencies or participating in specifically designed activities directed by a specialist. Similar procedures and programs have been developed for the adult offender who is either on probation or parole.

One approach used to meet community social problems is the formation of an interagency council that would usually meet monthly to share information and discuss problems of common interests in the community. Here the specialist can offer unique assistance in helping community agencies implement leisure services to meet leisure needs.

Where the size of the community and the funds available permit it, therapeutic recreation specialists have been employed by leisure service organizations, most often the municipal recreation agency. The specialist's role is usually that of supervisor of special services, although lack of funds may limit the number and kind of special population members actively served as well as the geographic area.

We cannot leave the community model without indicating that complications exist within the model relative to the development of recreation services for special populations. It takes time, effort, and a considerable amount of human service development to initiate recreation services. It takes planning, administration, community organization, consultation, coordination, and citizen participation. In the planning process alone, for example, it requires problem assessment, problem clarification, goal and objective setting, examination and decision among alternatives, and determination of strategy, as well as steps to take concerning the implementation of strategy, monitoring, and evaluation. In the end, provision of recreation service to special populations requires a commitment to the listening, sharing, and compromising inherent in the process of working with others and the requisite skills—communication, group process and organizational skills—necessary for meeting such a commitment.

SUMMARY

This chapter has provided an in-depth description of the therapeutic recreation process by examining the underlying rationale for this procedure and overviewing the various models where the process can be applied. By now, it should be evident that therapeutic recreation specialists employ a well-planned, systematic approach to meeting client needs through recreative experiences.

The chapters that follow will illustrate the use of the intervention in the various human service models.

NOTES

1. Doris Berryman, quoted in Virginia Frye and Martha Peters, *Therapeutic Recreation: Its Theory, Philosophy, and Practice* (Harrisburg, Pa.: Stackpole Books, 1972), p. 41.

2. Ibid., p. 42.

3. Edith L. Ball, "The Meaning of Therapeutic Recreation." *Therapeutic Recreation Journal* 4, no.1 (1978), 17–18.

4. Ibid., p. 18.

5. Frye and Peters, *Therapeutic Recreation*, p. 43.

6. Scout Lee Gunn and Carol Ann Peterson, *Therapeutic Recreation Program Design: Principles and Procedures*, 2nd ed. (Englewood Cliffs, N.J.: Prentice-Hall, 1984), pp. 53–62.

7. Gerald S. O'Morrow, *Therapeutic Recreation: A Helping Profession*, 2nd ed. (Reston, Va.: Reston Publishing Co., 1980), p. 123.

8. David Mechanic, *Politics, Medicine, and Social Science* (New York: Wiley-Interscience Publishers, 1974), pp. 227–48.

9. For a discussion about these procedures as they relate to reimbursement see Richard Patterson, "The Development of a Self-Sufficient Therapeutic Recreation Service," in *Expanding Horizons in Therapeutic Recreation III*, ed. Gary Robb and Gerald Hitzhusen (Columbia: Department of Recreation and Park Administration, University of Missouri, 1975), pp. 49–52.

10. *Webster's Third International Dictionary* (Boston: G. and C. Merriam Co., 1967).

11. Thomas R. Collingwood, "Therapeutic Recreation's Relevance to the Rehabilitation Process," *Therapeutic Recreation Annual* 7 (1971), 31.

12. Joanne Bridges, "Providing Therapeutic Recreation Services, the Two Way Stretch," *Therapeutic Recreation Annual* 7 (1971), 16.

13. David R. Austin, *Therapeutic Recreation: Processes and Techniques* (New York: John Wiley & Sons, 1982), p. 111.

14. Daniel D. Ferguson, "Assessment Interviewing Techniques: A Useful Tool in Developing Individual Program Plans," *Therapeutic Recreation Journal* 17, no. 2 (1983), 16–22.

15. Austin, *Therapeutic Recreation*, pp. 131–34.

16. Isaiah Ginsburg, "Therapeutic Recreation: A Modality for Rehabilitation of the Aged," *Therapeutic Recreation Journal* 8, no. 1 (1974) 42–46.

17. A partial listing of assessment instruments useful to therapeutic recreation specialists can be found in Gunn and Peterson, *Therapeutic Recreation Program Design*, pp. 298–318, and throughout various sections of AAHPER, *Physical Education and Recreation for Impaired, Disabled and Handicapped Individuals*.

18. *Therapeutic Recreation Journal* 14, no. 4 (1980). See also Christine E. Howe, "Leisure Assessment Instrumentation in Therapeutic Recreation," *Therapeutic Recreation Journal* 18, no. 4 (1984), 14–24.

19. Frederick J. MacDonald, *Educational Psychology*, 2nd ed. (Belmont, Calif.: Wadsworth Publishing Co., 1969), p. 253.

20. Abraham H. Maslow, *Motivation and Personality*, 2nd ed. (New York: Harper & Row, 1970).

21. Erik H. Erikson, *Childhood and Society*, 2nd ed. (New York: W. W. Norton & Co., 1963), pp. 247–74.

22. E. M. Duvall, *Family Development* (Philadelphia: J. B. Lippincott Co., 1971).

23. Frye and Peters, *Therapeutic Recreation*, pp. 99–100.

24. For additional help in writing objectives in behavioral terms see Robert F. Mager, *Preparing Instructional Objectives* (Palo Alto, Calif.: Fearon Publishing Co., 1962).

25. Dolores G. Musgrove, "The Application of System Analysis Theory to Therapeutic Recreation Service," *Therapeutic Recreation Journal* 5, no. 2 (1961), 60–62.

26. See NTRS, *Guidelines for Therapeutic Recreation Service in Clinical and Residential Facilities.*

27. See Suggested Readings at end of the chapter for various articles concerning evaluation tools.

28. Ray E. West, "Therapeutic Recreation Services as a Component of Optimal Health Care in a General Hospital Setting," *Therapeutic Recreation Journal* 13, no. 3 (1979), 3.

29. Kathleen J. Halberg, "Individualized Planning for the Aging Resident," in *Expanding Horizons in Therapeutic Recreation II*, ed. Jerry D. Kelley (Champaign: Office of Recreation and Park Resources, University of Illinois, 1973), pp. 107–12.

30. Joseph D. Teaff, *Leisure Services with the Elderly* (St. Louis: Times Mirror/Mosby College Publishing, 1985), p. 138.

31. Larry E. Decker, "Recreation in Correctional Institutions," *Parks and Recreation* 8, no. 4 (1969), p. 31.

32. Alfred H. Stanton, "Foreword," in John Cumming and Elaine Cumming, *Ego and Milieu: Theory and Practice of Environmental Therapy* (New York: Atherton Press, 1962).

33. David M. Rioch and Alfred H. Stanton, "Milieu Therapy," *Psychiatry* 16 (1953), 65–72.

34. Morris S. Schwartz, "What Is Therapeutic Milieu?" in *The Patient and the Mental Hospitals*, ed. Milton Greenblatt et al. (Glencoe, Ill.: Free Press, 1957), pp. 130–44.

35. M. Edelson, *Ego Psychology, Group Dynamics and the Therapeutic Community* (New York: Guno and Stratton, 1964), p. 93.

36. National Recreation Association, *Sheltered Workshop Project OVR 437* (New York: the association, 1961).

37. Haun, *Recreation: A Medical Viewpoint*, pp. 22–32.
38. John A. Nesbitt, "Special Recreation Digest," n.d., p. 3.

39. Ibid.
40. Fred Humphrey, "Therapeutic Recreation and the 1970s," *Therapeutic Recreation Annual* 7 (1970), 8–13.

SUGGESTED READINGS

ADAIR, BILL. "The Role of Recreation in Assessing the Needs of Emotionally Disturbed Youth." *Leisurability* 1, no. 4 (1974), 27–31.

ANTHONY, PATRICIA. "The Recreation Practitioner as Change Agent and Advocate for Disabled Persons." *Leisurability* 12, no. 1 (1985), 19–23.

AUSTIN, DAVID R. *Therapeutic Recreation: Process and Techniques.* New York: John Wiley & Sons, 1982.

CERTO, NICHOLAS J., STUART J. SCHLEIEN, and DAWN HUNTER. "An Ecological Assessment Inventory to Facilitate Community Recreation Participation by Severely Disabled Individuals." *Therapeutic Recreation Journal* 17, no. 3 (1983), 29–38.

COLLINGWOOD, THOMAS R. "The Recreation Leader as a Therapeutic Agent." *Therapeutic Recreation Journal* 6, no. 4 (1972), 147–52.

COMPTON, DAVID M. and DONNA PRICE. "Individualizing Your Treatment Program: A Case Study Using LIMT." *Therapeutic Recreation Journal* 9, no. 4 (1975), 127–39.

CONNOLLY, PEG. "Analyzing Program Cause as Well as Effect: A Model for Program Analysis." *Therapeutic Recreation Journal* 18, no. 1 (1984), 31–39.

CREWE, NANCY M., and others. "A Pilot Examination of the Use of Goal Attainment Scaling with a Physically Disabled Summer Camp Population." *Therapeutic Recreation Journal* 16, no. 3 (1982), 17–24.

DAVIS, WALTER E. "Motor Ability Assessment of Populations with Handicapping Conditions: Challenging Basic Assumptions." *Adapted Physical Activity Quarterly* 1, no. 2 (1984), 125–40.

ELLIS, GARY D., and SHARON NILES. "Development, Reliability and Preliminary Validation of a Brief Leisure Rating Scale." *Therapeutic Recreation Journal* 18, no. 1 (1985), 50–61.

HATFIELD, DICK. "Selected Bibliography and Glossary on DRG's Prospective Pricing." *Therapeutic Recreation Journal* 18, no. 4 (1984), 56–61.

HOFFMAN, MICHAEL B. "Recreative Therapy: A Prescriptive Approach." *Therapeutic Recreation Journal* 15, no. 3 (1981), 16–21.

HOWE, CHRISTINE Z. "Leisure Assessment Instrumentation in Therapeutic Recreation." *Therapeutic Recreation Journal* 18, no. 2 (1984), 14–24.

HUNTER, I. ROY, RONALD P. REYNOLDS, and M. LAURA WILLIAMS. "The Elaboration Model in Adapted Activity Research: Increasing the Programmatic Value of Program Evaluations." *Adapted Physical Activity Quarterly* 1, no. 1 (1984), 12–18.

JEWELL, DAVID L. "Documentation: Shibboleth for Professionalism." *Therapeutic Recreation Journal* 14, no. 1 (1980), 23–29.

KENNEDY, DAN W. "Using the Leisure Activities Blank with Spinal Cord Injured Persons: A Field Study." *Adapted Physical Activity Quarterly* 2, no. 3 (1985), 182–88.

——, and HERBERTA M. LUNDEGREN. "Application of the Discrepancy Evaluation Model in Therapeutic Recreation." *Therapeutic Recreation Journal* 15, no. 1 (1981), 24–34.

KREY, RUSSELL, and SHARON KREY. *Activity Therapy: An Innovative Approach to Individual Program Planning.* Provo, Utah: Dana Press, 1977.

KRUG, JAMES L. "A Review of Perceptual Motor/Sensory Integrative Measurement Tools." *Therapeutic Recreation Journal* 13, no. 3 (1979), 41–43.

LEVY, JOSEPH. "Behavioral Observation. Techniques in Assessing Change in Therapeutic Recreation/Play Settings." *Therapeutic Recreation Journal* 16, no. 1 (1982), 25–32.

MAGER, ROBERT F. *Preparing Instructional Objectives* (2nd ed.). Belmont, Calif.: Fearon Publishers, 1977.

——, *Goal Analysis.* Belmont, Calif.: Fearon Publishers, 1972.

MCDONALD, JESSYNA M. "Special Adaptive Recreation as Intervention in Vocational and Transitional Services for Handicapped Youth." *Therapeutic Recreation Journal* 19, no. 3 (1985), 17–27.

NAVAR, NANCY. "Leisure Skill Assessment Process in Leisure Counseling," in *Expanding Horizons in Therapeutic Recreation VI.* Ed. David J. Szymanski and Gerald L. Hitzhusen, pp. 68–94. Columbia: Department of Recreation and Park Administration, University of Missouri, 1979.

PARKER, ROBERT, and others. "The Comprehensive Evaluation in Recreation Therapy Scale: A Tool for Patient Evaluation." *Therapeutic Recreation Journal* 9, no. 4 (1975), 143–52.

PETERSON, CAROL A. "Application of Systems Analysis Procedures to Program Planning in Therapeutic Recreation Service." In *Therapeutic Recreation Service: An Applied Behavioral Science Approach,* ed. Elliott Avedon, Englewood Cliffs, N.J.: Prentice-Hall, 1974, pp. 128–55.

——, and SCOUT LEE GUNN. *Therapeutic Recreation Program Design: Principles and Procedures* (2nd ed.). Englewood Cliffs, N.J.: Prentice-Hall, 1984.

PLOWMAN, P. D. *Behavioral Objectives*. Chicago: Science Research Associates, 1971.

POPOVICH, D. *A Prescriptive Behavioral Checklist for the Severely and Profoundly Retarded*. Baltimore: University Park Press, 1977.

RILEY, ROBERT, ed. *Evaluation of Therapeutic Recreation through Quality Assurance*. State College, Penn.: Venture Publishing, Inc., 1987.

RUESCH, JURGEN. *Therapeutic Communication*. New York: W. W. Norton & Co., 1961.

STUMBO, NORMA J. "Systematic Observation as a Research Tool for Assessing Client Behavior." *Therapeutic Recreation Journal* 17, no. 4 (1983), 53–63.

TOUCHSTONE, WILLIAM A. "The Status of Client Evaluation within Psychiatric Settings." *Therapeutic Recreation Journal* 9, no. 4 (1975), 166–72.

VALE, WALLACE H., and SYLVESTER R. MLOTT. "An Assessment of Treatment Enjoyment and Effectiveness in Psychiatric Hospitalization." *Therapeutic Recreation Journal* 17, no. 1 (1983), 26–32.

7

Medical-Clinical Model

The medical-clinical model is in reality the general medical and surgical hospital (GM&S). Associated with this model/hospital, directly or indirectly, may be a medical or physical rehabilitation unit or facility as well as a psychiatric unit. It is the GM&S hospital that physicians in private practice turn to for the care and treatment of their patients. The model is primarily concerned with the alleviation or minimization through medical and/or surgical management of the acute disease process or trauma. The medical or physical rehabilitation unit provides services for those with altered levels of health and/or disability following the critical phase of treatment. As we noted in Chapter 3, such a unit may be an integral part of the model/hospital or may be a free-standing public or nonprofit facility designed to serve all physicians and all hospitals within a specific geographic area but have no direct affiliation with hospitals. (Consideration of the psychiatric unit, its philosophy, and its patients is found in Chapter 9.)

It is important to distinguish the orientation of medicine and surgery in general from that of rehabilitation medicine. Medicine and surgery are oriented primarily toward organic pathology, and their objectives are the treatment and the reversal of pathology to achieve cure. In incurable diseases the objective is the slowing down or remission of the pathologic process and the prolongation of life. On the other hand, medical or physical rehabilitation is concerned with the preservation and restoration of function of any part of the individual or the individual as a whole.

It is also important to recognize that a fine line exists in this orientation. Rehabilitation is an integral part of *all* phases of patient care and treatment; it is not a specific end product to be approached when the acute phase passes or where definitive treatment leaves off. Waiting until the acute phase passes before applying appropriate principles of rehabilitation care is contrary to the concept of quality care, often prolongs the acute-care phase, and exaggerates the concept of illness for the patient and family. Principles of rehabilitation therefore are applied in varying situations and are not confined to the specific rehabilitation unit or facility.

The course of events in this model/hospital resulting from an injury, disease, or congenital disorder as one moves from the medical and/or surgical service into rehabilitation is somewhat as follows. Usually, a severely injured person who first receives treatment in an emergency department proceeds to an intensive-care unit of the hospital or a unit for acute medical or surgical management. In the case of a person with a severe illness or congenital disorder, specialized diagnostic tests and other studies may be required initially. If the findings suggest surgical treatment, the next station is the operating room, followed by intensive care for a day or more. (The most common or frequently caused injuries, diseases, or congenital disorders are those associated with the nervous system, the musculoskeletal system, and the cardiopulmonary system.) In the larger and more comprehensive hospitals regardless of injury, disease, or congenital disorder, planning for rehabilitation is started prior to or immediately following the medical or surgical procedure. Such planning eventually leads to rehabilitative action that may start on the specific medical or surgical service and proceed to the more specialized rehabilitation unit or facility.

Basically, the candidate for medical reha-

bilitation following a medical or surgical procedure, either on the service unit or in the rehabilitation unit, usually needs three types of help:

1. Physical measures, such as active exercise, passive mobilization, and proper positioning
2. Mechanical devices, including splints, braces, prostheses, wheel-chairs, and many self-help devices
3. Education, counseling, and other psychosocial services[1]

Therapeutic recreation, as we will shortly note, may be involved in two of the three types of help.

With this brief introduction to the medical-clinical model, let us now consider the use of therapeutic recreation service in this model. Initially we will consider the delivery of therapeutic recreation service to two patients receiving acute care. Then we will follow the referral of one patient to the medical rehabilitation unit for continued treatment and rehabilitation.

ACUTE CARE AND TREATMENT

The delivery of therapeutic recreation service in acute care and treatment varies from hospital to hospital. In general, it is limited to specific services within medical and surgical services (i.e., orthopedics, pediatrics, obstetrics and gynecology, neurosurgery, cardiac/pulmonary surgery, oncology, general medicine and so on). Where therapeutic recreation service is provided, the program of services may be treatment oriented or diversional. In some hospitals the patient's physician may request therapeutic recreation service through a referral. Such a referral may be treatment-directed or diversional. In other hospitals the various medical/surgical services may have their own treatment team, which makes a referral for therapeutic recreation service. And in still other hospi-

tals therapeutic recreation service may be an ongoing diversional service on a specific service, e.g., pediatrics. In some settings all these approaches to services may be functioning. Regardless of who makes the referral, the approach to care and treatment or diversional services demands the therapeutic recreation specialist's ability to assess, plan, implement, and evaluate a plan of service that addresses the physical, emotional, social, and recreational needs of the patient jointly or separately.

ASSESSMENT

Assessment, as we have noted, is the gathering of data—subjective and objective to determine goals and objectives. The assessment begins with a referral.

Referral

The assessment of any patient receiving acute care begins with a referral from the physician or treatment team. No patient may be treated in a medical-surgical unit by a therapeutic recreation specialist without a medical referral. (This is also true for other allied health or activity therapists, namely, physical therapists, etc.) The referral may be a simple one for short-term treatment, or it may involve a complex and changing program for the severely ill person. In any case the referral should be concise, clear, specific, and individualized. The suitability of the referral and the effectiveness of the therapy are in large measure dependent on the physician's interest and knowledge of our field and the ability of the physician to work well with the specialist.

Referral Purposes. There are several important purposes of a detailed, specific referral:

It provides the therapeutic recreation specialist with basic aims and specific directions for treating patients.

It is designed to assure physicians that their orders will be followed and that misunderstanding between physician and specialist will not develop.

It provides a permanent record of the treatment prescribed and administered. (Such records are valuable for use in the future care of a patient and in insurance compensation.)

It serves to protect both physician and specialist in cases of medico-legal complications.

Referral Information. In general, the referral should include the patient's name, age, sex, and diagnosis. The medical history may be stated in brief, but usually this can be obtained from the patient's medical chart and sometimes in part from the patient. The physician will indicate the patient's present condition or problem. The objectives to be achieved may be specified. If not, consultation with the physician or treatment team will be necessary. Any precautions to be observed will usually be noted. The frequency and duration of treatment may also be included. It is not customary for the physician or team to indicate the activity or activities to be used to achieve the desired results; the activity or activities chosen are based on the professional knowledge and judgment of the specialist.

The referral will not include all the information needed to develop a treatment plan; therefore, the specialist will usually have to supplement knowledge of the patient's condition by reading the medical chart, by personal evaluation of the patient, and by discussion with other members of the treatment team. However, the referral should contain sufficient information for the specialist to proceed efficiently and with assurance.

The following two cases and discussion demonstrate, in a very limited fashion, the therapeutic recreation process in action. The initial discussion considers the basic knowledge the specialist has of the medical conditions presented in the specific cases, followed by an observation assessment of the patients. There are facts available to the specialist as a result of textbook and clinical knowledge, and these are areas that need to be investigated or discovered. The student should realize that many different and varied medical patterns and problems exist regarding the medical conditions presented here and that all such problems cannot be presented. Further, as information is gathered and analyzed, it is stored in a computer to be used eventually in the development of the treatment plan.

Case One

A fifty-seven-year-old male hemiplegia left side with minimal aphasia resulting from a cerebrovascular accident (stroke) is referred to therapeutic recreation services for activity to reduce intellectual regression and improve emotional feelings. Services are to be provided daily.

Case Two

A fifty-one-year-old male stricken with an uncomplicated myocardial infarction (MI) is referred to therapeutic recreation service for activities that will reduce anxiety associated with an increase of blood pressure causing increased cardiac work. Activity should be at the II level daily.

Data Collection

In data collection the specific physical, emotional, and social abilities and limitations of the patient are paramount for therapeutic recreation intervention on medical and surgical services. To assume certain abilities and limitations because of a stated pathophysiologic diagnosis is unfair to the patient. Few patients display a textbook picture; therefore, the abilities and limitations belong to the patient and not to the diagnosis.

Specialist's Knowledge—Case One. From the referral the specialist knows that a stroke is caused by an interruption of the blood supply to the brain due to a thrombus, an embolus, or a hemorrhage, and that the resulting symptoms reflect the location of the lesion. Further, the specialist knows that a careful assessment is necessary since the problems associated with a stroke are complex and include not only motor loss caused by the lesion and the physiological complications that develop secondary to the insult, but also problems having to do with sensorimotor function, intellectual function, communication and emotional function as well as family, social, and vocational adjustment. For example, five often complex neurological complications associated with hemiplegia (sometimes referred to as the Five As of hemiplegia) are aphasia, agnosia, apraxia, agraphia, and alexia.

The specialist knows that at the time of admission or shortly thereafter most stroke patients are helpless and may be in severe shock; however, their condition usually stabilizes within the first few days after the accident (although some get worse and die). Further, since the left side is affected in this case, it is not uncommon that aphasia occurs. General medical management in the acute phase is provided to maintain life, and as soon as the patient's condition allows, rehabilitation efforts will start. The specialist also realizes that the essential aim of early rehabilitation is to prevent complications. Unless appropriate preventive measures are initiated at the onset or within a day or two after admission, the patient may suffer severe and irreversible complications. If complications are not ameliorated, the patient's rehabilitation efforts could be permanently impeded. Further, preventive measures are directed not only toward the paralyzed muscles but toward the unaffected muscles to prevent atrophy in the uninvolved areas. In addition, the specialist is aware that there are emotional and psychological changes that take place as a result of sensory and motor disturbances, intellectual deterioration, and the general loss of self-respect and dignity. According to some authors, depression and self-concept are major psychological problems associated with conditions causing physical impairment, but the intensity will vary depending on the severity of the problem.[2]

The specialist knows that the reassurance and support that a stroke patient receives in the early phase and the measures taken to prevent complications are essential for long-term progress. Early care and treatment determines whether the patient later stands, walks, and is self-sufficient. The sooner rehabilitation measures are instituted, the greater the potential for eventual independence.

Specialist's Observation—Case One. As we have noted, the diagnosis, records, interviews, and observations supply the needed information for an assessment. The records provide a history of the medical problem, complications, and the action of other therapies. The interviews and observations, including a clinical evaluation of the patient's present behavior, provide baseline data for complete assessment and development of the plan. Observations of the patient, as previously noted, include an assessment of the patient's general appearance, interpersonal interaction, motor activity, and body language.

General Appearance. Regarding our stroke patient, the general appearance tells the specialist about the general condition of the patient; the specialist's work begins with observational evaluation. By viewing the patient, the specialist can determine any grossly apparent abnormalities as well as the emotional state.

The typical position assumed by our patient, as the specialist knows, is one in which the affected arm is held close to the body with the elbows and wrist in a flexed position and the fingers and thumb flexed to form a clawlike hand. The affected lower extremity is rotated outwardly at the hip, the knee is flexed, and the foot is in the plantar flexion. The emotional reaction will vary with each patient; fear and anxiety are quite typical.

Interpersonal Interaction. Observing the patient's interpersonal behavior tells the specialist about the patient's anxiety level, acceptance or rejection of present problem, motivation, and intellectual functioning. The emotional reaction of hemiplegic patients to the loss of control of their body is in many instances overwhelming. As soon as patients regain consciousness, they begin to react to the growing awareness of restrictions to their muscle control imposed by the brain injury.[3]

The presence of depression and a feeling of dependency in our stroke patient may be manifested in several ways, such as apathy, resentment, and loss of appetite. Further, interpersonal contact with the patient tells the specialist the degree of communication problems; however, such information will also be found in the patient's medical record. In varying degrees, patients who have lost their ability to communicate (expressive aphasia) as a result of a stroke have lost the ability to understand (receptive aphasia)

their environment, the ability to structure their thought process internally in a logical and meaningful order, and the ability to formulate language in a logical and meaningful order.[4] (When both forms of aphasia are present it is referred to as global aphasia.)

Motor Activity. Evaluation of motor activity in our patient includes the patient's agility, range of motion, and ability to manage himself in association with the involved and uninvolved extremities. Evaluation of this area also gives clues regarding the patient's ability to recognize his own body or its parts, left-right discrimination, spatial relationships, and other perceptual and sensorimotor problems that may in general affect the treatment plan.[5]

Our specialist knows that in order to move an object from one place to another, many functions must be integrated at various levels of the central nervous system. Some of these include interpretation of auditory instructions; recognition of an object through visual cues; decision on choice of color and size of object when this is relevant; estimation of distance between the object, the hand, and the receptacle for the object; prehension of the object by fingers and thumb; stereognostic perception of size, texture, and weight of object; determination of the amount of power needed to move the object; and coordination of prehension and motion to deposit the object in the receptacle.

Body Language. Along with interpersonal interaction and motor activity, body language lets the specialist know how our patient uses his body to communicate his needs. While the medical records will indicate the communication problems with our particular patient, it is worthy to note again that although a patient may stop talking, the patient does not stop communicating. In fearful situations hands shake and legs tremble; in painful situations the face becomes tense and the body becomes rigid; and in happy situations the body lets the world know. The real value of body language, however, remains in its blending with the spoken word to the extent possible to convey thoughts, ideas, and feelings.

Specialist's Knowledge—Case Two. The specialist is familiar in general with the various theories as to the etiology of heart disease, and further, that personality type is a highly controversial factor in the cause and effect of coronary disease. The specialist also knows that this specific patient is beyond the critical, postmyocardial infarction period and is being treated in the coronary-care unit. The specialist realizes that the patient's anxiety is undoubtedly the result of the process of adaptation to the illness. According to some investigators, physiological coping mechanisms give way to the more insidious psychological coping mechanisms of anxiety, regression, anger, apprehension, frustration, and dependency as patients begin the process of adaptation to the illness and acceptance of what the illness means to them.[6] The specialist may or may not know that extreme anxiety alone can cause increased adrenal stimulation, which in turn will speed up ventricular contraction, decrease diastolic filling of the heart, and demand more energy output of an already-taxed heart.[7] Therefore, activities allay many fears and anxieties that could be detrimental to cardiac function. When a heart patient is doing something, that patient is able to realize progress and thus alleviate undue tensions. Lastly, the specialist knows that treatment of the acute coronary by the armchair method has sound physiological principles. Studies have demonstrated that patients in a sitting position have less cardiac output than patients in a supine or semireclining position.[8]

Specialist's Observation—Case Two. The specialist is aware of the patient's present condition and prognosis through a review of the patient's medical record. Since more information is needed before a treatment plan can be developed, the specialist visits the patient in the coronary-care unit to gather data.

General Appearance. The physiological symptoms encountered by the specialist during the initial visit included some muscular rigidity, sweating, tremulousness, and restlessness. The specialist knows that such symptoms vary with each patient and are usually the result of psychological reactions to MI. The major reaction to MI is one of shock and disbelief, resulting in fear and anxiety. Manifestations of these reactions will vary with each individual under attack. The specialist also notes a disorientation on the part of the patient when he is asked how he is feeling. However, the specialist knows that this is not unusual and will pass in a few days.

Interpersonal Interaction. At the time the specialist interviews the patient, much disorganization may be occurring in the patient's life. Although the initial acute phase of the illness has ended, the patient's needs are as great as, if not greater than, before. The specialist realizes that during this period patients are only beginning to cope with their illness; they are still reacting to the crisis and its gravity. The specialist is also aware that a patient who is attempting to react to an MI may develop a multitude of defense mechanisms, such as regression, dependency, and denial.[9]

Interpersonal Interaction provides the opportunity to acquaint the patient with therapeutic recreation service and to allow the patient to express interest and concerns about specific activities. The specialist's concern is to assist the patient to identify and pursue behaviors that are consistent with the attainment of the well role, while at the same time reducing the anxiety and depression associated with the patient's grief.

Motor Activity. The amount or degree of motor or physical activity is determined by the physician. Today, as noted before, the hazards of prolonged bed rest are well documented, and patients with uncomplicated MI progress rapidly through a super-

TABLE 7.1. Approximate Metabolic Cost of Activities*

	Occupational	Recreational
1½–2 METs** 4–7 ml O₂/min/kg 2–2½ kcal/min (70-kg person)	Desk work Auto driving⁺ Typing Electric calculating Machine operation	Standing Walking (strolling 1.6 km or 1 mile/hr) Flying,⁺ motorcycling⁺ Playing cards⁺ Sewing, knitting
2–3 METs 7–11 ml O₂/min/kg 2½–4 kcal/min (70-kg person)	Auto repair Radio, television repair Janitorial work Typing, manual Bartending	Level walking (3.2 km or 2 miles/hr) Level bicycling (8.0 km or 5 miles/hr) Riding lawn mower Billiards, bowling Skeet,⁺ shuffleboard Woodworking (light) Powerboat driving⁺ Golf (power cart) Canoeing (4 km or 2½ miles/hr) Horseback riding (walk) Playing piano and many musical instruments
3–4 METs 11–14 ml O₂/min/kg 4–5 kcal/min (70-kg person)	Brick laying, plastering Wheelbarrow (45.4-kg or 100-lb load) Machine assembly Trailer-truck in traffic Welding (moderate load) Cleaning windows	Walking (4.8 km or 3 miles/hr) Cycling (9.7 km or 6 miles/hr) Horseshoe pitching Volleyball (6 person, noncompetitive) Golf (pulling bag cart) Archery Sailing (handling small boat) Fly-fishing (standing with waders) Horseback (sitting to trot) Badminton (social doubles) Pushing light power mower Energetic musician
4–5 METs 14–18 ml O₂/min/kg 5–6 kcal/min (70-kg person)	Painting, masonry Paperhanging Light carpentry	Walking (5–6 km or 3½ miles/hr) Cycling (12.9 km or 8 miles/hr) Table tennis Golf (carrying clubs) Dancing (foxtrot) Badminton (singles) Tennis (doubles) Raking leaves Hoeing Many calisthenics
5–6 METs 18–21 ml O₂/min/kg 6–7 kcal/min (70-kg person)	Digging garden Shoveling light earth	Walking (6.4 km or 4 miles/hr) Cycling (16.1 km or 10 miles/hr) Canoeing (6.4 km or 4 miles/hr) Horseback ("posting" to trot) Stream fishing (walking in light current in waders) Ice- or roller-skating (14.5 km or 9 miles/hr)

TABLE 7.1. *(Continued)*

	Occupational	Recreational
6–7 METs 21–25 ml O₂/min/kg 7–8 kcal/min (70-kg person)	Shoveling for 10 min (4.5 kg or 10 lb)	Walking (8.0 km or 5 miles/hr) Cycling (17.7 km or 11 miles/hr) Badminton (competitive) Tennis (singles) Splitting wood Snow shoveling Hand lawn mowing Folk (square) dancing Light downhill skiing Ski touring (4.0 km or 2½ miles/hr) (loose snow) Water skiing
7–8 METs 25–28 ml O₂/min/kg 8–10 kcal/min (70-kg person)	Digging ditches Carrying 36.3 kg or 80 lb Sawing hardwood	Jogging (8.0 km or 5 miles/hr) Cycling (19.3 km or 12 miles/hr) Horseback riding (gallop) Vigorous downhill skiing Basketball Mountain climbing Ice hockey Canoeing (8.0 km or 5 miles/hr) Touch football Paddleball
8–9 METs 28–32 ml O₂/min/kg 10–11 kcal/min (70-kg person)	Shoveling for 10 min (6.4 kg or 14 lb)	Running (8.9 km or 5½ miles/hr) Cycling (20.9 km or 13 miles/hr) Ski touring (6.4 km or 4 miles/hr) (loose snow) Squash racquets (social) Handball (social) Fencing Basketball (vigorous)

10+ METs
32+ ml O₂/min/kg
11+ kcal/min
(70-kg person)
	Shoveling for 10 min
	(7.3 kg or 16 lb)
		Running 6 mph = 10 METs
		  7 mph = 11½ METs
		  8 mph = 13½ METs
		  9 mph = 15 METs
		  10 mph = 17 METs
		Ski touring (8+ km or 5+ miles/hr) (loose snow)
		Handball (competitive)
		Squash (competitive)

SOURCE: S. M. Fox, J. P. Naughton, and P. A. Gorman, *Modern Concepts in Cardiovascular Disorders* 41, no. 6 (June 1972). By permission of the American Heart Association, Inc.

*Includes resting metabolic needs

**1 MET is the energy expenditure at rest, equivalent to approximately 3.5 ml O /kg body weight/minute.

+A major excess metabolic increase may occur due to excitement, anxiety, or impatience in some of these activities, and a physician must assess his patient's psychological reactivity.

vised program of increased activity. While bed rest usually continues for three to four days following admission, some physicians will allow their patients up in a chair as soon as twenty-four hours after the infarction. In general, it is felt that if the patient is medically stable at that point, the patient is ready to begin chair-bed activities.[10] (Chairs are equipped with cut-out tables in order to carry out hand tasks.)

Activity is based on METs, a term used to describe the energy expenditure for an activity. A MET is a metabolic equivalent that can be assigned to activities regardless of a person's weight. One MET represents the energy expenditure of a person at rest; it equals approximately 3.5 ml/O_2/kg of weight per minute. The MET range according to the American Heart Association (AHA) is 1½ to 10+. However, a hospitalized MI patient is usually limited to activities with low MET levels (1 to 3 METs).[11] Table 7.1 indicates the metabolic cost of occupational and recreational activities.

Although the MET is the primary scale used, it is not the only one. Some hospitals, organizations, and physicians have developed their own or modified the one developed by the AHA. Tables 7.2 and 7.3 reflect therapeutic and functional classifications that are used in some settings.

Body Language. What is noted through body language may also be a reflection of general appearance. Our MI patient may react in a negative fashion to any suggestion about activity because of the fear associated with any activity and the possibility of pain. Anxiety, if unrelieved, will usually increase pain by increasing musculoskeletal contraction and decreasing the threshold of pain. Our patient may look and act disinterested or listless, be relatively nonverbal, talk pessimistically, and even cry. Such behaviors, as our specialist knows, are reactions to depression, which is a common symptom observed in MI patients. In males sexual aggressiveness, verbally and nonverbally, may be noted. It is a response to the patient's per-

TABLE 7.2. Functional Capacity

Class I:	Patients with cardiac disease but without resulting limitation of physical activity. Ordinary physical activity does not cause undue fatigue, palpitation (rapid beating) of the heart, dyspnea (difficult labored breathing), or anginal (suffocating) pain.
Class II:	Patients with cardiac disease resulting in slight limitation of physical activity. They are comfortable at rest. Ordinary physical activity results in fatigue, palpitation, dyspnea, or anginal pain.
Class III:	Patients with cardiac disease resulting in marked limitations of physical activity. They are comfortable at rest. Less than ordinary activity causes fatigue, palpitation, dyspnea, or anginal pain.
Class IV:	Patients with cardiac disease resulting in inability to carry on any physical activity without discomfort. Symptoms of cardiac insufficiency or of the anginal syndrome are present even at rest. If any physical activity is undertaken, discomfort is increased.

SOURCE: Jay S. Shivers and Hollis F. Fait, *Special Recreational Services: Therapeutic and Adapted* (Philadelphia: Lea and Febiger, 1985), p. 138.

ception of the illness as a threat to his masculinity. Another matter is the level of fatigue, as noted earlier, when involved in any type of activity. Fatigue can lead to pain, which increases cardiac output. The beginning signs of fatigue include increased pulse rate, dysnea, and palpitation.[12]

After the specialist has collected the needed data, the information is analyzed through the computer to complete the assessment. In these two particular cases the assessment supplies information for developing the individualized treatment plan.

PLANNING (GOAL DEVELOPMENT)

The formulation of a plan is the second phase of the therapeutic recreation process. It occurs after the assessment, yet it is definitely uppermost in the specialist's mind

TABLE 7.3. Therapeutic Classification

Class A: Patients with a cardiac disorder whose ordinary physical activity requires no restriction.

Class B: Patients with a cardiac disorder whose ordinary physical activity needs no restriction but who should be advised against severe or competitive efforts.

Class C: Patients with a cardiac disorder whose ordinary physical activity should be moderately restricted and whose more strenuous habitual efforts should be discontinued.

Class D: Patients with a cardiac disorder whose ordinary physical activity should be extremely restricted.

Class E: Patients with a cardiac disorder who should be at complete rest, that is, confined to bed.

SOURCE: Jay S. Shivers and Hollis F. Fait, *Special Recreational Services: Therapeutic and Adapted* (Philadelphia: Lea and Febiger, 1985), p. 138.

during the assessment phase. As the specialist gathers data, consideration is being given to the barriers that may prevent intervention and the activity or activities that may be used to attain the goal. It also needs repeating that the ability of the specialist to identify any barriers that stand in the way of goal attainment rests on the accuracy and completeness of the assessment. Since the goals are known because of the referral in both cases, the concern of the specialist is with identifying what stands in the way of goal attainment by examining clues to determine what action is needed to eliminate or work around the interference, thereafter, with what activity or activities can be used to reach the respective goals.

A question such as, "What are the potential barriers that may prevent Mr. X. (Case One) from participating in an activity to limit further intellectual regression?" clearly indicates what needs to be considered. Problems that are clearly stated, are unambiguous, and indicate the obstacle that prevents goal attainment provide the specialist with a definitive statement and an idea of how to approach a solution.

Taking into consideration goal development and barriers to goal attainment, let us now consider these two factors in relation to our case studies.

Goal Setting—Case One

In this case the goals, according to the referral, are reduction of intellectual regression and improvement of emotional feelings. We noted, as a result of data gathering, that a number of barriers may exist. One barrier to goal attainment may be the involved side if eventual consideration is given to an activity that incorporates the use of both arms and hands. Another barrier is limited communication as a result of the aphasia, which may affect any activity that involves communication. Still another barrier is the intellectual regression that is occurring at present. And still another barrier is the anxiety that is associated with the stroke and is reflected in depression and apathy. In addition, the case is further compounded by time. In some situations like this one, the goal must be acted upon immediately, or additional problems may develop. It is a rare problem situation that can stand too long without resolution, especially in light of DRG procedures today. Such a situation taxes the ability of the specialist where barriers exist and solutions are expected quickly.

After the specialist has analyzed the goals in relation to the obstacles, the goals or needs are recorded as the first step in developing the treatment plan (even though goals are already known).

An initial treatment plan in relation to our stroke patient may read as follows:

Assessment: Hemiplegia left side
Problems: Loss of physical functioning (paralysis) left side
             Limited aphasia with ability to understand commands and gestures although speech is slurred and hesitant
             Intellectual regression

Goal: Depression and apathy resulting from anxiety about condition
To reduce intellectual regression
To increase positive emotional feelings

After giving attention to the problems and goals, consideration is given to activity or activities that will be used to achieve goal attainment. The use of specific activities in a treatment-oriented plan requires the specialist not only to critically analyze the considered activities in relation to their basic requirements and demands in association with the illness, but also to determine the risk, value, and consequence of the activity as a means of meeting the intent of the referral and the problems identified by the assessment. Such a situation offers a great challenge.

Although past experience and/or knowledge provide guidelines to suggest what will lead to the desired activity or activities, such activity or activities are in the end influenced by (1) various behavioral areas (physical, emotional, mental, and social); (2) accomplishing the preferred intent; (3) the absence of harmful side effects or aftereffects; and (4) the most efficient and appropriate way to meet the preferred goal. Such so-called guidelines as these provide the specialist with a means for making a decision.

After a review of the assessment problems and goals, as well as an analysis of the activities that may contribute to goal attainment, the specialist selects the activity or activities. For the stroke patient the following activities have been selected to meet the goals of the referral:

Goal: To reduce intellectual regression
Activity: Audio cassette "NewsCurrent"[13]

Goal: To increase positive emotional feelings
Activity: Checkers

As we noted in the previous chapter, once the activity or activities have been selected and deemed the best approach to meeting the need or goal of the referral, a means of evaluating the delivery of therapeutic recreation service is necessary. In brief, the final phase of the planning process is the creation of specific behavioral objectives. If the specialist's plan of action is to help the patient meet a need, then the expected outcome of the plan describes how the patient will look, feel, or be after the plan has been implemented. Relative to the stroke patient, the specialist is concerned with seeing the patient demonstrate behavior that reflects an increase in intellectual behavior and an improved emotional feeling. Having determined those behaviors that are appropriate for the stroke patient, the specialist is ready to write the terminal behaviors into the plan.

Goal: To reduce intellectual regression
Activity: Audio cassette "News-Current"
Behavioral objective: After listening to one of three current-event cassettes each day for three days, the patient will verbally respond correctly to five of the seven questions asked at the easy level on the first day and at the intermediate level on the second and third days.

Goal: To increase positive emotional feelings
Activity: Checkers
Behavioral objective: The patient will complete one game per day with the specialist for three days using the uninvolved arm and hand.

Goal Setting—Case Two

During the assessment of our MI patient, the specialist recognizes the patient's strong psychological reactions to his MI, including the use of various defense mechanisms. The specialist realizes that regression or withdrawal into helplessness can lead to total dependency on others, and further, that such behavior can lead eventually to chronic invalidism; likewise, that denial may become pathological. The display of these behaviors interferes with rehabilitation. Lastly, the specialist is quite aware that the patient is expending considerable energy in coping with his anxiety and coming to grips with reality. But at the same time the specialist knows that activities started early in the recovery phase can do much to prevent the development of problems such as regression and anxiety.

As in the previous case, even though goals are known and obstacles noted, the specialist begins to formulate a treatment plan as follows:

Assessment: Myocardial Infarction (intramural/posterior)

Problems: Anxiety associated with attack
Fear of the unknown
Limited disorientation
Limited muscular rigidity
Restlessness
Communication depressing

Goal: To reduce anxiety
To increase positive communication
To stimulate him to take part in his recovery and rehabilitation
To assess potential leisure experiences for future planning and rehabilitation
To assist the patient to begin to identify leisure behaviors that are consistent with attainment of well role

The reader will note that more goals have been proposed than were indicated by the physician in the referral. This is not uncommon and is usually encouraged if the additional goals do not distract from the overall treatment plan for the patient. The additional goals are the result of the assessment, wherein the specialist uncovered additional needs associated directly and indirectly with the patient. They are also the result of the specialist's knowledge about the care, treatment, and rehabilitation of the patient in the unit. The specialist is aware that the DRG for an uncomplicated MI patient is approximately 9.8 days, and that the patient will be discharged directly to his home with a referral to a cardiovascular wellness exercise program.[14] Prior to the discharge, the specialist knows that the patient will participate in a teaching-learning care program that will cover medications, diet, activity graduations and restrictions, and risk factors and teach him how to monitor himself.

What the specialist has done relative to the referred goal and those uncovered is to set priorities. Priority setting refers to the act of giving preferential attention to one thing over competing alternatives. Priority setting enables the specialist to organize and plan the treatment program to meet those goals that are most urgent and to consider ways of handling the goals of lesser urgency. Priority setting does not negate the importance of the lower-priority goals; it simply puts goals into a realistic framework for consideration and solution. As high-level goals are met, lower-level goals shift upward. Many factors, unfortunately, affect priority setting: people, policy, money, time, and goals. These factors, the specialist knows, often determine the priority of goals in a treatment plan.

Turning our attention to the activity selection for our MI patient, the specialist knows that activity for this patient needs to be very limited and will incorporate intellectual or passive activities with frequent rest periods. Activities that use upper-body movement, although requiring only a limited range of motion, use too much motion, strength, and pressure. As the patient improves and the internist revises the referral, a program of increased activity can be gradually initiated.

The activities planned by the specialist to meet the goals of the MI patient are as follows:

Goal: To reduce anxiety
Activity: Leather-belt assembly (kit)

Goal: To increase positive communication
Activity: Leather-belt assembly (kit)

Goal: To stimulate him to take part in his recovery and rehabilitation
Activity: Leather-belt assembly (kit)

Goal: To assess potential leisure experi-
            ences for future planning and reha-
            bilitation
Activity: Leather-belt assembly (kit)

Goal: To assist the patient to begin to iden-
            tify leisure behaviors that are consis-
            tent with attainment of well role
Activity: Leather-belt assembly

Having determined the goals and activities to reach goal attainment, it now becomes necessary for the specialist to devise
a plan for evaluation. This plan, as noted
earlier, is composed of a description of the
terminal expectations. It is well to remember that the use of measurable criteria for
evaluation of therapeutic recreation services
provides predictability to the therapeutic
recreation actions and reliability to the evaluation. When the criteria for performance
are stated in behavioral terms, evaluation is
relatively simple. Further, other health personnel can recognize the desired behavior
when it is stated in behavioral terms,
thereby providing additional objectivity to
the evaluation. In sum, the more measurable and objective the criteria, the more reliable the evaluation will be; and the more
clearly the criteria are stated in behavioral
terms, the more probable it is that the specialist will be able to evaluate the therapeutic recreation service and action quickly.

Goal: To reduce anxiety
Activity: Leather-belt assembly kit
Behavioral   The patient will assemble a belt
objective: within three days after initiating
             the activity.

Goal: To increase positive communica-
             tion
Activity: Leather-belt assembly
Behavioral   The patient during the activity will
objective: engage in appropriate conversation
             with the specialist as judged appro-
             priate by the specialist.

Goal: To stimulate him to take a part in
             his recovery and rehabilitation

Activity: Leather-belt assembly
Behavioral   The patient will complete the
objective: leather belt within three days as
             well as cooperating in other treat-
             ment procedures as deemed appro-
             priate by staff.

Goal: To assess potential leisure experi-
             ences for future planning and reha-
             bilitation
Activity: Leather-belt assembly
Behavioral   The patient during the activity will
objective: discuss with the specialist activities
             he has engaged in since adoles-
             cence.

Goal: To assist the patient to begin to
             identify leisure behaviors that are
             consistent with attainment of well
             role
Activity: Leather-belt assembly
Behavioral   The patient will identify ten be-
objective: haviors that are consistent with the
             well role as judged appropriate by
             the specialist.

The selection of a leather-belt assembly
kit as an activity while the patient is sitting
goes along with the concept of protecting
the patient against excessive myocardial effect in the acute and postacute stages of his
disease. The performance of small hand activities at the "minimal," or 1.25 METs,
level while the patient is sitting assist in decreasing anxieties associated with the disease and reduces the work of the heart. During the first week the patient's exposure to
cardiac work is usually kept minimal. As the
patient begins to move into the convalescence stage and predischarge planning, the
progression from minimal to light activity
for increasingly longer periods can be initiated.

The selection of the leather-belt kit also
has the advantage of allowing the specialist
to discuss with the patient a variety of topics
once the patient has learned the assembly
procedures. Other activities, such as listening to music or working a crossword puzzle,
could have been used but they require concentration and might interfere with gather-

ing information for use in leisure counseling and discharge planning. However, such activities can be recommended for use to reduce boredom while patients are alone in their room or between tests or therapy sessions.

Before moving on to the implementation phase, it is important to refer to why therapeutic exercises as activities were not incorporated into the plan since it was quite obvious that exercises, even though they may have been limited, would be excellent activities for both patients. In the critical acute stages of treatment, therapeutic exercises, unless contraindicated, fall into the realm of nursing responsibility—if not nursing, then physical therapy and possibly occupational therapy when concerned with the upper extremity. This is not to say that the therapeutic recreation specialist does not know range-of-motion exercises, cannot learn the exercises, or does not provide such a service; rather, it is founded on tradition of treatment responsibilities of the respective disciplines. In some settings specialists do provide the service, but such a service is limited. However, therapeutic recreation specialists become more involved in exercise programs as the patient becomes less bedfast.

IMPLEMENTATION

As we begin consideration of implementation we must keep in mind that implementation involves more than just implementing a plan. There are any number of dimensions to the plan, which greatly increases its effectiveness. This section therefore identifies and discusses dimensions or factors and conditions associated with implementation. Coupled with the dimensions considered in Chapter 6 under implementation, these dimensions enhance the application of the total implementation phase. These additional dimensions include continuity of care, communication, and intervention strategies.

Continuity of Care

When more than one person or discipline is involved in the delivery of care and treatment, more than one treatment plan is developed. A written treatment plan by each of those involved in the treatment is absolutely essential if duplication, omissions, and errors are to be avoided. In relation to the two case studies, four or five disciplines will be involved. When the nurse, physical therapist, therapeutic recreation specialist, occupational therapist, and inhalation therapist, for example, have developed their respective treatment plans and entered them in the chart, continuity of care and treatment can be expected. Unless a unified approach is used, patient treatment, energy, comfort, and dignity may not be preserved, the patient may become confused, and a lack of progress will be noted in the patient. When all disciplines involved are aware of the treatment plan, the patient is provided with consistent approaches, and goals for all therapies are more likely to be met.

It must also be remembered that if more than one person or discipline are involved in treatment, a sequence of treatment must be established. Otherwise, all therapists may decide to provide treatment at the same period of time. Timing and synchronizing schedules, conveying information, and making proper preparation for treatment affect the success of the treatment plan. However, in order for sequence of treatment to occur, systematic communication must be practiced among those involved.

Communicating the Plan

One of the most important and vital purposes of the treatment plan is its use as a communicative tool. The treatment plan conveys accurate information about the status of the patient and is therefore one way of alleviating hearsay and distortions in verbal communication. The written plan of the specialist provides information to many persons: the physician, the nurse, other team members, and all other personnel involved in the patient's care and treatment. In turn, the plans of these others provide the specialist with information about the patient. A glance at the respective plans orients all involved to the situation. From one perspective, the plans act as a relay system; the plans indicate the goals, the kinds of approaches to treatment used in the therapies, and the patient's response to treatment, and they record changes in the patient's condition (through charting or separate progress notes).

Whenever possible, a dialogue among those involved in treatment strengthens the treatment process and helps ensure continuity of care. When therapists pool data to identify new problems or to modify approaches, a sense of satisfaction develops as contributions are accepted and ideas incorporated. By listening and conferring with one another to further develop and implement the treatment plan, each therapist begins to see how the pieces fit—how the approach of one therapist coupled with the scientific knowledge of another provides a more comprehensive picture. Such sharing of ideas, observations, and suggestions creates a sense of responsibility in the various therapists for the delivery of services. As a result, the patient benefits. But for this to occur, the plan must be available—oral and written.

Intervention Strategies

The effectiveness of the therapeutic transaction between specialist and patient may well depend upon how well the specialist understands and functions in the intervention. Understanding a given patient becomes grounded in the critical, evaluative perception of the patient as that patient functions in relation to the particular limitations and as the patient interacts with those who occupy his or her social world.

Patient Attitudes. Few of us stop to consider how well adapted our bodily design is to the functions it performs. Indeed, so dependent upon the accomplishment of seemingly ordinary skills and functions do we become that we have great difficulty in adapting to any limitations of these functions. To lose or be threatened with the loss of a complex, coordinated, and controlled functional activity which has been achieved and integrated into our personal system is to lose or be threatened with the loss of self. According to Rubin, the loss, or threat of loss, of self is equivalent to loss of life. Emotional responses serve as warning signals of the extent of danger, and we immediately mobilize energies for self-protection and self-preservation.[15]

In the case of the MI patient, when he is asked to move about in the early stages of his illness we may very well expect weakness, but rarely do we expect such a person to be unable to marshal energy to turn from side to side or to sit up. This is a fearsome regression; if a person loses so much functional control, how much more will he lose? With every bit of functional control lost from the available personal resources, a bit of personal life space is lost.[16]

It is difficult to relay a feeling of being trapped through discussion. Many of us who enjoy photography are familiar with the work of Margaret Bourke-White, who besides her technical competence, was able to convey illuminating insights, perspectives, and viewpoints on her subjects. In order to take her pictures, she often had to strap herself into some preposterous position—under the wing of a moving airplane or at the top of a slightly swaying skyscraper. This active, competent woman was stricken with a degenerative disease that immobilized and confined her to the restricted life space of her bed for several years. When she started to recover, she wrote about her experiences with the same insight and capacity for graphic portrayal that had characterized all her work. One phrase she used to describe her feelings about the situation stands out: "I felt trapped, trapped within the boundaries of my own body."

We cannot underestimate the indispensability of motion. Each organ has a function, a movement, an action. Motion is essential for physical survival; movement is essential for physical and mental well-being. But movement, action, or function is not enough; we must be able to control it. Our stroke patient who is paralyzed on the left side is distressed and anxious. It is very nice to survive a stroke, to exist, but in itself it is not enough.

Loss of control produces shame. There is nothing shameful about any function of the body, per se. It is the inability to control it for appropriateness in time and place that produces shame. If the stroke patient inadvertently soils himself, his clothing, or his bedding, he is ashamed. If the same patient cries, he is ashamed. We expect to be in control of ourselves, especially in the simplest functions.

Enabling another to achieve control of function through activities is an important role for the specialist. The ability to function with control, to achieve what we intend, gives us a sense of high accomplishment. It is important that the specialist assist patients to find initial success. If activities are unattainable in patients' eyes, then those activities are worse than useless; they simply force the patients to recognize how far they are expected to go. The way may appear to be too long and too hazardous, and they may develop feelings of humiliation or anger.

Patient Communication.   How does the specialist talk to patients? What do we say when patients tells us that they cannot move an arm, a hand, or fingers to play a game? What do we say when they tell us that to move a particular extremity causes pain? If specialists listen, they may be helpful; the specialist may learn how to make patients comfortable or assist them to move body parts. To brush their comments aside with a routine "Yes you can, just try" is not always worthy of us. Could we say instead, "Tell me what the problem is with your arm.

Perhaps together we can consider a better body position that will help you to move your arm," or "I thought you might have trouble. Will you let me suggest a different way of moving the arm and tell me if it helps?" Then your patient knows you are sincerely interested. Assured by your manner, some of the tensions decrease, and success in participating is found.

When we as specialists respond to patients with false assurance, we are, in effect, saying their concerns are trifling, that we, in similar circumstances, would not be affected by the problems that are affecting the patients. Belittling any human being is inappropriate. Even if the concerns expressed seem groundless to us or neurotic in origin, as sometimes they are, we must remember that those concerns are just as sound and logical to the person experiencing them as any derived from actuality. The important thing to understand is that the concern *is* real to the patient.

Our role as professionals is to be kind in a thoughtful way. Sometimes a simple remark, "It must be hard" or "I can see that this isn't easy for you," is sufficient, for this in no way robs patients of their dignity. We are telling them they are not complainers; they are not bores; they are just patients with concerns.

Refusing to listen to patients describe their feelings by rushing away, interrupting, kidding, or diverting them may be done from good motives, but it is not always effective. Everyone needs an audience. To listen attentively may sound like elementary advice, but when we let our patients relieve themselves through talking, we help them more than we know. Through sharing, we dilute their misery. Is there any one of us who hasn't experienced this in some way? If someone has hurt or ridiculed you, doesn't it ease the pangs to tell your best friend about it? Conversely, try to remember a time in your life of deepest trouble. Would it have helped you then to have had someone tell you a joke? We think you know the answer.

Specialist Intervention. The never-ending challenge of coping with the many parameters of human behavior constantly stimulates and motivates specialists to improve their methods of intervention. The reader is encouraged to review the two cases and provide additional dimensions to the recorded comments.

Case One

The initial interaction of presenting the "News Current" activity was met with some confusion on the part of the patient, even though the patient had responded with a "Hello" when the specialist entered the room. As the specialist spoke to the patient about the first activity, she saw an anxious, frightened man with tense, taut muscles. However, as she began to explain the activity and to adjust the sitting position of the patient in bed, she noted that the patient had relaxed a bit and had accepted the audiophone. Even though the patient was anxious, he answered correctly five of the seven questions. Because of speech limitations the specialist had come prepared with pencil and paper and had even revised the questions so they could be answered verbally or nonverbally in a yes-or-no fashion. Noting the fatigue of the patient following the initial activity, she did not begin the second activity.

On the second and third days of treatment both activities were conducted successfully. During these two days the patient became more independent in his participation. Throughout the entire effort the specialist encouraged the patient to participate actively and continually evaluated his response to the activities. In addition, the specialist continued to listen to him regarding any regression in intellect or physical state.

Following each day's treatment program, the specialist noted the reaction and progress of the patient to treatment in the patient's chart. Over the next few days the behavior of the patient improved and he was no longer preoccupied with fear and pessimism but saw himself as increasingly capable of handling the demands of his situation. Moreover, treatment plans were revised, and eventually the patient was referred to the rehabilitation department.

The rationale for our use of a hemiplegic patient as a case study is quite easy to explain. It is one of the more frequent neurological disabilities that a therapeutic recreation specialist will encounter in a GM&S hospital or a long-term care facility (nursing home). It affects all age groups although it occurs most often in later life. Hemiplegia also offers the most complex problems of rehabilitation because brain involvement often gives rise to many additional disabilities, because prognosis is difficult to assess, and because elderly patients often have few resources and little to motivate them positively toward recovery.[17]

Case Two

As the specialist entered the room, the nurse was in the process of trying to transfer the patient from the bed to an armchair. However, the patient indicated he did not need help since the physical therapist had taught him how to transfer to a chair. Both the specialist and nurse praised the patient for his successful transfer. Thereafter, the nurse left the room, and the specialist adjusted the cut-out table to the chair.

The introduction of the activity presented no problem, and the patient participated freely and with some enthusiasm, even though he frequently asked about the potential harmful effects of the activity on his heart. During the activity the specialist noted any signs of fatigue, expressed either verbally or nonverbally, and initiated rest periods. Following the activity, the patient commented about how good he felt. In the opinion of the specialist, the treatment visit was profitable and revealing. Of particular note for all therapists was that the patient indicated he was accustomed to being independent but at the same time was aware of future limitations. The specialist encouraged him to participate to the best of his ability in all therapies, as well as informing him that before discharge the specialist would be involved with him in the teaching-learning program which would explore postdischarge leisure experiences. In addition, the patient began to indicate his leisure interests during this treatment session.

As the patient improved, the various treatment programs of gradually increased activity enabled him to regain strength and confidence. Encouraged by his increasing ability, he accepted more readily the various therapies while reducing his aggression; he became more accepting of his illness and the required restrictions and generally took on the glow of successful recovery. Prior to discharge the patient became involved in the predischarge teaching-learning program. At that time the specialist discussed his leisure interests, allaying anxieties and emotional fears about the activities, and provided a list of community resources with activities of interest to him. During the time allocated for leisure counseling the patient gave many clues to the fact that his leisure concern was whether or not he would be successful in returning to his golf game and when he could do so. Since the patient was being referred to the local cardiac rehabilitation wellness center, the leisure information gathered about him was sent there. Although his progress to complete recovery will be long, the successful participation in the various therapies is in a positive direction, promising to all team members but especially to the patient.

Those who provide therapeutic recreation service to individuals with cardiovascular problems need to keep in mind that the capacity of the normal heart to do work far exceeds the work requirement under basal conditions or during ordinary light activity. In persons who are not in good physical condition because of illness or age, the maximal working capacity of the heart is greatly reduced.[18]

The difference between the capacity of the heart to do work and the demand for cardiac work is called the *cardiac reserve*. With age and heart disease the cardiac reserve is reduced. During prolonged extensive physical activity above light levels the cardiac capacity to do work is reduced by fatigue in proportion to the intensity and the duration of the activity.[19] Therefore, the conditions of work or leisure activities and the intervals of rest as well as the condition of the myocardium influence cardiac reserve.

Successful management of the patient with cardiac disease depends upon keeping the load imposed upon the heart below the cardiac capacity so that the patient maintains an adequate cardiac reserve.[20]

In myocardial disease fatigue during muscular effort, regardless of how little, occurs more rapidly than it does in a heart in good condition. Consequently, the amount and duration of effort must be less, and the period of rest during which recovery can occur must be longer.

For the patient who has just experienced a MI, a program must be planned that will eventually restore the patient to the greatest usefulness possible with a damaged heart. The initial care of the cardiac patient will include the beginning steps of the rehabilitation program anticipating the return of the patient to his or her home, work, and leisure activities. This program of restoration is long and involved. While the physician will make decisions during the acute and convalescent stage of the illness regarding activity limitation, it is imperative at the same time that the therapeutic recreation specialist know the relative cardiac stresses imposed by various activities not only in relation to those used in the treatment plan but in counseling the patient against activities that cause excessive cardiac stress.

EVALUATION

Evaluation, as we have noted, is an ongoing process. Evaluation involves a reflecting or looking back at the actions taken to determine how effective they were in terms of patient behavior change; it identifies the specific changes in the patient's behavior patterns as they relate to the patient's ability to overcome problems and satisfy needs. Further, unless evaluation takes place, no one will know which actions produced the desired effects.

Because therapeutic recreation service is just beginning to provide such service in medical-surgical departments, evaluation models are not available; therefore, the therapeutic recreation specialist must become an astute observer, a purposeful listener, and a communicator, verbally and nonverbally. In fact, structured evaluation models as such may be difficult to develop since time is an important element relative to treatment and length of stay (DRG) of patients in some medical-surgical departments. Relative to the three elements of observation, listening, and communication in Case One, the interactions suggest that the approach used by the specialist was effective in obtaining patient participation. The specialist was prepared for the challenge of communicating with one who might not be able to or want to communicate. The fact that the patient progressed to a point where he could handle demands of the situation illustrates the effectiveness of the approaches used by those caring for him, including the therapeutic recreation specialist. The patient's referral to the rehabilitation department also indicates obvious progress as a result of successful treatment.

Case Two is a good illustration of how subjective feelings about participating tell the specialist how one aspect of the treatment plan is progressing. Further, by the patient's demonstrating desired behavioral changes, the specialist and other health personnel have evidence that the behavioral objectives are in the process of being met. This case also shows the importance of coping with problems of a physical and psychosocial nature that affect the patient after discharge. Astute listening to the patient's fears and concerns as he prepares to go home from the hospital will provide the specialist with cues that can help the specialist plan with the patient for anticipated eventualities.

It bears repeating that there is no stereotyped, *one way only* to proceed through the phases of the therapeutic recreation process, nor is there a definite pattern to follow in moving back and forth between different phases. These are factors that are determined according to the needs of the patient in each situation and the abilities of the specialist.

MEDICAL REHABILITATION DEPARTMENT

Medical rehabilitation, according to Rusk, has frequently been termed the third phase of medicine, following preventive medicine and curative medicine and surgery.[21] There are, of course, elements of medical rehabilitation in preventive medicine and in curative medicine and surgery, as we have noted, just as elements of the latter are present in medical rehabilitation.

There are many definitions of medical rehabilitation. A review of these definitions, for the most part, would lead to a definition as follows: Medical rehabilitation is a clinical process designed to help disabled persons make maximal use of their residual capacities and to enable them to obtain satisfaction and usefulness in terms of themselves, their families, and their community. Although medical rehabilitation is especially concerned with the disabled, the concepts and the techniques of rehabilitation, as we have noted in this and previous chapters and will continue to note, are also applicable in every phase of care and treatment of the acutely and chronically ill.[22]

The practice of physical medicine and rehabilitation has grown rapidly during the past four or five decades because of the changing concepts with regard to the approach modern physicians take in treating their patients. Today physicians realize that they must be concerned not only with the physiological process of the disease but also with the psychological, social, and vocational problems of the patient.

ACTIVITIES OF DAILY LIVING

Rehabilitation medicine strives to develop whatever potential abilities a person may have, regardless of physical or psychological impairment. Therefore, methods have been developed for the disabled to appraise and to improve those activities that are generally carried out by normal persons in their daily routine. In the terminology of rehabilitation these are called Activities of Daily Living (ADL). It is impossible to consider in any depth the elements associated with the concept of ADL. In brief, they include mobility, self-care, and communication.

The achievement of mobility is of considerable importance in rehabilitation. Patient mobility serves at least three purposes: (1) a physiological purpose, namely, to prevent disease phenomena; (2) a psychological purpose, namely, to stimulate and motivate the patient; and (3) a rehabilitative purpose, that is, to enable the patient to carry out activities of daily living, including those activities required for recreation and for work.[23]

Students working in rehabilitation need to become familiar with transfer techniques—the displacement of the patient from one piece of furniture or equipment to another (bed to chair or bed to wheelchair), wheelchair locomotion, ambulation aids including crutch gaits, and the various types of prostheses. Publications containing this information are found in the Suggested Readings following this chapter. However, a quicker method of obtaining the information is to request it from your local community hospital if they have a rehabilitation department or physical/occupational therapy department, since they usually have instructional material that they give their patients upon discharge. If the rehabilitation facility is freestanding, regardless of type, they will usually have instructional material for their clients. You might want to consider inviting a staff member to give a demonstration to your class in these matters.

Self-care is the ability to carry out unassisted the ordinary activities of personal care, such as feeding, dressing, and bathing. The various methods used to restore a patient to self-care include physical conditioning techniques to increase strength and range of motion, training instructions in self-care methods by circumventing disabil-

ity, use of assistive devices, and use of adapted equipment and modification of living arrangements.[24]

One of the greatest challenges in rehabilitation, according to Porch, are the patients who desire to communicate but are unable to do so because of a serious breakdown in their communication system. In such cases it requires great diligence and creativity to reestablish communication.[25] Communication defects, including speech and hearing, often are difficult to analyze and require specialized services.

REHABILITATION TEAM

Effective rehabilitation depends upon the skills and services of members of many professions. In the more comprehensive health-care facilities that have a medical rehabilitation department or unit, a physician who has specialized in physical medicine and rehabilitation is usually in charge. The designation *physiatrist* is the term commonly applied to the specialist in this field. This term derives from the Greek words *physikos* ("physical") and *iatros* ("physician"). The term signifies that the specialist is a physician who employs physical agents for the evaluation of the extent of disability and for the rehabilitation of patients.

It is interesting to note that if we compare the surgeon, the internist, and the physiatrist from the standpoint of the tools that are employed, in general the surgeon uses the scalpel and other surgical instruments, the internist uses drugs, and the physiatrist uses physical agents and activity therapies. From the standpoint of disease, with which we are concerned, in general the surgeon deals primarily with acute and chronic diseases in which surgical excision, surgical repair, or some similar use of the instruments employed will be helpful; the internist is concerned primarily with those diseases, acute and chronic, that respond to the pharmaceutic and biologic agents that are commonly used; and the physiatrist is concerned primarily with acute and chronic diseases in which physical agents and procedures, frequently employed by a team of medical and allied health workers, will be of benefit. However, the parameters of these specialties are somewhat blurred, and each may at times employ procedures used by the other.

The number of members on the total team is often governed by the personnel policies and financial limitations of the healthcare facility, as well as by the availability of personnel within a geographic area; therefore, the size, scope, and productivity of the team may vary from facility to facility. This does not imply that a large team is more productive than a small team.

Team Function

Although varied functions can be ascribed to the total rehabilitation team, evaluation, collaboration, and communication appear to be the essential functions.

Evaluation. Each team member provides a written assessment of the patient for the permanent chart records and indicates areas of improvement as the patient makes gains. Specific therapies and approaches to therapy are suggested and modified throughout the program. The patient begins with simple functions and progresses to more difficult integrated actions. Therapy begins when the point of difficulty is determined. However, the evaluation and where therapy begins vary with the specific discipline and the goals and objectives of the rehabilitation plan.

Collaboration. Collaboration among team members is essential in providing a coordinated approach. The extent to which any one person can collaborate with another person or with a group is directly affected by the individual's self-concept, professional identity, and vested interest in personal abilities and professional expertise. Trust in our own abilities and in the abilities of others develops over a period of time.

Communication. Frequent contact for verbal interaction is important in maintaining open communication channels. Team conferences afford the opportunity for free expression of thoughts and ideas when a democratic atmosphere prevails. Communication through written records and reports promotes sharing of information and is a necessity.

REHABILITATION PROCESS

The rehabilitation process starts with an *evaluation* of the patient's medical status, disabilities, assets, and psychosocial circumstances. This is followed by the application of an appropriate *rehabilitation program* designed to bring the patient to optimal functional ability. Next comes *discharge planning,* followed by *follow-up care* to assist the discharged patient with any physical, psychosocial, or vocational problems.

Basically, the rehabilitation process just described remains the same wherever rehabilitation is carried out. However, the degree to which it is carried out and the tasks and techniques involved will differ depending upon the comprehensiveness of the facility.

Evaluation

Prior to the actual transfer of stroke patients to the rehabilitation department, they attend one of the rehabilitation department's semiweekly evaluation clinics, where problems are analyzed and discussed by the rehabilitation team. Decisions as to the feasibility of transferring patients to the rehabilitation department are then made on the basis of the department's ability to contribute to a patient's overall physical, emotional, social, and vocational rehabilitation. Prior to this evaluation, the physiatrist and other members of the rehabilitation team may have been involved with the patient. It is not unusual for such involvement to occur, as it did with our stroke patient.

It is essential to stress that evaluation during rehabilitation is the process of determining the functional status and the functional potential of the patient. It must be distinguished from diagnosis, which determines the pathologic status, and from prognosis, which estimates the course of the pathologic process. Obviously, evaluation cannot be divorced completely from diagnosis and prognosis since the functional potential is often determined by the nature and the course of the disease.[26] Evaluation requires all the basic information obtainable by general medical examination, namely, history, physical examination, and laboratory studies. In addition, careful appraisal of strength, motor function, range of motion, self-care, and communication abilities is necessary. Also, the individual must be assessed as a social being. The home, family, work, and general environment must be considered. To this a formal or informal assessment of personality, attitude, and adaptability must be added to complete the evaluation.

The way in which evaluation is achieved differs from case to case and depends largely on the complexity of the disability and the individual problem. In sum, the total patient evaluation consists of three parts: (1) medical evaluation, (2) disability evaluation, and (3) the psychosocial evaluation.

Specifically, the medical evaluation is carried out by the physiatrist. It is frequently supplemented by data furnished by the rehabilitation team. The disability evaluation consists of four phases: (1) evaluation of the physical disability or impairment, including primary, secondary, and preexisting disabilities; (2) assessment of physical assets including general physical strengths and residual strengths; (3) evaluation of activities of daily living capabilities including mobility, self-care, and communication; and (4) evaluation of vocational abilities. The psychosocial evaluation considers (1) educational and social history of the patient; (2) present social and economic status; (3) present and past leisure interests; (4) present emotional state including reaction to the disability and expectations; and (5) opinions and feelings about present medical and rehabilitation care.[27]

With all of the above-mentioned data available, the team in an evaluation conference formulates a prognosis, establishes goals, and develops a rehabilitation program plan. The plan considers each problem that has been noted by the team. The plan succeeds when each problem is solved to the highest degree obtainable by available therapeutic techniques. In general, this conference team prepares a plan not only for the present but also for discharge and follow-up when the patient returns home.

The formulation of the rehabilitation goals has two steps. The first step is to determine the physical rehabilitation potential of the patient. It is based upon the diagnosis, the prognosis, and the expected permanent disability. The prognosis for spontaneous recovery from physical disability varies with the disease. In hemiplegia, for example, few patients recover full muscle strength. The hemiplegic usually becomes ambulatory and self-caring but does not regain the full use of the hemiplegic arm. The second step is associated with the patient's motivation to work at rehabilitation and become as independent as possible.

There are cases where the diagnosis and prognosis cannot be made with certainty, nor is it always possible to assess the patient's motivation initially. In such instances intermediate or temporary goals are set, and the final goals are made later in a reevaluation conference.

With this brief introduction to the rehabilitation department and the rehabilitation process, let us now return to our stroke patient who was referred to the rehabilitation department. The need for referral to a rehabilitation program for our stroke patient arises from the functional deficits that followed the stroke. The evaluation of the patient at the time of transfer to the rehabilitation department was as follows:

. . . partial self-sufficiency with residual difficulties in the use of the involved upper extremity and in standing and walking. Speech evaluation reveals mild expressive aphasia and moderate receptive aphasia. No visual problems. Leisure experiences limited as a result of vocational pursuit. Psychological tests indicate no problem in orientation, concentration and memory, perceptivity and emotional liabilities; however, patient does have a fear of falling when standing. Emotionally, the patient has a positive, cooperative, receptive learning attitude about his rehabilitation; he wants to become self-sufficient again and return to work. Family reaction positive. The prognosis, while guarded, is good to excellent.

The reader needs to keep in mind that this evaluation is in reality a brief summary of what would be presented and recorded at the conference.

Therapeutic Recreation, Rehabilitation, and Evaluation. The purpose and role of therapeutic recreation service and the role of the specialist in medical rehabilitation in a clinical setting or in a nonmedical setting have not been clearly defined, although they may very well incorporate the two domains—rehabilitation and education of the leisure ability model.[28] It is sufficient to say that the purpose and role of both elements—service and specialist—will vary in nature and intensity in medical rehabilitation according to the degree of disability and the general condition of the patient at the time the patient is referred or admitted to rehabilitation. The rehabilitation in such settings ranges from short-term activities of daily living training or outpatient rehabilitation to intense rehabilitation that may take weeks, if not months, to enable the individual to become independent or to be prepared for attended care outside the hospital.

In the opinion of Carter, Van Andell, and Robb, therapeutic recreation programming as related to the physically impaired should focus on assisting the individual in "(1) psychologically and socially adjusting to the impairment, (2) developing realistic leisure and activity goals based on functional abilities, and (3) developing optimal independence in life skills via participation in recreation and leisure activities. A concomitant purpose should be to enhance the rehabilitation

goals directly associated with the physical impairment, where appropriate."[29]

The initial rehabilitation goals for our patient as developed by the therapeutic recreation specialist might read as follows:

> To increase physical functioning in association with other therapies
>
> To assist in expressive and receptive language development
>
> To increase feelings of worth and accomplishment
>
> To increase personal awareness of importance of leisure experiences[30]

Rehabilitation Program

While some tasks associated with the rehabilitation program can be carried out simultaneously, other rehabilitative measures must be carried out in a special place, with special apparatus, or in a group or individual teaching sessions. Naturally, this leads to the establishment of a daily schedule for each patient. The basic schedule will reserve time for maintenance of vital functions, such as toileting, bath, and meals, which usually integrate with some rehabilitation measures. For example, during mealtime our patient can have a short period of training in left-handed eating. Such an activity leads to strengthening the left upper extremity. Following the meal, the patient may be given a face cloth and asked to wash his face with his left hand. This activity again offers the opportunity to strengthen the left upper extremity and hand while at the same time offering a good opportunity to talk with the patient about his concerns.

The special sessions in addition to the scheduled therapeutic recreation program for our patient would include, but are not limited to, prevention of secondary disabilities mainly due to disuse, improvement of physical fitness relative to the nondisabled side, training in activities of daily living, and psychosocial counseling.

In association with the other therapists and therapies, the therapeutic recreation specialist has assessed the information from the evaluation conference and indicated rehabilitation goals for the stroke patient. The next step for the specialist is to develop individual objectives relative to the goals, select specific activities for their therapeutic outcome relative to the goals, and formulate behavioral objectives. The therapeutic recreation rehabilitation program plan for our patient might read as follows:

Goal:	To increase physical functioning in association with other therapies
Objective:	Increase sensorimotor functioning in upper extremity
Activity:	Checkers
Objective:	Increase upper extremity functioning of the affected side
Activity:	Checkers and shuffleboard
Objective:	Increase skills in the upper extremity unaffected side
Activity:	Checkers and shuffleboard
Objective:	To increase muscle strength, coordination, balance, and endurance
Activity:	Checkers and shuffleboard
Goal:	To assist in expressive and receptive language development
Objective:	To encourage functional speech
Activity:	Checkers, shuffleboard, and leisure counseling
Objective:	To provide stimulation and support to participate in verbal communication
Activity:	Checkers, shuffleboard, and leisure counseling
Goal:	To increase feelings of worth and accomplishment
Activity:	Checkers and shuffleboard
Goal:	To increase personal awareness of importance of leisure experiences in the individual's own lifestyle
Activity:	Leisure counseling

The rationale for the selection of the activities that will be initially provided in a one-to-one relationship to meet goals and objectives is fairly obvious. Checkers and shuffleboard require fine motor and gross motor movement respectively. They also increase muscle strength, body coordination, and endurance of upper and lower extremities, all of which are a major problem with our patient. In addition, shuffleboard provides the opportunity to work on endurance and balance. The specialist can request the patient to shift from one arm and hand to the other in playing the activities, thereby increasing functional ability in the affected extremity while at the same time strengthening both the upper and lower involved and uninvolved extremities.

The two proposed activities also allow the specialist to support the speech therapist's efforts. As the patient increases functional ability, a feeling of worth and accomplishment will occur. The leisure counseling activity finds the patient in a formal group setting wherein personal leisure attitude and awareness, leisure decision making, leisure activities relating to the disability, and leisure-resource information are considered.

The values associated with these two activities and this patient are not complete. There are many other activity values and characteristics that the specialist would consider in the physical, cognitive, and affective behavioral areas. Further, these activities along with the objectives will change over the next few days as the patient's overall functional behavior changes.

In preparing the rehabilitation treatment plan for our patient and in the personal approach to the patient, including activity direction, the specialist would be aware of various characteristics associated with a left-side hemiplegic patient. While it is impossible to consider all of the postacute characteristics here, the abridged list does offer some insight about some factors that may affect the success or failure of the plan. (All diseases have characteristics that can affect the success or failure of the treatment plan. The specialist working in rehabilitation needs to be especially aware of them in developing the plan and in approaching the patient.) Some characteristics for our specialist to consider are as follows:

The patient may have a fear of falling when participating in shuffleboard. This fear is not particularly unusual since patients with left-side hemiplegia have problems with depth perception.

The patient may complain of his left shoulder hurting (or it may be the right shoulder if the hemiplegia is on the right side). Again, this is not unusual, but should be brought to the attention of staff for specific exercises.

The patient with left-side hemiplegia will profit more from verbal instruction as opposed to nonverbal instruction.[31]

The patient may have a tendency to perform activities too quickly, impulsively, and erratically.

Dysarthria and aphasia are common speech disorders found in hemiplegic patients. In our particular patient, relative to expressive aphasia, the specialist is careful to give the patient sufficient time to express himself and not display impatience or anticipate every need so that the patient does not talk. Regarding the receptive aphasia, the specialist speaks in short simple sentences and gives only one direction at a time.[32]

Some left-side hemiplegia patients show more concern for the development of their upper extremity than they do for their lower extremity. The cause is unknown.

Be familiar with goniometric terminology (range of motion).[33]

Keep in mind that each time patients are helped they are reminded of their disabilities. But each time they can carry out the activity unaided, their morale is boosted.

Since the rehabilitation program must be adjusted and advanced according to the response and progress of the patient, it is imperative to record the date and the patient's status in order to evaluate progress. Reporting through progress notes need not be a chore. As we pointed out in an earlier chapter, recording the treatment plan and noting the progress of the patient are really tools that verify and augment the activities of the profession at work. Regarding progress per se, Beddall and Kennedy, in a small sample study of practitioners, found that "progress notes were the most frequently utilized method of determining client progress within a therapeutic recreation program."[34]

It is not an overstatement to say that recording treatment plans and progress notes is equally as important as the treatment itself. In this day of specialization and with rehabilitation relying on a team approach in working with individual patients, communication becomes an essential tool. Further, for fiscal accountability, liability concerns, reimbursement purpose, and DRG auditing, documentation of progress or delay is not only needed but required. In a recent article about fiscal accountability, risk management, and therapeutic recreation service Touchstone had this to say about documentation:

TR documentation should be a component of the medical record and include referral, assessment, treatment plan and evaluation. A physician referral to the TR should suggest approaches and outline medical precautions. Assessment procedures should include interviews, observations, and testing results which contribute to the treatment plan. An individualized treatment plan should list specific treatment goals and objectives, target dates, precautionary measures, therapists, and schedules. An evaluation should encompass documenting treatment outcome measures, writing progress notes, and proposing discharge plans and follow up.

TR documentation should be clear, precise, and objective. This is important because it establishes guidelines for treatment intervention, involves realistic and relevant goal setting, individualizes treatment, and provides treatment interpretations for the third party/payers, regulatory agencies, families, and courts.[35]

A progress note for our stroke patient after a few days of treatment might read as follows:

7/12/86 Patient is cooperative and continues to increase strength in affected and unaffected arms and hands. No pain in shoulder. Improvement in endurance and balance noted with increased ambulation and coordination. Some fatigue evident following shuffleboard. Patient talking more in leisure counseling but frustration still present. Positive attitude continues about rehabilitation.

Discharge Planning

At the initial rehabilitation evaluation conference a determination is made regarding the approximate length of time it should take to rehabilitate the patient, with discharge planning starting immediately following the evaluation. This planning is carried on throughout the rehabilitation program and terminates when the patient is discharged or referred to another facility for continued rehabilitation. With some patients, the rehabilitation goals are achieved in a reasonable length of time, and the patient is discharged. On the other hand, some patients will not reach their goals and will need continuous and permanent assistance with their vital functions and activities of daily living. In such cases patients do not become independent and are discharged or transferred to other facilities for further rehabilitation and for care (extended care facility, skilled nursing facility, etc.) or discharged home with home-care follow-up.

If the patient is discharged home, the home is usually evaluated in terms of how well suited it is for a person with a disability. This evaluation may be done by staff from the rehabilitation facility or by personnel from a home health-care agency or the visiting nurses' service. Special attention is naturally given to stairs, ramps, and stairways inside the house, the width of doorways and accessibility of areas to a wheelchair, and to special adjustments needed for the use of the bed and bathroom.

In the more comprehensive rehabilitation centers and depending upon the patient's progress, a discharge conference may be held when all discharge planning has been accomplished. During the conference the patient and family are present. Each team member usually outlines measures taken during the rehabilitation program and what should be done following discharge. In fact, if everything is well prepared, it is simply a matter of going down a check list to make sure nothing has been forgotten. This conference with its review provides the material to be incorporated in the discharge summary report.

Regarding our stroke patient and discharge planning, we note that one of the objectives of the rehabilitation treatment plan was to increase the patient's awareness of the role of leisure in his life through leisure counseling. This objective focuses on the future. Discharge planning is closely interwoven with treatment since treatment is directed toward the eventual independence of the patient.

Because the period of rehabilitation time for our patient is necessarily limited (efficiency, economics, and so on) the specialist responsible for leisure counseling may not be able to cover all of those elements suggested by Peterson and Gunn in the leisure education part of their therapeutic recreation service model.[36] However, the time would be sufficient to consider problems connected with the patient's past leisure participation and attitude, new and old leisure activities, appropriate use of present leisure time, and where to find community leisure resources.[37] If time does not permit the consideration of all of these matters, scheduled outpatient visits may be in order. On the other hand, if the individual lives in a community where a referral program has been developed between the rehabilitation department and the community recreation department, aspects left out of the leisure-counseling rehabilitation program can be continued with the therapeutic recreation specialist working through the community agency.[38]

Follow-Up

The weakest link in most rehabilitation programs is follow-up care after discharge. Failure in this respect is responsible for much regression and development of preventable disabilities. Regularly scheduled outpatient visits or periodic home visits by home health-care agency personnel are the means to assure maintenance of the level of functional improvement achieved by rehabilitation. Individuals are by no means assured satisfactory adjustment to family, friends, or general environment by reason of having successfully accomplished a rehabilitation program. Any sort of disruption may precipitate a problem that the patient will need assistance in solving. Therefore, it is important that the individual be assured at the time of discharge of the availability of a willing ear and help during readjustment.

In the case of our particular patient, it would be hoped that he will continue to improve and achieve capacities far beyond any predicted levels. Relative to leisure experiences, it would be anticipated that he will return to participation in those activities within the limitations of his disability that were a part of his life patterns prior to the CVA. In fact, as a result of participation in leisure counseling, it would be further anticipated that he will participate more in leisure activities and be more knowledgeable about leisure and leisure resources.

We might hope that he has been referred to a community recreation agency or another agency offering leisure services. However, that might not be true for him or for other disabled individuals completing a rehabilitation program. A major obstacle to participation in leisure experiences following discharge is the poor link between the rehabilitation facility and community recreation agencies, especially in smaller commu-

nities. Very few rehabilitation departments in GM&S hospitals or even freestanding rehabilitation facilities have developed a referral system. Today more community recreation departments are aware of the disabled and not only are making an effort to make their facilities accessible, but have developed specialized programs for the more severely disabled. While changes are occurring slowly in agencies and in communities, barriers still exist—some social, some physical, and some programmatic. Consideration of the disabled in the community is explored in greater depth and detail in Chapter 11.

REHABILITATION CONCLUSION

It is difficult to determine with certainty a recovery timetable for our patient as well as for other stroke patients. According to the literature, the positive outcome of rehabilitation for the hemiplegic patient is dependent largely on psychological matters rather than physical factors if physical management and treatment are adequate and all benefits of rehabilitation achieved.[39]

Further, in the rehabilitation of our patient or any other patient no one discipline or method by itself can assume the total responsibility for member management if optimal results are to be achieved. A comprehensive rehabilitation program can be compared to a symphony orchestra. If you were to listen to a single instrument playing its part in a symphony, the tones produced would be meaningless and ineffective in most cases. It is only in the total harmonious well-integrated and properly conducted efforts of all the necessary instruments that the beautiful and distinctive harmony of the musical theme is created. On the other hand, occasionally and at an appropriate time a single musical instrument is selected to play a solo. Similarly, it is in a well-integrated and properly directed team approach that the rehabilitation of the member is best accomplished. At times selected methods or disciplines may play the predominant role in helping members find their proper places in society. Also, the emphasis on a particular type of therapeutic approach may be different at the beginning of a member's treatment than during the period of convalescence, when the major responsibility changes from one segment of the therapeutic team to another.

SUMMARY

This chapter described in brief the role of a therapeutic recreation specialist in implementing the therapeutic recreation process in a traditional medical-clinical model (GM&S) of service as well as in an inpatient medical rehabilitation service that is affiliated with the model. The use of two case studies demonstrated the process and the action of the specialist. Throughout the chapter, knowledge, techniques, and processes used by the specialist to develop and determine the individual treatment plans were described. General information about medical-surgical services, rehabilitation services, and the rehabilitation process were also discussed.

NOTES

1. Howard A. Rusk, *Rehabilitation Medicine* (St. Louis: C. V. Mosby Co., 1964), p. 28.

2. R. D. Adams and M. Victor, *Principles of Neurology* (New York: McGraw-Hill Book Co., 1977), pp. 79–83, and Marcia J. Carter, Glen E. Van Andel, and Gary M. Robb, *Therapeutic Recreation: A Practical Approach* (St. Louis: Times Mirror/Mosby, 1985), p. 255.

3. Adams and Victor, *Neurology*, p. 82.

4. Helen Broida, *Coping with Stroke* (San Diego: College-Hill Press, 1979), p. 16.

5. Adams and Victor, *Neurology*, p. 117.

6. Barbara M. Dossey, "Acute Myocardial Infarction," in *Critical Care Nursing*, 2nd ed., ed. Cornelia V. Kessner, Cathie E. Guzzelta, and Barbara M. Dossey (Boston: Little, Brown & Co., 1985), pp. 513–14; and Franklin C. Schontz, *The Psychological Aspects of Physical Illness and Disability* (Philadelphia: W. B. Saunders Co., 1977), pp. 116–22.

7. Dossey, "Acute Myocardial Infarction," *Critical Care Nursing*, p. 515.

8. L. L. Trigiano, "Move That Cardiac Early," in *Rehabilitation Nursing*, ed. Victor A. Christopherson, Pearl P. Coulter, and Mary O. Wolanin (New York: McGraw-Hill Book Co., 1974), p. 378.

9. Wilma J. Phipps, Barbara C. Long, and Mary F. Wood, *Medical-Surgical Nursing*, 2nd ed. (St. Louis: C. V. Mosby Co., 1983), pp. 796–804.

10. P. D. White, *Rehabilitation of the Cardiovascular Patient* (New York: McGraw-Hill Book Co., 1978), p. 21.

11. S. M. Fox, J. P. Naughton, and P. A. Gorman, *Modern Concepts in Cardiovascular Disorders* 41, no. 6 (1972), pp. 53–59.

12. Ibid., p. 55.

13. "NewsCurrent" is a product of "NewsCurrent," P.O. box 52, Madison, Wis. 53701.

14. "DRG's Today," *Synopsis* (supplement, University of Alabama Hospital, November 14, 1983), pp. 64–75.

15. Reva Rubin, "Body Image and Self-Esteem," in *Rehabilitation Nursing*, p. 52.

16. Ibid.

17. Gerald G. Hirschberg, Leon Lewis, and Patricia Vaughan, *Rehabilitation* (Philadelphia: J. B. Lippincott Co., 1976), p. 221.

18. Dossey, "Acute Myocardial Infarction," *Critical Care Nursing*, pp. 512–13.

19. Ibid.

20. Ibid.

21. Rusk, *Rehabilitation Medicine*, p. 11.

22. See definitions in various rehabilitation publications found in footnotes and Suggested References.

23. Hirschberg, Lewis, and Vaughan, *Rehabilitation*, p. 69.

24. Hirschberg, Lewis, and Vaughan, *Rehabilitation*, p. 94.

25. Bruce E. Porch, "Communication," in *Rehabilitation*, pp. 100–101.

26. Hirschberg, Lewis, and Vaughan, *Rehabilitation*, p. 162.

27. Ibid., pp. 163–65.

28. Carol A. Peterson and Scout L. Gunn, *Therapeutic Recreation Program Design: Principles and Procedures*, 2nd ed. (Englewood Cliffs, N.J.: Prentice-Hall, 1984), pp. 1–10.

29. Carter, Van Andel, and Robb, *Therapeutic Recreation*, p. 263.

30. The reliable, valid assessment and evaluation instruments that can be used by the therapeutic recreation specialist with patients in physical rehabilitation are rare. However, the Goal Attainment Scale (GAS), which considers behavior or problems of patients regardless of diagnosis or setting, offers some promise. See William A. Touchstone, "A Personalized Approach to Goal Planning and Evaluation in Clinical Settings," *Therapeutic Recreation Journal* 18, no. 2 (1984), 25–31, for a discussion of the instrument.

31. Roberta Chapey, *Language Intervention Strategies in Adult Aphasia* (Baltimore: Williams & Wilkins, 1981), p. 82.

32. A. Holland, "Observing Functional Communication of Aphasic Adults," *Journal of Speech and Hearing Disorders* 47 (1982), 50–56.

33. Students who plan to find employment in physical medicine and rehabilitation departments need to become familiar with goniometric terminology even though they will not be specifically involved in the use of goniometry. *Goniometry* is the measurement of joint motion (range of motion); it is an essential step in the evaluation of function in a patient with muscular, neurological, or skeletal disability. The terminology will be found in reports and records, physicians may make reference to physical functioning through their referrals, and the specialist may refer to the joint measurement form found in some patient's charts in considering various activities. A list of the terms and their definitions is found in Appendix A.

34. Therese Beddall and Dan W. Kennedy, "Attitudes of Therapeutic Recreators toward Evaluation and Client Assessment," *Therapeutic Recreation Journal* 18, no. 1 (1985), 62–70.

35. William A. Touchstone, "Fiscal Accountability through Effective Risk Management, *Therapeutic Recreation Journal* 18, no. 4 (1984), 24.

36. Peterson and Gunn, *Therapeutic Recreation*, pp. 22–44.

37. Ibid.

38. See Christine Z. Howe, "Leisure Assessment Instrumentation in Therapeutic Recreation," *Therapeutic Recreation Journal* 18, no. 4 (1984), 14–24, for review of instruments that measure leisure interest and attitudes in leisure counseling.

39. Hirschberg, Lewis, and Vaughan, *Rehabilitation*, p. 243.

SUGGESTED READINGS

Note: Publications concerned with transfer techniques, wheelchairs, ambulation aids, etc. are indicated by an asterisk.

*ANDERSON, MILES H. *Upper Extremities Orthotics.* Springfield, Ill.: Charles C Thomas, Publishers, 1979.

AUSTIN, DAVID R. *Therapeutic Recreation: Processes and Techniques.* New York: John Wiley & Sons, 1982. Chaps. 3, 4, and 5.

BERNSTEIN, LEWIS, ROSALYN S. BERNSTEIN, and R. H. DANA. *Interviewing: A Guide for Health Professionals* (2nd ed.). New York: Appleton-Century-Crofts, 1974.

BERRA, KATHY. "Cardiac Rehabilitation Update." *Critical Care Update* 12, no. 3 (1983), 362–67.

BIRKERSTOFF, E. R. *Neurology* (3rd ed.). New York: Arco Publishing, 1982.

BOROCH, R. M. *Elements of Rehabilitation in Nursing: An Introduction.* St. Louis: C. V. Mosby Co., 1976.

BRILL, NAOMI I. *Working with People: The Helping Process* (3rd ed.). Philadelphia: J. B. Lippincott Co., 1984.

COATS, HEATHER, and ALAN KING. *Patient Assessment: A Handbook for Therapists.* New York: Churchill Livingstone, 1983.

COMPTON, DAVID M. "Research Priorities in Recreation for Special Populations." *Therapeutic Recreation Journal* 18, no. 1 (1984), 9–17.

CONNOLLY, PEG. "Analyzing Program Cause as Well as Effect: A Method for Program Analysis." *Therapeutic Recreation Journal* 18, no. 1 (1984), 31–39.

DOWNEY, JOHN A., and NEILS L. LOW, eds. *The Child with Disabling Illness: Principles in Rehabilitation.* Philadelphia: W. B. Saunders Co., 1974.

*FORD, J. R., and B. DUCKWORTH. *Physical Management for the Quadriplegic Patient.* Philadelphia: F. A. Davis Co., 1974.

*FLAHERTY, P. T., and S. J. JURKOVICH. *Transfers for Patients with Acute and Chronic Conditions.* Rehabilitation publication no. 702. Minneapolis: American Rehabilitation Foundation, 1970.

GOLDENSON, ROBERT M., et al. *Disability and Rehabilitation Handbook.* New York: McGraw-Hill Book Co., 1978.

HAMILTON, HELESA, and MINNIE B., ed. *Cardiovascular Disorders.* Springhouse, Pa.: Springhouse Publishing Co., 1983.

"Letters to Editor" (regarding the articles of Charles D. Sylvester and Kenneth E. Mobily, respectively, which appeared in the *Therapeutic Recreation Journal* 18, no. 1 [1985]). *Therapeutic Recreation Journal* 20, no. 1 (1986), 89–92.

Lower-Limb Prosthetics (rev. ed.). New York: New York University Medical Center, Post-Graduate Medical School, Prosthetics and Orthotics, 1980. Pp. 187–238.

MAGER, ROBERT F. *Preparing Instructional Objectives.* Belmont, Calif.: Fearson Publishers, 1962.

*MINOR, SCOTT D., and MARY A. MINOR. *Patient Care Skills: Positioning, Range-of-Motion, Transfers, Wheelchairs and Ambulation.* Reston, Va.: Reston Publishing Co., 1984.

MOBILY, KENNETH E. "A Philosophical Analysis of Therapeutic Recreation: What Does It Mean to Say 'We Can Be Therapeutic?'" Part 1. *Therapeutic Recreation Journal* 18, no. 1 (1985), 14–26.

*NAGLER, WILLIBALD. *Manual for Physical Therapy Technicians.* Chicago: Year Book Medical Publishers, 1974. Pp. 85–110 and 129–72.

*NIXON, VICKLE. *Spinal Cord Injury: A Guide to Functional Outcomes in Physical Therapy Management.* Rockville, Md.: Aspen Publication, 1985. Pp. 77–106.

O'MORROW, GERALD S. "Team Practice and the Therapeutic Recreation Specialist," in *Expanding Horizons in Therapeutic Recreation.* vol. 2, ed. Jerry D. Kelley. Champaign: University of Illinois, Office of Recreation and Park Resources, 1973.

*PERRY, JACQUELIN, and HELEN J. HISLOP. *Principles of Lower Extremity Bracing,* Washington, D.C.: American Physical Therapy Association, 1972.

PETERSON, CAROL A., and PEG CONNOLLY. *Characteristics of Special Populations: Implications for Recreation Participation and Planning.* Washington, D.C.: Hawkins & Associates, 1978.

PETERSON, CAROL A., and SCOUT L. GUNN. *Therapeutic Recreation Program Design* (2nd ed.). Englewood Cliffs, N.J.: Prentice-Hall, 1984.

PURTILO, DONALD. *Human Survey of Diseases.* Reading, Mass.: Addison/Wesley, 1979.

SCHULMAN, EVELINE D. *Intervention in Human Services* (2nd ed.). St. Louis: C. V. Mosby Co., 1978.

STOLOV, W. C., and M. A. CLOWERS, eds. *Handbook of Severe Disability.* Seattle: University of Washington, 1981.

STUBBINS, J. *Social and Psychological Aspects of Disability: A Handbook for Practitioners.* Baltimore: University Park Press, 1977.

SYLVESTER, CHARLES D. "Freedom, Leisure and Therapeutic Recreation: A Philosophical View." *Therapeutic Recreation Journal* 18, no. 1 (1985), 6–13.

Therapeutic Recreation Journal 14, no. 4 (1980). Entire issue addresses assessment.

TUBBS, STEWART L., and SYLVIA MOSS. *Interpersonal Communication.* New York: Random House, 1978.

VAN RIPER, CHARLES, and LOU EMERICK. *Speech Correction: An Introduction to Speech Pathology and Audiology* (7th ed.). Englewood Cliffs, N.J.: Prentice-Hall, 1984.

WEST, RAY E. "Therapeutic Recreation Services as a Component of Optimal Health Care in a General Hospital Setting." *Therapeutic Recreation Journal* 13, no. 3 (1979), 7–11.

*WOOD, LUCILE A., ed. *Nursing Skills for Allied Health Services.* Vol. 1. Philadelphia: W. B. Saunders Co., n.d. units 14 and 15.

8

Long-Term Care Model

It is exceedingly difficult to generalize in one chapter about therapeutic recreation service and its process in relation to long-term health care facilities. If for no other reason, the diversity of characteristics associated with such facilities as the nature of the auspice (sectarian, governmental, non-profit, profitmaking), the goals of the varied facilities, the philosophy of care and treatment in the facilities, the characteristics of the individuals found in the facilities, and the kinds of programs and services provided by each facility prevent an orderly discussion. However, as an introduction to this chapter we will look at some similarities and will consider them relative to the model.

The young, the old, the sick, the weak, the bright, the dull, the rich, the poor, males, females, whites, blacks, foreign-born, native-born—all of these can be found in long-term health-care facilities. They typically come from a stressful situation or crisis, or as the result of disease or disability. Regardless of the situation, all are in need of help or rehabilitation.

Some health-care facilities are similar in nature to the custodial model of earlier years in which little attention was paid to care and treatment needs, even though standards exist today that outline a higher level of service. The situation is further compounded in that funding for social and recreational services may be grossly inadequate or nonexistent.

Facilities that have this kind of overall internal life are what Goffman referred to in the early 1960s as *total institutions.*[1] All aspects of life—sleeping, eating, working, and playing—are carried out in a very routine and controlled manner. Associated with this concept is *institutional neurosis,* a problem resulting from particular loss of contact with the outside world and complete submersion in the institutional or facility routine. The patient becomes highly dependent as the personality is gradually eroded, and apathy and withdrawal result. Typically the posture of older patients in such facilities shows the effects; slumped in a chair, head bowed, and with little facial expression, they take no interest in events happening around them.

While some long-term health-care facilities have moved forward slowly, many others have taken a more progressive approach. Such facilities offer diagnostic, preventive, therapeutic, rehabilitative, supportive, and maintenance services for individuals of all age groups who have chronic physical, developmental, or emotional impairments. The goal in these facilities is the promotion of the optimum level of physical, social, and psychological functioning. Between the extremes are a great variety of facilities in all stages of development.

This chapter is structured on the basis of the therapeutic recreation process followed in the previous chapter, except the concern here is with individuals in long-term care facilities, primarily the nursing home and its elderly residents. The process and concepts discussed here can be applied to any number of congregated residential settings. In addition, in a limited fashion, other matters associated with the management, programs, and services of nursing homes are considered. (To foster sensitivity to some of the special problems of the aging, a number of sensitivity-training modules are presented at the end of this chapter.)

Regarding therapeutic recreation service, the student should keep in mind that although reference is made to this service in the nursing home, such service may in fact be called Patient Activity Service. Also, the service or activities provided may be of a therapeutic nature rather than therapy, although many nursing homes try to provide both types of programs. The activity approach taken depends on many factors, including type of facility (skilled, intermediate, etc.), size, location, finances and reimbursement programs, personnel, and administrative philosophy.

The student also needs to recognize that a therapeutic recreation specialist is not the only one qualified to be employed as an activity or patient activity director, even though the services are activity or recreational in nature. Others who are employed to provide activity services are registered occupational therapists, certified occupational therapy aides, social workers, and individuals who have worked in patient activities for two years or who have completed a state certified training program of 32 hours or more in this area.

CHARACTERISTICS OF THE NURSING HOME

A clarification is needed initially regarding a nursing home. The term *nursing home* is relatively imprecise, being used to describe several different types of facilities. As noted in Chapter 3, a nursing home is for the accommodation and care of convalescents or other persons who are not acutely ill and not in need of hospital care but who do require nursing care and related medical services. Since nursing homes have a large resident population of individuals sixty-five years of age or older, the public tends to include all residential-care facilities for the elderly under the term nursing home, but distinctions do exist based on several factors, including ownership (profit versus nonprofit), participation in federal reimbursement programs (Medicare and Medicaid), levels of care provided, and regulation by state licensing authorities.

RESIDENT PROFILE

Although nursing homes are designed for the convalescence and long-term care of the seriously ill of all ages, their population consists primarily of the elderly. Moreover, these elderly residents have a variety of physical, mental, and emotional conditions that affect their functional behavior and abilities. According to one source, 90 percent of the residents in nursing homes are sixty-five years of age or older.[2] This represents about 5 percent of the 1.2 million residents of the United States who are sixty-five and older.[3] However, this percentage rises to 20 percent for those eighty-five and older,[4] and the 1.2 million is projected to increase to 2.2 million by the year 2020.[5] It is also documented that the chance of admission to a nursing home increases with advancing age, and with advancing age, the length of stay increases because of increasing impairments and disabilities.[6] Current information about Medicare beneficiaries indicates an average of 4.4 illness conditions during 1980 for each person sixty-five years of age and older.[7]

Residents in nursing homes suffer from mental and physical disabilities, often in combination with each other. Most of these impairments are chronic in nature. By definition, a chronic illness is one that is not curable.[8] Treatment attempts to limit the further progress of the illness or disease and its complications and to maximize the functional capacities of the patient. The salient fact about these multiple chronic health problems for nursing home care is that they result in functional disabilities. In other words, the problems impair people's capacity to care for themselves in normal living situations.

According to many investigators and surveys, there are three major types of physical impairment that afflict residents in nursing homes. First are circulatory and/or neurological disorders such as heart disease and stroke, compounded by speech disorders associated with a stroke. Next are arthritis and other disorders affecting the skeletal system. And last are digestive disorders such as diabetes. In addition to physical impairments, mental disorders are extremely prevalent among the residents, especially older residents. While no exact data are available, various surveys indicate that at least half of all older residents have one or more mental conditions. Many other studies make reference to the large proportion of confused and disoriented older residents. In recent years, as a result of the increase in the number of mentally retarded individuals in the community who have lost close supportive relatives plus those discharged from training schools and hospitals, there has been a gradual increase in the number of such individuals placed in nursing homes.

How do these multiple mental and physical impairments affect the way residents function? In nursing homes the most commonly noted disabilities are in the spheres of ambulation and personal self-care. The most frequently cited required aids are wheelchairs, walkers, and crutches, in that order. Estimates vary regarding the amount of help needed in activities of daily living as a result of being either mildly or severely disabled or incontinent. The vast majority appeared to need help in bathing, dressing, toileting, and eating. While these surveys are open to discussion, a visit to a nursing home may very well confirm many of these findings.

Additional evidence of the overall functioning problem of older people is found in a community study conducted by the federal government (Table 8.1). While the study is now nearly ten years old, the findings probably would change little if conducted today. The study asked questions in five areas of human functioning: social, economic, mental, physical, and activities of daily living. The results in each area are combined to form a picture of the state of well-being of those sixty-five years of age and older who are institutionalized. The scale begins with "Unimpaired," which means excellent to good in all five areas of human functioning. At the other end of the scale "Extremely impaired" means mild or moderate impair-

TABLE 8.1. Status of Well-Being in Institutionalized People Over 65

Impairment Level	Percent of Institutionalized People
Unimpaired	1
Slightly	1
Mildly	2
Moderately	5
Generally	4
Greatly	11
Extremely	76

SOURCE: U.S Department of Health, Education and Welfare, Federal Council on Aging, *Public Policy and the Frail Elderly* (Washington, D.C.: U.S. Government Printing Office, December 1978), p. 28.

ment in four areas and severe or complete impairment in the other, or complete impairment in two or more areas. The study also reported a dramatic increase in the age level as one moved down the impairment level.[9]

DIMENSIONS OF CARE

There are many dimensions of care we could consider, but for our purpose we will address only a selected few: philosophy of care, levels of care, and Medicare and Medicaid.

Philosophy of Care

The newer philosophy that underlies the development of care stems from the recognition that individuals in need of nursing home management are already victimized by a variety of problems: emotional, social, nutritional, economic, medical, and surgical. Moreover, the nursing home is becoming aware of its potential for meeting the medical, social, and psychological needs of the resident. Implicit in these comments is the rejection of the notion of custodial care in favor of a positive philosophy of active treatment and rehabilitation. This philosophy is supported by federal regulations (Health Care Financing Administration, Division of Long-Term Care, "Conditions for Participation for Skilled Nursing and Intermediate Care Facilities") and voluntary organization accrediting standards (Joint Commission on Accreditation of Hospitals, *Accreditation Manual for Long-Term Care Facilities*).

The objectives of the modern nursing home are of a positive and challenging nature. They may be stated as follows:

1. To provide continuing care for those recovering from surgical or medical disorders

2. To assist the resident in reaching optimal physical and emotional health through medical and nursing care, rehabilitation, and nutritional programs

3. To provide the care that residents' disabilities prevent them from providing to themselves such as dressing, feeding, toileting, grooming, bathing, and transportation

4. To provide for the total needs of residents—physical, emotional, social, and spiritual[10]

From another view, the objectives are not to cure (as opposed to the acute and episodic care and treatment rendered in a general hospital) but to help residents cope with impairments, to decrease their dependence on others, to diminish their disability, and to help them function at the highest level.

The importance of attention to these objectives is self-evident. The latter objective is of importance to therapeutic recreation specialists especially from the psychosocial perspective. The concern here is with (a) a physical and social environment designated to communicate a view of each resident as a unique, dignified, and respected individual, and (b) life-enriching and life-enhancing services to help each individual live with full realization of his or her potential for well-being and enjoyment.

A philosophy of care recognizes not only the needs of the residents but also the relationships between the staff and residents. It is known that physical dependency and mental confusion increase when staff have negative, disrespectful, or belittling attitudes. Conversely, more positive mental attitudes are related to permissive, friendly staff attitudes and positive expectations.[11] Studies have also shown the favorable effects of freedom and encouragement of competent behavior, opportunities for choice, social responsibility, and social interaction with other residents and with people outside the facility.[12]

Too often the "good" residents are the ones who don't assert themselves. The regressed, brain-damaged resident, incontinent, confused, and disoriented, may be treated as a child rather than as a dignified adult. It is often easier to "do for" than to encourage residents to do for themselves, simpler to use nursing home clothes than to use the residents' own clothes, easier to keep them quiescent through drug "therapy" than to initiate programs of stimulation and activity, less trouble to overuse geriatric chairs for the elderly resident than to have the old people "wandering about" or in "danger of falling."

In nursing homes offering a low-program level of care, investigators have found dramatic improvement in residents when attention was given to basic medical and psychosocial care. Activity programs with apathetic elderly resulted in new interest of the residents in personal grooming, conversational interaction, initiation of activities, and a desire to work. In facilities providing a high level of care to begin with (excluding rehabilitation service), even the most regressed older residents improved when individualized programs were tailored to their unique life experiences, personalities, and needs.[13]

Basic to all the clinical and research findings is the clear message that the impaired individual in the nursing home retains the "whole person" needs that characterize all human beings. It is paradoxical that increased specialization has often resulted in fragmentation and compartmentalization. While individuals in nursing homes may share some characteristics, they vary widely in behavior, personality, socioeconomic background, types of mental and physical disabilities, and level of functioning, and they represent different generations.

Decisions regarding care and the participation of residents in activities require careful consideration. With the best intentions in the world, an overprotective staff can infantilize and humiliate residents, especially elderly residents, through deprivation of the rights and privileges due all adults in exercising choice about their own lives. A delicate balance must be struck between providing quality care on the one hand and using power vested in staff to control every aspect of existence.

Levels of Care

There are two types of nursing home facilities or levels of care, both of which may at times be found within one facility. The first of these facilities is the *skilled nursing facility* (SNF), where twenty-four-hour nursing care is available under the supervision of a medical director and a registered nurse. The nursing care found in SNFs includes assessing needs, providing services, and evaluating care services. The other type or level of care is the *intermediate care facility* (ICF), where nursing care also is available but supervision is less comprehensive, as is the level of care.

Other extended-care facilities such as retirement homes, personal-care homes, and homes for the aged do not provide round-the-clock specialized medical or nursing care, nor are they eligible to participate in the Medicare or Medicaid programs. Further, they are often unregulated by the state in which they operate, although in recent years an effort has been made to regulate such facilities. They normally provide group living arrangements and some assistance with such daily needs as bathing, food preparation, and eating.

Medicare and Medicaid

State regulations or standards have been promulgated extensively for skilled nursing and intermediate care facilities. Since many of these facilities choose to participate in the federal Medicare and Medicaid programs, they also must meet the additional standards of the Health Care Financing Administration and the Joint Commission on Hospital Accreditation, as noted earlier in this chapter. Although these standards address the physical environment and the medical and nursing requirements, including treatment programs, staffing patterns, and psychosocial needs, the psychosocial needs have not always been fully considered by the facility or the intent of the regulations and standards fully met.

Medicare is operated uniformly across the nation by the federal government, and

Medicaid is a joint federal-state program whose benefits vary from state to state. Medicare covers only skilled nursing facilities and pays only a total of 2 percent of the nation's nursing home bills.[14] Even this small amount inhibits significant expansion of long-term care services. Meanwhile, the costs are being driven up by high inflation, demographic trends, and utilization of services.[15] Moreover, Medicare is keyed to recuperative and rehabilitative services, not custodial and chronic care. In brief, Medicare will pay for up to one hundred days of care for a single illness. The person must have been hospitalized for at least three days and transferred to a nursing home within fourteen days after being released from the hospital. Following the one hundred days, the patient must be rehospitalized or assume the full cost of care in the nursing home. To assure a proper level of care for the resident, a utilization review committee functions to periodically review the resident's continued need for the level of care being provided. Medicaid, on the other hand, is available only to persons whose income and assets are limited. Applications generally are processed by state and local welfare departments. If the individual in need of nursing home care has moderate resources, that person must first exhaust them and then apply for Medicaid. As opposed to Medicare, there are no duration limits on Medicaid-reimbursed care.

Residents' Rights. In order for nursing homes to participate in Medicare and Medicaid programs, they must establish residents' rights policies. These regulations were established by the federal government as the result of the failure of other sources of protection for nursing home residents. The policies speak to safeguards in certain designated areas such as handling of resident funds, use of physical and chemical restraints, confidentiality of resident records, participation by residents in medical decision making, assurances that residents are entitled to file complaints, assurances that

residents can participate in religious activities, and limitations upon the ability of facilities to require residents to perform work for the facility.[16] In addition, a few states (New York and Maryland), have adopted their own nursing home residents' rights provision.

Another program concerned with promoting and protecting resident concerns is the ombudsman program. *Ombudsman* is a Scandinavian word to denote a government official who investigates complaints of citizens against the government or its bureaucrats. There are various forms of the program in all states, and both paid and nonpaid volunteers are used to investigate complaints. Since there are so many nursing homes in each state, volunteers are used frequently to supplement government surveys of a nursing home. The ombudsman investigates complaints and seeks recommendations from nursing home residents during weekly or monthly visits. These problems are then taken up with the nursing home administrator. Alleged complaints may include, but are not limited to, the following: nature of institutional life, quality of program services, quality and quantity of staff, financial matters, legal problems, nursing home rules and policies, dietary matters, and physical facilities.

STAFFING AND SERVICES

The staff of a nursing home consists of an administrator, director of nurses and/or a supervising nurse, registered nurses, licensed practical nurses, attendants, activity director, social worker, food supervisor, office workers, and maintenance and kitchen personnel. Each resident has a personal or attending physician. Homes usually have a consulting dietitian, an occupational therapist, and a physical therapist. Volunteer workers are usually in attendance.

Services provided in a nursing home usually consist of room and board, medical care, nursing care, transportation, counseling, therapeutic recreation, physical therapy, occupational therapy, social service, and religious services.

Volunteers

During the past three to four decades we have noted that volunteer services are no longer performed only by members of the leisure class. Average citizens with new-found leisure time volunteer to assist those who need help. Not only do average citizens in the modern community have more leisure, but they are also better able to take advantage of new opportunities for volunteer contribution.

The emerging role of volunteers, especially in nursing homes, in providing services means that volunteer services are an integral part of the overall program of services. According to one source, the purposes of the volunteer in settings for older persons (for that matter in any long-term care facility) are:

1. To bring the warmth of human personality to the elderly
2. To help arrange new experiences to promote the mental, physical, emotional, and social growth of older people
3. To assist in retaining and restoring the function of older people to a level at which they can continue their lifestyles
4. To encourage a milieu in which older people feel self-confidence and self-worth
5. To motivate older people to look forward happily to tomorrow because of today
6. To strengthen meaning and purpose in the lives of older people[17]

It is not unusual for the specialist to be assigned the additional responsibility of recruiting, orienting, assigning, supervising, and evaluating volunteers in the nursing home. Regular contact with volunteers—both individuals and groups—and recognition of services rendered is necessary to reinforce their relationship with the nursing home.

A major factor to be considered in the function of a volunteer service program is the vital importance of staff understanding that volunteers supplement staff services. At no time should volunteers take the place of staff. Further, staff should understand the demands that volunteers and their program will make on them, as well as the value of the volunteer program to residents. The primary justification is better service to the residents. It takes a nursing home staff who can recognize and appreciate the true contribution that volunteers make in the care, treatment, and rehabilitation of residents to train and use volunteers effectively.

The concept of this chapter and space does not permit an extensive discussion of the selection and use of volunteers and the administration of their services. However, it is extremely important to comment, before moving on, that a special aptitude for drawing residents out and for working with them on an individual and group basis is more crucial than the volunteer's ability to engage in specific craft and recreational pursuits. The specialist can always recruit volunteers with specific technical skills, but the volunteer must have the human skills. Further, the development of an effective volunteer program requires an investment in time and effort, and the nursing home must be committed to the idea that the values to be derived from the program are worth the investment.

PSYCHOSOCIAL INTERVENTIONS

This section introduces some of the better-known basic group-interventive techniques used with nursing home residents. In fact, the techniques can be found in many types of long-term care facilities. The techniques have value in that they offer the potential for improving the resident's behavior, well-being, and functioning. They are of a verbal/nonverbal nature, and activities may be used to achieve specific aims. However, these techniques are not solely under the direction of any one discipline. They are presented here because in some nursing homes and other long-term care facilities therapeutic recreation specialists are responsible for their direction.

The following four group-interventive techniques by no means constitute an exhaustive survey; they are simply examples of popular programs that have evolved in recent years.

Reality Orientation

Reality orientation (RO) as described by its founders, Folsom and Taulbee, "is a basic technique in the rehabilitation of persons having a moderate to severe degree of memory loss, confusion, and time-place-person disorientation."[18] There are two parts or phases to RO. One is the twenty-four-hour reality orientation phase for any confused resident. This phase incorporates an RO board, which is usually located in a central area of the facility. The board spells out such common information as the name of the facility, the weather, the date, the year, and information on activities that will take place that day, including the names of on-duty staff by shifts and of volunteers. Other environmental aids that might be used throughout the facility are large calendars and clocks and color coding of key places and doors.

Residents invariably are told where they are going (to the doctor, to the activity room), what will happen when they arrive, and what is expected of them. Staff are expected to be patient, to address older residents by last name, to repeat directions, to reward the resident for correct responses, and to gradually decrease direct assistance when the resident is able to be more self-directing. As the name of the program suggests, all conversation and activities must be reality oriented. The atmosphere should be quiet and friendly.

The other phase, classroom RO, as the name implies, takes place in a special room and is aimed at those who require more intensive work in a structured environment because of being grossly confused. Meetings are half an hour long and are usually held five days a week for a minimum of ten weeks. The group consists of four to six residents. The program supplements the twenty-four-hour approach. The approach can vary from the usual orienting procedure (time-place-person) to memory games. These sessions also may include grooming, exercise, and sensory training.[19]

RO is not a panacea. It works only if there is total cooperation and the staff is committed and involved in the functional improvement of the resident. Further, RO is not to be confused with reality therapy, which is a specific type of psychotherapy initially developed by William Glasser for use with delinquent adolescents.

Remotivation Therapy

Remotivation, like RO, is a structured type of approach that focuses on simple, objective aspects of day-to-day living. Its goals are to stimulate residents to become involved in thinking about the real world and to help them relate to others. In other words, the emphasis is on resocialization. Remotivation is often used after a resident has successfully completed RO.

Remotivation therapy sessions are usually conducted two or three times a week for approximately thirty minutes to one hour for a period of about three months with a group of five to twelve residents. In preparation for each meeting, the remotivator gathers materials on a particular topic. Visual aids such as pictures, articles, or props are used so that a high level of attention, interest, and reaction will be maintained. The subject matter always relates to the world from which the group member comes, and individuals are encouraged to participate in discussion about it. Topics dealing with residents' problems and family relationships are avoided.

Each session follows a pattern of successive stages: creating a climate of acceptance (greetings and establishing rapport); building a bridge to reality through introduction of the topic; detailed discussion of the topic and use of the previously prepared visual aids; discussion of work, particularly work the group members used to perform; and lastly, summary of the session as well as expressions of appreciation for the group's attendance, and a reminder of the time and place of the next meeting.[20]

According to some group leaders, the second stage may present problems, since poor vision or the inability to read may interfere with the use of the particular prop when a subject is introduced.[21] One author also found that substituting leisure for work in stage four has greater appeal for some residents. A major concern is developing a diverse selection of topics that appeal to and are of interest to a wide range of residents.[22]

Reminiscing Therapy

Reminiscing therapy is a group approach that uses the concept of reminiscing as a treatment modality. It is an approach being used more and more with elderly persons, especially those who are depressed. Evidence indicates that by reminiscing, residents are helped to accomplish the developmental tasks of older age and achieve a new sense of identity and a more positive self-concept.[23] Other studies of a more general nature suggest that reminiscing "enhances self-esteem, increases enjoyment of social relations, promotes intergenerational understanding, and helps individuals maintain a consistent self-concept."[24]

A traditional group-work approach is used in the sessions. Meetings are held once or twice weekly for approximately one hour. Goals for the residents include increasing self-esteem, increasing socialization and the ability to share meaningful memories with others, and increasing the awareness of the uniqueness of each participant.[25] Within the group the leader encourages the sharing of memories that may range from happy to sad, relaxed to sober and run through all

stages of life. Any sort of subject can be discussed in the session.[26]

Group Psychotherapy

This form of group therapy is another preferred treatment procedure found in nursing homes. Not all nursing homes can provide this form of therapy however, since it requires the leadership of an individual educated in psychiatric theory and group dynamics. On the other hand, there are many groups that use a psychotherapy approach and are conducted by a variety of personnel representing various disciplines. Group psychotherapy with residents is a very difficult technique because the attempt to solve problems through the group is difficult. The group is often slow to develop into a "group," and group continuity is threatened because of disabilities, tests, relative visits, and so on. When groups are successful they decrease the sense of isolation, facilitate the development of new roles or reestablishment of familiar roles, and afford group support for changes and enhancing self-esteem.

Other Interventions

Other interventive therapy forms that have had limited success in changing the behavior of residents in nursing homes include attitude therapy (a specific attitude to take toward each resident is decided upon by staff), which is used independently or in conjunction with RO; various behavior-modification techniques, such as positive reinforcement, desensitization, aversive procedures, modeling, and token economics, which aim to effect change in specific behaviors; contract therapy (agreement about behavior); sensory retraining; resocialization; and self-image therapy.

Like all therapy interventive techniques, the techniques considered in this section require training, some only limited, others extensive. Special skills and judgment are necessary in the selection of behaviors to be treated and in implementing the rather complex programs. Certain techniques may work with some residents with particular problems and not with others. In some situations success is achieved, but if the sessions are not sustained, success is limited or there is a return to former behavior. Although all of the techniques have produced favorable results, none is an unqualified success. All require sensitivity and judgment in their application. Further, they require a commitment of the total staff.

THERAPEUTIC RECREATION SERVICE (PATIENT ACTIVITY SERVICE)

As we begin this section, it is well to remember that the nature of the setting, its social structure and normative patterns, and its organizational hierarchies and behavior will strongly influence therapeutic recreation practice in any long-term care facility. While this is also true in other settings, it is especially so in the long-term care facility. The zealous, albeit well-intentioned, therapeutic recreation specialist who attempts to bypass any of the above factors and conduct independent group activities will encounter conflict or abandonment or isolation of the program from the rest of the home. To be effective, therapeutic recreation service must be understood and supported by all significant nursing home units or divisions.

The delivery of therapeutic recreation services (or patient activity services) represents a key segment of the total care and treatment program in a long-term care facility, primarily a SNF, by encouraging residents to function physically, emotionally, and socially in pursuit of a meaningful way of life. The therapeutic recreation program is directed toward meeting the needs of (1) those residents who are involved in a therapy-oriented program with specific treatment plans, and (2) those residents who participate in a planned and diversified schedule of therapeutic activities. These activities are designed to promote, sustain, and meet therapeutically the residents' physical and psychosocial needs as well as to assist residents in becoming adjusted to the nursing home environment, to the staff, and to resident peers.

Group Programming Considerations

Before considering the therapeutic recreation process, it is important to take into account some general factors that have an impact upon the process but are not necessarily a part of it.

Group Formation. The group can serve many needs for residents, from giving them peer support to developing a sense of self-esteem, to helping them develop new modes of functioning. But before this can happen the group has to come into being; it has to begin.

The specialist realizes there is no hard and fast rule or criterion that dictates the formation of a group. The specialist also recognizes that there may be seven or more different types or groups of residents to be considered:

1. The physically, emotionally, and intellectually intact
2. The physically disabled and intellectually intact
3. The ambulatory resident with advanced organic brain syndrome
4. The severely physically disabled with organic brain syndrome
5. The intellectually intact, ambulatory terminal resident
6. The terminal resident who is intellectually intact but severely debilitated
7. The mentally retarded or developmentally disabled person with or without various physical deficits

The specialist is further concerned about the diminution in perceptual and sensory perceptions of the elderly resident. In addition to visual losses, there are those losses related to auditory acuity and sensitivity found in many residents. And last, the specialist is aware of those who are nonambulatory or immobile because of such conditions as contractures, decubitus ulcers, incontinence, and weight loss resulting in malnutrition. These physical problems may impose severe behavioral characteristics, including depression, social withdrawal, apathy, and even stupor on the already bedfast resident.

In the final analysis, it is the purpose or goal of the proposed group that determines the thoughtful selection of residents in association with their functioning level. For example, the purpose of a particular group might be to facilitate orientation and social adjustment of newly admitted residents. Though all such residents could benefit from such a group experience, it would be inappropriate to mix severely brain-damaged residents with those whose cognitive functioning is intact. The nature, pace, and content of the group process, as the specialist knows, is different for different types of residents.

To inventory all activity groups that can be formed in a nursing home or any long-term care facility is an impossible task. Similarly, any classification of groups by type would be incomplete and beyond the focus of this section. Nevertheless, for illustrative purposes, a limited taxonomy will be offered:

1. *A group to focus on experiences relating to entry into the nursing home.* The very process of entry into a nursing home is often a very traumatic event for individuals of any age, one that is accompanied by loss of relationships and distortion of bonds between individuals, loss of possessions, feelings of loneliness, fear of death occasioned by a catastrophic illness, and general anxiety. The situation is further compounded because new residents may very well know they are probably relinquishing their independent living for the remainder of their lives. An activity group can enable residents to share experiences while participating in an activity. Such a group can be the vehicle for building new relationships and for orientation to the facilities, services, and staff.

2. *A group to focus on residents with emotional problems.* Therapeutic gains can be achieved via the activity group process with groups composed of residents who are depressed, those who exhibit behavioral problems, or those who appear withdrawn and isolated. Such persons may also be involved in other types of groups.

3. *A group to focus on residents and their family members.* It is wise to develop and maintain a group activity program that focuses on the residents and their families. Family members themselves often have reactions to the admission and residence of a loved one. Activities directed toward reliving past experiences help the resident to gain a reality perspective.

4. *A group to foster socialization.* There are an infinite variety of group activities that foster socialization. Such groups go a long way toward combatting anhedonia (loss of capacity for pleasure) and promoting social interchange and close friendships.

5. *A group to offer opportunities for creating new roles and continuity of previous roles.* Like socialization groups, these groups provide opportunity for roles that offer status and foster individuality, self-esteem, and a sense of mastery. Groups formed to plan or implement activities can include the production board of the nursing home's newsletter and groups to plan special events for holidays and parties.

6. *A group for self-actualization and personal growth.* In this category are activity groups with an emphasis on new learning and new skills—painting, sculpture, music playing, and the like.

7. *A group to link the nursing home and community.* Residents generally are deprived of the kinds of activities that keep people in "normal" living situations connected with the community outside their own dwelling. All needs are met in the nursing home, resulting in isolation and a sharply constricted world. No matter how benevolent the administrator of the home is, it is essential for residents to feel part of the total community. Groups that take residents out of the home and bring the community into the home are extremely desirable. Groups that create involvement with younger adults and children are particularly useful for those who live in a world of elderly people.

As emphasized earlier, every effort should be made to keep family ties viable. Further, community groups of which residents have been members should be invited and encouraged to visit and to make it possible for the respective residents to attend their meetings and special events in the community.

In conclusion, suggested criteria for forming a group might include the following:

Level of health

Degree of vision and hearing loss

Goals for particular residents

Relevance of the activity to resident's interests

Relevance of the activity to specialist's estimate of the resident's unconscious motivation

Resident's level of ability in relation to the requirements of the activity

Amount of affect shown in resident contact with specialist

Ability to handle interpersonal contact as seen in resident's reaction to group

Number and quality of present group affiliations

The Value of Group Activities. The quality of life in a nursing home or in any long-term care facility is largely reflective of the activities program. Considering that most of a resident's day is spent in free time, the nature of the activities program can be critical to the value of the overall nursing home program of services. Further, the activity program is the key to creating a therapeutic milieu that provides all residents with stimulation, meaningful roles, choices, social interaction, opportunity to express individuality, and ties with the community. Many activities can be provided to achieve goals relating to the milieu or the entire group of residents. For example, a recreational family night might be designed to help residents experience community spirit and belonging, maintain previous roles and family ties, and improve feelings of self-worth.

For an activity program to be therapeutic, it must result in positive changes that will last. Thus, for an activities program to be therapeutic, residents should not only enjoy and benefit from attending the activities, but they must also be affected in some way that carries over to other aspects of their lives. Activities must do more than produce an occasional bright spot of entertainment in an otherwise dull existence; activities must help residents learn new information, skills, and behaviors or improve their feelings of self-esteem and independence.

Activity groups can also provide an arena and opportunity to develop mastery in negotiating the environment of the home. Residents tend to feel very small, meek, and obedient in the face of the rather complex, frightening milieu in which they find themselves. Collective efforts, as well as efforts on the part of residents that are shared and supported by other residents, can be uplifting. Thus, an activity group can be a source of strength for facing the larger world, the nursing home.

There is a positive relationship between good physical, emotional, and social health and participation in activities. Without purposeful activity the motivation to maintain health may wither away. Day and evening activities can be organized for and with residents to utilize their time productively. Activities of all kinds can prevent or reduce chronicity of symptoms, regression, isolation, apathy, and withdrawal, as well as listlessness, milling around, and the excessive reminiscing about the past too often observed among older residents.

Lastly, the activity group can become a unit for satisfying mutual needs. The specialist is not an authority figure representing the home, but rather assumes various roles depending upon the activity and the level of functioning of the residents. Thus, the role the specialist projects within some specific activities allows residents in that activity to achieve a sense of control and mastery of their participation. It also gives the specialist room to provide support and protection to residents, taking into account their dependency needs.

Group Participation. While activities can help overcome many problems of a personal nature associated with the nursing home, they can be helpful only to the resident who participates. If a resident will not participate, obviously that resident cannot be helped. The nursing home staff and interdisciplinary team of which the specialist is a member must resolve the dilemma of whether a resident must participate or has the right *not* to participate, even though such participation would be helpful to the resident. Sometimes a resident just wants to be left alone. This is related to the resident's need for privacy, emotional as well as physical. Considering individual cases over a period of time, the specialist begins to determine whom to encourage a little more and whom to leave alone. Yet the question of participation versus nonparticipation is not one to be taken lightly. There is a fine line between urging and forcing residents to participate in activities.

Associated with participation is the need to identify and capitalize on the resident's strengths while not neglecting physical, emotional, social, and intellectual needs or focusing on losses and deficits. Existing and latent strengths in many instances constitute the foundation on which constructive therapeutic activity programs can be built. The specialist and other nursing home staff, including volunteers, who might participate with residents in activity programs should be supportive, even at times demanding of a resident's performance. Satisfaction with poor performance will more than likely guarantee continued poor performance. Making demands on residents may, in fact, encourage achievement.

Group Scheduling. Assuming that communication with the nursing home staff has taken place regarding the scheduling of the various activity groups, the nature of staff involvement, and the purpose of the activity group, a calendar needs to be developed, preferably on a weekly or monthly basis. It is desirable for the calendar to include all group activity services planned during the month, as well as provide the staff with a list of the residents participating in the various group activities.

However, the scheduling of activity groups can present a number of problems. In many nursing homes it is not unusual for only one specialist, and even in large nursing homes no more than two specialists, and maybe an aide to be employed. Therapies, treatments, individual and group activities, meals, housekeeping duties, and so on, are all competing for the residents' time. All of these matters are further compounded by the limited energy the resident has to spend in the full range of daily activities. It is no wonder some residents want to rest or nap after lunch or in the middle of the afternoon.

Some of the problems associated with scheduling and resident participation can be reduced if a recreation council or committee is established. Where possible, and within the limitations of residents, participation of residents in the program-planning process is at times an essential component of program development. The specialist should meet with council members monthly to review the upcoming month's schedule and discuss new programs or the elimination of current programs that are poorly attended.

One final note about participation. There is always concern about how the death of a resident affects the day-to-day program schedule. To some extent it depends on the popularity of the resident and the length of the illness. Generally speaking, death does not seem to affect residents as much as we might think; residents seem to be able to adjust better than staff. The only thing that can or should cancel a program is a medical quarantine. However, a department policy should be formulated to handle this matter. The authors' experience has been to acknowledge the death and allow residents in the activity to talk about it. If it is an individual in the group, the fact that the person will be missed can show others that they will also be missed if they die.

Group Activity Space. The physical environment of the nursing home and the setting where activities are conducted also are important in planning and implementing an activity program.

The physical structure of many older and some newer nursing homes were not designed with activity programs in mind. Planners did not envision the myriad of services that would be needed; thus, space is at a premium. Even in many new nursing homes, with costs high, appropriate spaces for activities often do not exist.

The physical comfort and needs of the activity-group participants need to be considered to the fullest possible extent. Spaces that are too vast are as undesirable as overly crowded quarters. Other considerations are doorways that permit access by wheelchairs, nonslippery floor surfaces, chairs that do not tend to tip, and appropriate temperatures and lighting. The various activity rooms need to be made comfortable and inviting.

In the main, the specialist must be prepared for the constraints of physical space. Often the activity program will be a second or even third use of space. Dining areas, a chapel, a staff or visitors' lounge, or a conference room may have to be used as an activity room. Careful scheduling and clearances, of course, are critical. In good weather access should be available to an outdoor area.

A summary of the factors considered in this section plus other general factors associated with leadership and programming are found in Figure 8.1 on p. 206.

THE THERAPEUTIC RECREATION PROCESS

In this section we consider the therapeutic recreation process in action in a nursing home. Two case histories are provided to demonstrate the process. The initial one is carried out to completion (assessment, planning, implementation, and evaluation), including a brief discussion of the usual procedure used in admitting an individual to a nursing home. We describe the eventual referral of that individual to an interdisciplinary team conference to formulate a care and treatment plan. The second case is interrupted after the goals are stated in the planning process to allow the student, with guidance from the instructor, the opportunity to complete the care plan for the resident as well as to determine how it would be implemented and evaluated.

CASE EXAMPLE ONE

Case History of Mrs. O.

Mrs. O., age seventy-two, is slightly over five feet tall and weighs nearly two hundred pounds. She has a fifteen-year history of orthopedic difficulty resulting from an automobile accident. A spinal disc had been removed several years earlier to prevent complete immobilization. Fol-

FIGURE 8.1. Leadership Techniques and Program Concepts with Elderly Clients

1. Enunciate clearly. Stand directly in front of the client, and make sure you gain the client's attention before speaking. Speak in a lower voice tone, since upper frequencies are more difficult to hear.
2. Address clients by preferred title and name. Show respect by using Mr., Miss, Mrs., or Dr.
3. Plan rest intervals, and encourage conversation as a form of social interaction during these time periods.
4. Intersperse motivators such as food, familiar "old" song, companionship, or responsibility in the program format.
5. Listen to the trivial conversation and accept the signs of affection, whether they be a handshake, pat on the shoulder, or eulogy to younger generations. The need to receive and give with "touch" is as necessary as always, yet the elderly frequently receive less.
6. Schedule activities with daily routines in mind. Consider weather, traffic patterns, amount of daylight remaining, transportation routes, and the availability of additional supportive services.
7. Activities in the program should allow for various levels of participation. Clients should feel comfortable dropping into and out of activities.
8. Design activities so clients receive peer recognition and are encouraged to improve by competing against personal performance levels.
9. Avoid experiences that might prove embarrassing. Examples of such situations are a client dropping out of an activity that is too physically demanding, or a therapeutic recreator completing a project so that it resembles a "model" for clients.
10. Schedule intergenerational activities to encourage participation with persons in the mainstream of community affairs.
11. Compensate for lessened visual discrimination by using contrasting colors and sizes.
12. Include such experiences as volunteering, developing a resource, or providing a service, to allow clients to experience a "meaningful role."
13. The student who chooses to work with aging persons must bring to the helping process several qualities. Patience, humor, consistency, firmness, and a willingness to confront resistive clients are musts. This may involve repeated reminders and ignorance of excuses. Other needed qualities include being a good listener, maintaining a positive attitude, being frank and at the same time sincere, and willingness to motivate and share enthusiasm.
14. Cost analysis occurs in the planning of all programs but is most critical with aging persons as their incomes may be fixed or of necessity limited. When a coffee hour asks for a "twenty-five-cent donation" per cup, some persons will not attend.
15. Accommodate the potential heterogeneity of the group. The chronological age span may be from five to twenty years or more.
16. Rules, procedures, directions should be explicit and precise.
17. We do not automatically improve with age. Habits and attitudes are carried through the aging process. A person who lacked musical ability as a child will probably be the same as an adult.
18. Plan carefully around the physical environment. Restrooms and parking lots should be close and accessible. Entries and exits should be well lighted and marked. Voice amplifiers and controls for heat, lights, and temperature should be available.
19. Permit clients to pursue activities for short time periods to allow for memory loss and decreased attending skills.
20. Realize and consider the importance of feelings. Fear of crime, failure, loss of health, financial dependency, death and dying, and physical changes associated with aging are realities of becoming "old." Recognize the desire to leave something meaningful, to share a special memento, to "get things in order," to eat certain foods, or to follow a specific routine.

SOURCE: Reproduced by permission from Marcia Jean Carter, Glen E. Van Andel, and Gary M. Robb, *Therapeutic Recreation: A Practical Approach* (St. Louis: Times Mirror/Mosby College Publishing, 1985), p. 375.

lowing rehabilitation, she was ambulatory with the assistance of two canes but subsequently regressed to the point of being confined to a wheelchair. A brace was fitted, and Mrs. O. received training in the use of a quad cane but complained of the pain when walking and returned again to her wheelchair. Although the pain was real, it was aggravated by her obesity and arthritic knee (osteoarthritis). As a result of her inability to ambulate, she resigned herself to a passive state and withdrew from contact with relatives and friends and from partaking of social events to the degree she would have liked. She defended herself against this withdrawal and the anxiety it created by a bitter humor, and an underlying depression was noted. A mild hearing loss was also noted.

Admission Phase and Referral

Individuals are usually admitted to a skilled nursing facility only on the recommendation of a physician. However, if the individual's family physician does not plan or follow the individual into the nursing home, the individual, the family, or sponsor can be assisted by the social service department in appointing an appropriate attending physician.

At the time of admission the physician provides the nursing home with medical information about the incoming resident. If the resident is coming from a hospital, a transcript of the resident's hospital record is provided, including a description of the resident's functional status. If the resident is coming from home, medical information is provided prior to or on the day of arrival. If such information is not provided, a medical history and physical examination must be performed within forty-eight hours of admission at the nursing home.

Within a few days following admission and, depending on the size, scope, philosophy, and staffing pattern of the facility, the resident is referred to the interdisciplinary team (sometimes called a multidisciplinary team) for assessment. The referral to the team may come from either the personal or attending physician of the resident, or there is a blanket referral. The team is responsible for exploring, developing, planning, and coordinating a resident-care plan and discharge plan. Ideally, the resident's physician, attending physician, or medical director of the nursing home (each nursing home is required to have a medical director employed either full or part time or as a consultant) is present at the interdisciplinary meeting. When the doctor does not attend, the nursing director or social worker assumes responsibility for the direction of the meeting.

The meeting furnishes an opportunity for various department or unit heads (medical, nursing, dietary, social service, therapeutic recreation service, occupational therapy, etc.) to become familiar with the medical and psychosocial history of the newly admitted resident, to discuss the current functional status of the resident, to consider treatment procedures and realistic goals for overcoming various problems of the resident, and to identify the resident's potential for returning to the community or for transfer to another setting. If discharge is not in the foreseeable future, that will be noted. In addition to considering newly admitted residents, the team also reviews the progress of residents already participating in their specific care plan. Moreover, consideration may be given to discharge planning for appropriate residents.

In addition to the interdisciplinary conferences concerned with formulating a care plan and reviewing progress, there may be preadmission case conferences, problem-oriented conferences (to deal with special difficulties that have arisen with a particular resident), and even unit, floor team, or area team conferences to coordinate the care of residents in a particular area of the home. Such conferences provide the opportunity to discuss not only residents but problems and situations concerning the entire unit.

While interdisciplinary conferences are a well-established method of diagnosing, developing plans, or evaluating, they are ineffective unless thorough preparation takes place. In preparation for a conference, the therapeutic recreation specialist needs to evaluate the resident as everyone else does, from the vantage point of his or her particular expertise. Discussion should result in consensus about the approach and the care plan. Some method of spelling out goals and procedures and evaluating achievements needs to be employed.

ASSESSMENT

As noted in the previous chapter, the specialist has knowledge about problems associated with individuals who enter nursing homes from personal experience, education, and the interdisciplinary conference. One nursing home administrator has pointed out: "It is essential for the activity coordinator to be aware of the nature of the patient population to be served including the patient's ability to adapt to disability, to congregate living and to separation from home and family."[27]

Regarding Mrs. O., the specialist realizes that the very process of entry into the home is a traumatic event, one that is accompanied by a loss of relationships and distortion of bonds between individuals, loss of possessions, feelings of loneliness, and general anxiety, and further, that Mrs. O. is relinquishing her independent living. The specialist knows that entering a new group, particularly a closed group with the strict boundaries of the home, creates considerable anxiety. To resolve these problems and to reduce the practical difficulties to a minimum, the specialist helps Mrs. O. to feel accepted and welcome not only to the home but to the various activity groups through introductions. By considering the entry needs of Mrs. O., the specialist reduces the fears and fantasies that Mrs. O. may have about the home and acts in such a manner as to support psychosocial functioning.

Unfortunately, the nursing home environment in many instances fosters dependency and engenders feelings of loss; the very nature of the setting helps reinforce the societal myths and stereotypes of the ill, the disabled, the aged, and the fears that are associated with each of these problems. In consideration of life in a nursing home, we are reminded of an article by Nelida Ferrari, written some years ago but still fresh today, that discussed the unique aspects of groups and individuals in a nursing home. She pointed out that individuals living in such a setting are already living as a group, "united not by their past experiences, but by a common presence of need and discomfort, of frustration and anxieties . . . together, but lonesome. They [have] solitude, but not privacy. They [are] alone, but without the chance to be themselves. A group yes, but a lonely group, with its members unidentified in a big gray mass."[28]

Data Collection

In order to develop a resident's therapeutic care plan it is necessary to have as accurate and complete an assessment as possible. Ideally, the assessment begins shortly after the resident has been admitted and before the interdisciplinary team meeting. The goal regarding assessment is to elicit recreation and leisure-interest information, as well as probing and exchanging general health information with the resident through an interview. The initial contact with the resident involves a greeting to make the resident feel comfortable, provide structure, and indicate the goal of the interview. The interview should incorporate the following empathic characteristics:

1. Establishing trust
2. Building rapport
3. Helping the person to identify recreation and leisure interests
4. Paraphrasing for clarity of interest
5. Discussing abilities to pursue activities within limitations
6. Keeping questions to a minimum
7. Allowing freedom of expression

This list of desirable characteristics may be demanding, but it includes items that any involved, caring, helping specialist does intuitively.

Taking information from the resident, as the specialist knows, may involve more than the ordinary amount of skill because of (a) sensory deficits, which may make communication difficult; (b) the need to establish rapport by building trust and allaying anxiety; and (c) the increased requirement of feedback.

In gathering information in the interview, the specialist uses an interest survey from whose format follows a question-and-answer interplay. An open-ended questionnaire elicits more information than a closed-ended questionnaire. Excluding specific recreation and leisure-activity interest questions, open-ended questions usually begin with the following words: how, when, where, who, why, and what. Interviewing skills enhance the interview process, since there is usually difficulty in administering any type of self-taking interest form with the disoriented and/or disabled resident.

While interviewing has its place in the assessment procedure, observation also has its place, as noted earlier. Observation may be of an objective nature—that which can be seen, felt, or heard—or of a subjective nature—that which is reported by the resident. Behavior is what is known to exist because it has been observed; it is seen, heard, or even sensed as it happens, but it is not inferred or deduced. Further, observation need not always be associated with the interview situation; accurate observation may be made during all interactions. In many respects, observation may be more useful, especially for the therapeutic recreation specialist in an activity environment.

Interview. In the interview the specialist follows a semistructured format with Mrs. O. that is designed to avoid stress and allow for a friendly conversation that flows from one topic to another on the activity-interest form. The specialist is interested in knowing, in addition to activity and leisure experiences and physical abilities and limita-tions, about problems associated with memory, communication, socialization, self-concept, self-reliance, judgment, senses, and the like. (See Figure 8.2.) The responses in all these areas are helpful in selecting appropriate activities and approaches to be used with Mrs. O. in meeting her physical and psychosocial needs. If the interdisciplinary team has not previously met, this information is added to Mrs. O.'s record for inclusion and discussion at the team meeting.

As a result of the interview with Mrs. O., the specialist identified and recorded the following:

ACTIVITY INTEREST

Listens to semiclassical music

Likes reading—newspaper and suspense novels

Knits

Sews

Needlepoint (learning a new activity)

Watches TV—soap operas

PROBLEMS

Overweight

Depressed over changes associated with living arrangement compounded by feeling that family has abandoned her

Preoccupied with events in an earlier period of time

Feeling of dependency and helplessness because of restriction to wheelchair

Limited mobility because of restriction to wheelchair

Fear that arthritis will affect wrist and fingers resulting in inability to pursue sewing interest and so-called hobby

Complains of pain and tenderness associated with movement of arthritic knee, of pain in back when bending forward, of being fatigued after limited personal self-care, and of being lonely (but has made no effort to leave room)

FIGURE 8.2. Therapeutic Recreation Service Assessment

Name: _____   Medical Number: _____

Birthdate: _____   Age: _____

Admission Date: _____   Place of Birth: _____

Diagnosis: _____

Religious Preference: _____

Education: _____

Occupation: _____

PHYSICAL

Ambulatory _____   Wheelchair _____   Walker Cane _____

Paralysis _____   Hearing _____   Vision _____

Continent _____   Feeds Self _____   Dresses Self _____

Communication Skills _____

Observations _____

_____

MENTAL

Alert _____   Disorientation: Person _____   Place _____   Time _____

Depression _____   Wanders _____

Observations _____

_____

SOCIAL (Hobbies/Interests)

1. _____   5. _____

2. _____   6. _____

3. _____   7. _____

4. _____   8. _____

Completed by _____ Date _____

OTHER

No contact with other residents except roommate

No visitors since admission

When questioned about her ability to do ADL and leisure activities, responded with hostile humor about her problems

Appears to be quite aware of worldly events

PLANNING

Following the assessment, the specialist analyzes the information so as to develop a care plan that includes meeting the physical and psychosocial needs of Mrs. O. Likewise, other disciplines are in the process of developing their respective plans. In addition, Mrs. O.'s medical examination record, which is now available on the unit, indicates that her functional ability is limited until such time as her weight is brought under control so as to reduce the stress on her right knee. Further, antiinflammatory medication is ordered for the knee, physical therapy is prescribed, and exercise for both knee and back are recommended. Since residents are automatically entered into the therapeutic recreation program at the time of admission unless otherwise noted, the specialist proceeds with developing goals and considering activities to achieve goal attainment.

In preparation for developing a care plan for Mrs. O., the specialist must now consider those physical and psychosocial factors that are associated with her problems or obstacles. Space prevents an in-depth analysis of each problem and its related elements, but it is important, nevertheless, to highlight a few of these obstacles and strategies for their resolution.

The specialist realizes that for many individuals with arthritis the greatest fear is to be wheelchair bound, totally dependent, and confined to a nursing home. However, they also know that they may avoid that fate with adequate physical therapy and exercise. Still, the response to discomfort, limitation, and fatigue can easily cause isolation and confinement. The specialist knows that Mrs. O. needs to become involved in various activities.

The specialist further recognizes that the verbal hostility expressed through humor is probably Mrs. O.'s reaction to her disability, seeing it as an unfair act of fate. Further, it reflects her need to strike out at the unknown force that has changed her life. Such hostile humor may be an unconscious way to crystallize feelings in a socially acceptable manner. Thus the specialist knows to be alert to such behavior during activities, while at the same time being tolerant and attempting to understand what forces are behind Mrs. O.'s behavior.

The specialist is also aware that the problems associated with pain—depression, dependency, and anxiety—are the result of any number of physical and psychosocial factors, such as: (1) lack of opportunity for back muscles to relax because Mrs. O. is bending forward; (2) cumulation of physical and emotional stress and strain (It is known that emotional stress contributes to some forms of arthritis. Symptoms may appear after a crisis—Mrs. O.'s automobile accident—and develop further during times of emotional stress—accident, removal of disc)[29]; (3) lack of a state of balance among bones, discs, muscles, tendons, and ligaments as well as back alignment; (4) inflammation of arthritic knee; (5) coping with problem of self, back, and knee is in itself a source of tension, depression, and fatigue;

(6) overweight; and (7) uncertainty about the course of the affected joint and back in relation to her daily performance.

Taking into consideration the problems of Mrs. O., the following goals or needs are noted and recorded with no priority being given. (The reader needs to realize that a lengthy list of goals could be developed; however, the focus will be on the more obvious problems and goals.)

Problems: Overweight
Fear, depression, and anxiety resulting from present living arrangement, arthritic knee, and painful back
Pain resulting from fear, anxiety, overweight, fatigue, and general body condition
Verbal abuse of individuals through negative humor
Limited mobility

Goals: To improve body image
To assist in reduction of pain
To develop ability to relax
To increase socialization
To acquire appropriate conversation skills
To acquire new leisure interests
To improve self-concept

Following the determination of goals, the specialist considers what activities are best suited to reach goal attainment. In some nursing homes this process is completed after the specialist attends the interdisciplinary team meeting. Thus the specialist can gather additional information relative to needs prior to the final decision. In other nursing homes the therapeutic recreation care plan is decided on before the team meeting and adjustments made thereafter if necessary. For our situation, we will follow the latter procedure.

After careful analysis of the current group activities and their value or purpose, the specialist is ready to consider the goals in relation to activities. Regarding Mrs. O., the following group activities have been selected by the specialist to meet the goals:

Goal: To improve body image
Activity: Exercise (wheelchair group)

Goal: To assist in the reduction of pain
Activity: The various activity groups as noted

Goal: To develop the ability to relax
Activity: Music-listening group

Goal: To increase socialization
Activity: Current events club, recreation council, exercise group, and music-listening group

Goal: To improve conversation skills
Activity: The various activity groups as noted

Goal: To acquire new leisure interests
Activity: Sewing class (needlepoint) and residents' monthly newsletter (writing)

Goal: To improve self-concept
Activity: The various activity groups as noted

Considering Mrs. O.'s condition, the reader is undoubtedly concerned about the exercise program. Let's step back a moment and consider the wheelchair exercise activity. The activity has a purpose of providing opportunities for wheelchair-bound residents to improve health and fitness. The goals of this activity are as follows:

To improve physical fitness
To increase physical functioning
To release physical tension
To prevent physical deterioration
To increase socialization
To stimulate affective responses

Prior to the assignment of Mrs. O. to the wheelchair exercise group activity, the specialist will make a more complete assessment of Mrs. O.'s physical limitations so that unnatural or discomforting positions are avoided. This is important since joints become less flexible and bones more fragile with age. The value of the activity for Mrs. O. is that the loss of movement increases tension, and tension produces pain; in addition, extra weight on the joint and indirectly on the back also causes pain.

Meanwhile, the physical therapist will be developing a care plan centering on therapeutic exercises as prescribed to maintain maximum range of motion in the joint. A program of a like nature will also be developed to strengthen back muscles. Muscle weakness impairs the stability of the joint and back and predisposes both problems to additional trauma and pain.

Regarding the music-listening activity, music has long been known as an effective tool in changing behavior. Studies have demonstrated very clearly that music stimulates the entire body, producing physical sensations and causing subtle physiological changes.[30] In addition, music has been used to deepen the relaxation process, to change moods, to help individuals move with more freedom, and to develop group cohesiveness.[31] As most specialists know, music is an easy way to encourage social interaction and an integral part of exercise programs. New residents who are withdrawn, hostile, and depressed usually react favorably to music because it creates a nonthreatening environment. It also provides an atmosphere for expression of feelings—fear, anxiety, and so on. Thus the assignment of Mrs. O. to a music-listening activity should be beneficial. The reason for the assignment of Mrs. O. to the current events club and residents' council plus the other two activities is self-evident. All require some form of socialization. Residents can contribute to current events or topics can be presented by the specialist with residents' opinions discussed. Any sort of news—national, community, and nursing home—can be included. Topics or events help residents to discover common interests and experiences among themselves; this can lead to strong friendships and increased interaction. In addition, factual information that relates to personal health can help Mrs. O. and others adapt to the changes that accompany the aging process, and they can benefit from each other's support in addition to the socialization value.

In addition to the current-events club and other activities having a socialization value, the assignment of Mrs. O. to the residents' recreation council provides the opportunity for Mrs. O. to have some control over her life in the facility. It allows her to feel somewhat confident that her needs will be met by the specialist; it is a vehicle through which Mrs. O. can express her wishes and share in decision making, thus reducing powerlessness. It further allows her the opportunity for playing an adult role rather than the constant role of resident, of the helpless one who must always take and never be the giver or the helper.

Mrs. O.'s interest in learning needlepoint is pursued by scheduling her for a sewing class, a resident-led group that meets informally two afternoons a week in the lounge. Such an activity could quite possibly develop into a hobby, and a hobby can be not only a source of personal pleasure but a powerful distractor from pain.[32]

The specialist also suggests that Mrs. O. might want to join the resident's newspaper staff because of her reading interest. The resident who formerly covered the specific wing that Mrs. O. is living in was discharged. It would also give her the opportunity to develop writing skills since she would be responsible for developing the articles about the unit for the newsletter. Further, it would allow her to write on current events taking place in the home. The opportunity would provide Mrs. O. with recognition—a sign of individual worth to many residents.

If Mrs. O. follows the care plan that is being recommended to the interdisciplinary team, it would be anticipated that her self-concept would improve. Moreover, participation in the group activities would provide Mrs. O. with the opportunity for success and achievement, which would assist her to change her self-concept about her arthritic knee. As you know, a person's body image is changed when hands, feet, shoulders, or knees are deformed. At the same time, the care plan is also directed toward the relief of pain. More time alone or being inactive means less distraction from pain and makes all aspects of one's life less bearable. Thus coping with the depression, tension, anxiety, and fatigue associated with the arthritic knee and painful back can be alleviated to a large degree through various relaxation techniques and participation in social activity.[33] The long-term goal for Mrs. O. is eventual discharge; however, if that is not feasible, then to assist Mrs. O. to become as independent as possible in the home.

Having determined which activities will meet Mrs. O.'s goals, the specialist must now develop a plan for evaluation, which in reality becomes a description of terminal expectations for each goal. The goal, activity, and behavioral objectives for Mrs. O. are as follows:

Goal: To improve body image
Activity: Exercise (wheelchair group)
Behavioral Objective: Following three weeks of participation in the wheelchair exercise group activity, Mrs. O. will have lost seven pounds. (The specialist is aware that Mrs. O. will be put on a diet and participate in a physical therapy program.)

Goal: To assist in the reduction of pain
Activity: The various activity groups as noted
Behavioral Objective: Following three weeks of participation in the various scheduled activity groups, Mrs. O. will demonstrate a reduction in pain by:
verbally indicating a decrease in pain
indicating a desire to participate more frequently in scheduled activities
moving body more freely

Goal: To develop ability to relax
Activity: Music-listening group
Behavioral Objective: Following three weeks of participation in the music listening group activity, Mrs. O. will demonstrate the ability to relax by:
verbally indicating a decrease in pain

requesting records for private listening

measuring pulse rate before and after listening to music

verbally communicating feelings about relaxation

Goal: To increase socialization

Activity: Current-events club, recreation council, exercise group, and music-listening group

Behavioral Objective: Following three weeks of participation in the various scheduled activity groups, Mrs. O. will demonstrate increased socialization by:
> verbally recognizing other residents voluntarily
> showing a willingness to engage in conversation
> indicating a positive responsiveness to participate in activities
> participating actively in activities

Goal: To improve appropriate conversation skills

Activity: The various activities as noted

Behavioral Objective: Following three weeks of participation in the various scheduled activity groups, Mrs. O. will demonstrate improved conversation skills by:
> maintaining an appropriate conversation with staff and other residents
> refraining from inappropriate humor
> responding in an appropriate manner to comments or questions by specialist, staff, and other residents

Goal: To acquire new leisure interests

Activity: Sewing class (needlepoint) and newspaper (writing)

Behavioral Objective: After three weeks Mrs. O. will be participating in the sewing class and interviewing seven or more residents in the unit.

Goal: To improve self-concept

Activity: The various activities as noted

Behavioral Objective: Following three weeks of participation in the various scheduled activity groups, Mrs. O. will demonstrate improved self-concept by:
> refraining from inappropriate humor
> interacting more frequently with staff and residents
> remarking about weight loss

After the specialist has developed the care plan, it is taken to the interdisciplinary team meeting and discussed with other disciplines. In this way a list of strengths, problems, needs, and goals are developed for Mrs. O., resulting in a comprehensive plan of care for meeting her needs and achieving her goals. In addition, Mrs. O.'s care-plan review date will be noted. Federal regulations require that Mrs. O.'s plan be reviewed and revised, if necessary, at the end of ninety days. Prior to the date changes, additions, and notes regarding the progress of Mrs. O. toward goal achievement are indicated in her record or chart. Such charting is important because Mrs. O.'s needs, like other residents needs, can change quickly. Naturally, all changes, additions, and progress notes are dated.

Resident Record. It is wise at this juncture to discuss the purpose of the resident's health record and the documentation of this record. While the resident's health record serves a number of purposes, a most important one is that it is a basis on which to plan for and evaluate the care given and communicate the results of that care and treatment to all team members.

The content of health records will be facts, opinions, conclusions, observations, and hearsay (unfortunately); each comment must be carefully worded to indicate its essence.

Health records are either source oriented or problem oriented. In keeping source-oriented records, which are the more traditional format, each person on the health-care team uses separate forms. This method of documentation can become unwieldy since it usually requires the reading of every form in order to get the whole picture of the individual resident.

More recently many skilled nursing facilities (and other health facilities) have gone to the problem-oriented record, which contains four basic components: the *data base* (medical and social history); the *problem list* (self-explanatory, but each problem is assigned a number, which ensures that progress notes relate to specific problems); the *initial care plan* (each problem has its own care plan with time-related goals); and *progress notes*. Progress notes contain the progress of the resident with respect to each problem and include narrative notes and flow sheets. On a flow sheet dates are recorded in the left margin of the page, and observations and treatments are written across the page, thereby producing a graphic picture of the care that the resident received. The flow sheet may also be designed to indicate progress with each specific numbered problem.

IMPLEMENTATION

Implementation of the plan incorporates those dimensions discussed in the previous chapter—*continuity of care, communicating the plan,* and various *intervention strategies.* Continuity of care, as noted earlier, can be expected when all disciplines involved with Mrs. O. have completed their respective care plans and each has implemented its plan. Further, it is absolutely essential that members of each discipline concerned with Mrs. O., as well as with any of the other residents, communicate their plan with the others so that all disciplines involved are aware of all the goals in order to ensure consistency. Continuity of care and communicating the plan cannot be emphasized enough. Successful adjustment and care and treatment of Mrs. O. and others depend on thorough orientation by all health-care personnel, including therapeutic recreation service, to the functions of other disciplines and an awareness of their approaches and their specific goals.

Intervention is a painstaking task in a nursing home, even when the prognosis is optimistic for residents. Working with elderly residents like Mrs. O. demands of the specialist patience, minimal expectations, and a high degree of tolerance to both frustration and irritation. If specialists expect to observe immediate change in working with the elderly residents, they will encounter extreme disappointment.

Because the success of any care plan is in large part dependent upon the patient's willingness to participate, time must be devoted toward helping Mrs. O. make the effort to get involved. Working with residents in nursing homes can be exhausting since many residents require constant stimulation and individual attention. The demands of the group, regardless of its composition, require a sharp attention to details, the observation of each resident, and sensitivity to the environment at all times.

Prior to Mrs. O.'s entry into her various assigned group activities, the specialist will have met with her to explain the various activities, the purpose of the activities, and where and when the activities meet. At the same time the specialist is preparing Mrs. O., the specialist is informing the other group participants that a new resident will be joining their group. As the specialist knows, when an older new resident joins a particular activity group, he or she is generally a passive participant, and the activity is most often seen as a threat rather than a challenge. Therefore, it is important for Mrs. O. to see the various activities as something in which she can participate and that will serve her needs rather than an something planned and imposed on her by the specialist and others. According to one source, activities are not ends in themselves but are "settings for interpersonal relationships among members that produce feelings of approval and recognition."[34]

The specialist's contact with Mrs. O. and

other residents in any of the group activities enables the specialist to observe the effect of the activity on each individual. The specialist needs to be alert to the ways in which the activity hinders or fosters the goals developed for Mrs. O. and the other participants. Group activities cannot be simply considered as a means of filling time; groups are effective therapeutic media.

The interpersonal relationship of the group activity participants provides opportunities for meeting psychosocial needs. It is the specialist's responsibility to guide these relationships so that performances and achievements are positive, realistic, and can instill a sense of mastery; this is important since residents like Mrs. O. have met much frustration in the outside world. From one perspective, the specialist directs intervention activities in a way that helps residents find the coping strengths and resources within themselves to produce the necessary change for accomplishing the goals.

Let us now return to Mrs. O. and her care plan with a brief illustration of her participation and progress:

In the course of the first few weeks, Mrs. O. was reluctant and then hesitant about participation in any of her scheduled group activities, although the specialist did review with her on a number of occasions her care plan. Eventually, Mrs. O., with gentle prodding, responded to the specialist's request to attend various group activities.

At first her behavior verbally and physically disrupted group activities. However, when other group residents, assisted by the specialist, indicated their disapproval and ignored her behavior, Mrs. O. gradually modified her behavior to be more acceptable. Thereafter, she moved slowly into the group life in the various activities, while at the same time working through her feelings of isolation and the limitations of nursing home living. She indicated to the specialist and staff that although she missed her family and friends, she enjoyed the friendships she was making. Moreover, she was beginning to take pride in her accomplishments in the exercise program and the current-events club. After

starting her exercise program and her diet, Mrs. O. lost seven pounds.

The resident recreation council involvement has been partially successful. Since the council meets only monthly, Mrs. O. has yet to become involved. At the first meeting she did express her opinion about some activities; however, she was still upset about being a resident, and her comments were mostly negative. The council did not meet the next month.

The music activity emerged as a most important medium. Mrs. O. sang songs with the other group participants, and because she had a pleasant voice she began to respond to requests from participants for special songs. This led to her anticipating every music activity session.

Another activity she enjoyed was her needlepoint class, although it took some time before she became involved. When she was first introduced to the group participants, she sat quietly near the exit and simply watched and listened to the group conversation without comment or committing herself. After observing the group for over a week, she asked if she could join the group. Since her active participation she has made a number of small gift decorations. As a result, she anticipates the sessions and enjoys the social interaction that takes place.

There was less success in interviewing other residents on the unit for the newsletter. This may have been more the residents' fault and lack of additional knowledge by the specialist about Mrs. O. and other residents before suggesting this activity, since a number of the residents on the unit had visual and hearing limitations. Mrs. O. lost interest in pursuing the activity even though the specialist and staff encouraged her to continue.

Staff comments have been positive, especially as they relate to her verbal behavior. Her fears and anxiety have declined, and she comments less and less about the pain in her knee and back.

EVALUATION

Evaluation is based on criteria or goals whether the evaluation is in relation to the group activity or to the individual within the group. Although we have focused primarily on Mrs. O. within the group and meeting her goals, it is important to comment briefly about group evaluation before proceeding.

In group activities, the emphasis is on the needs of the group as a whole, although the specialist will be aware of the personal needs of each resident as a member of the group. The focus of attention by the specialist is on helping each resident achieve his or her needs through the group. As a result of such an approach, group activity goals must be sufficiently specific and concrete to be measurable. Only in this way will the specialist be able to know if the goals have been accomplished and the needs of the residents as a group met.

Many times broadly stated goals are meaningless. Preference must be given to goals for which there is a reasonable chance of attainment. Group goals, like individual goals, are influenced by the setting and its administrative structure. In the end, group goal formulation is a process that is dependent upon feedback mechanisms and responds to changing signals, cues, and conditions.

There are a number of methods that can be used to evaluate group activities. Formal and informal discussions with the nursing home staff on the unit or in the interdisciplinary team meeting can be effective. Formal narrative reports and various kinds of checklists completed by the staff and/or specialist are also possibilities, likewise, the case study method. Their effectiveness or value will again relate to the home, its purpose and organizational and administrative structure.

In evaluating various group activities, the following factors, which are not all-inclusive should be considered:

To what extent have the expressed purpose and goals of any specific group been met?

How fully are individuals participating in the group activities, and with what results?

Are attitudes and behavior of individual group members being carried over into other spheres of social interaction in the facility?

Are activities appropriate for adults, and do residents see themselves as participating in a dignified way?

Do residents respond to the activities and seem to comprehend what is going on?

How adequate are cues being provided to help residents maintain their orientation to time and place?

Is preparation and orientation for the group sufficient to allow residents to receive personal attention without disrupting the continuity of the activity for other residents?

Do residents have an opportunity to contribute to the group?

Evaluation determines if the therapeutic recreation service interventions were effective. From another perspective, resident-centered objectives that were established to meet specific goals determine the criteria. Evaluation reflects on the end behaviors of the resident in response to the care plan. In the case of Mrs. O., and for that matter any other resident, did she meet her respective behavioral objectives? This information is charted and becomes a part of the personal medical record of Mrs. O. The specific format or style used to record progress toward goals or changes in the care plan or even regression from goals is usually dictated by the nursing home, but the specialist's or department's own preference may also be used. Charting should be done as soon as possible following the activity, when observations are still fresh. A progress note on Mrs. O. after sixty days might read as follows:

12/8 Is attending all scheduled activities. Participation as a volunteer with resident newspaper discontinued. Positive verbal behavior with increased cooperation and socialization continues. Fear and anxiety continue to decrease. Comments about less pain in knee and back and feels generally better. Keeps asking about when family will visit. Overall improvement noted since 11/10.

In the final analysis, therapeutic recreation care plans should be suitably molded and evaluated in accordance with the maintenance of health, dignity, enjoyment, family relationships, sustained care and treatment, and realistic goals.

CASE EXAMPLE TWO

Our second case provides the reader with the opportunity to finalize a therapeutic recreation care plan. Assessment information is provided, including the diagnosis for the specific resident, and goals are determined. It is the responsibility of the reader to consider the activities, the group assignment, the behavioral objectives, and the evaluation procedures.

Imagine not knowing what day of the week it is or whether you just finished eating breakfast, lunch, or dinner. Imagine not recognizing your family or friends. Imagine living with a person who forgets to turn the stove off or cannot remember that he closed the door or turned off the light when he has just done so. Imagine living with, and taking care of, a person with these memory problems.

Memory loss is just one of the many signs of *dementia*, a drop in intellectual functioning frequently associated with old age. For 1.5 million elderly people the gradual loss of memory is the first sign of Alzheimer's disease, a chronic, irreversible form of dementia that eventually leads to death. In 1981 the disease was the fourth most common cause of death in the United States. It accounted for more than 50 percent of all nursing home admissions and for $10 billion spent annually for nursing home care. The annual average personal cost in 1984 was $17,000 plus health insurance.[35]

Case History of Mr. H.

Mr. H., age seventy-three, widowed, and formerly living with his older son's family, was recently admitted to the nursing home three-and-a-half years after being diagnosed with senile dementia, Alzheimer type (SDAT or Alzheimer's disease). His social history indicates the typical symptoms: initial minor memory loss, which gradually became worse; disorientation in time; flattening of personality; loss of sense of humor; confusion and restlessness. His son reported that lately his father had changed his hours all around, so that he was up half the night. What finally convinced the son to bring his father to the nursing home was that last week Mr. H. said he was going to the mall but showed up at his younger son's house instead, talking about ice skating in Shaw Park a long time ago. When questioned about this activity, he became very hostile toward his son although he recognized he was confused. And just two days ago Mr. H. put his dentures in the waste basket because he did not recognize the waste basket for what it was. As a result of the varied problems, the son's family has had little time for themselves and their obligations.

The family physician made the necessary arrangements for Mr. H. to be admitted and provided the medical information. During the next interdisciplinary team meeting Mr. H.'s case was considered.

ASSESSMENT

In preparing for the team meeting, the specialist is aware that there is no known cure for the disease and that care and treatment is basically environmental, keeping Mr. H. as healthy and as safe as possible.[36] Drug related therapies are currently focused on two areas: attempts to slow down or reverse the disease process and symptom relief. Neither has yet met with much success, according to researchers.[37] At the same time, the specialist knows that routine is essential since it increases predictability in a life that usually feels unstructured and amorphous. Further research indicates that exercise provided on a regular daily basis has a calming effect on such residents. It helps them sleep better, prevents stiffness, maintains a resident's mobility, and provides a pleasurable activity. In exercise routine is very important, including time of day and the type and sequence of the exercises. The activity should be quiet and orderly so as not to add to the possible agitation of the resident.[38]

The specialist also realizes that until the last stages of the illness Mr. H. will undoubtedly retain his ability to take pleasure in simple activities. He will continue to enjoy simplified versions of the same activities he appreciated in the past. Music will be a pleasurable activity, especially songs he learned long ago. He will enjoy automobile rides and pet therapy. On the other hand, the specialist knows that activities that require decision making, including the capacity to choose between two alternatives, will only add to Mr. H.'s confusion and disorientation. As the illness progresses toward the final stages, evidence shows that music, holding something that feels nice and is comforting, and being hugged and touched continue to be important.[39]

Interview and Data Collection

The initial interview with Mr. H. to collect leisure-experience information starts off with polite conversation. However, he soon insults the specialist and begins to complain about being in the nursing home. Even though the specialist attempts to reassure Mr. H. that there is warmth, caring, and understanding in the nursing home for him, the specialist must eventually disengage herself from the situation quietly. After the interview, the specialist recalls that interaction with strangers by individuals with Alzheimer's can be difficult, although each will respond differently. A panic reaction is not unusual when such a resident finds himself or herself in strange surroundings and is made anxious by the situation. When this occurs, the resident may overreact by shouting accusations at anybody who is nearby.[40]

The specialist further makes note that any future conversations need to be at a simple level and must not include any double entendres or meanings behind words. Also, the specialist should keep activity instructions on an elementary level and not become upset if the resident overreacts by shouting, accusing people nearby, refusing to move, or even striking out. If any of those situations do occur, it will be best to respond in a firm and comforting way so as not to escalate the reaction.[41]

PLANNING

During the interdisciplinary team meeting it is reemphasized that the staff needs to be alert to their facial expressions and other nonverbal behavior since Mr. H. may be more sensitive to people's manner than to the meaning of their words. Also, meals, baths, activities, bedtime, and any outings should be regularly scheduled. To help Mr. H. maintain contact with self, staff, and reality, the staff will encourage him to do as much as he can for himself so that his self-concept through independency and skill will remain for as long as possible. Further, praise and encouragement by others of his activities needs to become a part of his daily routine. Moreover, he must be allowed to make as many decisions as possible for himself as long as he can; this to be accomplished through simple alternatives of yes or no rather than open-ended questions. And most important, staff should remember the basic need to be assured, to be comfortable, and to feel safe.[42]

In preparing the therapeutic recreation care plan, the specialist realizes that it is not particularly wise to attempt to improve the ability levels of Mr. H. regardless of activity, due to the progressive nature of the disease. Further, the key to providing activities, as the specialist knows, is to keep activities simple but challenging while utilizing existing skills.[43] In addition, once the activity program has been developed, Mr. H. should be provided with a daily activity schedule, which notes the particular activities and their time and place. In this way his confusion may be decreased and participation increased or at least maintained.

Following the team meeting and a reading of Mr. H.'s social history (which indicated a childhood and adolescent interest in swimming, ice-skating, stamp collecting, table games, and piano playing) the following goals were established:

To maintain positive self-esteem/self-worth

To maintain participation in activities

To decrease confusion when possible

It now becomes the student's responsibility to further develop the care plan.

MODULAR SENSITIVITY TRAINING FOR STUDENTS DEALING WITH THE ELDERLY

Students may encounter problems in working with older individuals in long-term care facilities. To assist students in becoming more comfortable, a variety of activities can be performed in the classroom to sensitize them to the needs and problems of the elderly. The following activities address the areas of loneliness, sensory deprivation, learned helplessness, invasion of privacy, and territoriality.

MODULE 1: LONELINESS

Objective:	To promote insight into the causes of loneliness and to experience the outcome of sharing loneliness with others.
Exercise:	In a circle, students will recollect their single most lonely time and relive the feelings alone, with closed eyes, for several moments. Then each student will write a brief account of the situation and share it with other students.
Discussion:	(a) What emotions were evoked while students relived their own experience and while others were describing their own experiences?
	(b) What similarities were observed in the loneliness situations?
	(c) How might loneliness be more common or less common for the aging than for younger individuals?
	(d) How do loneliness and social isolation differ, and which most accurately characterizes the aging?

MODULE 2: SENSORY DEPRIVATION

Objective:	To provide experience of sensory deprivation.
Materials:	A blindfold.
Exercise:	Students form dyads. Partner A is blindfolded; Partner B will take A on walk for twenty minutes, during which time there should be no verbal interaction. Partner B must indicate positive aspects of environment to be experienced by Partner A as well as dangers. Roles are reversed.
Discussion:	(a) What specific anxieties were experienced by blindfolded Partner A?
	(b) Were the nonvisual aspects of the environment experienced differently?
	(c) What were some of the nonverbal cues used by Partner B to direct blindfolded Partner A?
	(d) As time passed, did Partner A's degree of comfort increase or decrease?

MODULE 3: LEARNED HELPLESSNESS

Objective:	To promote understanding of the interactions between dependency behavior and infantilization.
Exercise:	Sometime prior to classroom meeting two students are instructed to alternate in feeding each other an entire meal. The receiver may not use hands or arms. The meal should encompass different food textures.
Discussion:	(a) Was it more difficult to be on the giver or the receiver end?
	(b) How did the rate of feeding affect the enjoyment of the food?
	(c) While being fed, were instructions communicated to the

giver, and if so did giver heed the instructions?

(d) What feelings were evoked for the giver concerning the experience of feeding an adult a whole meal?

MODULE 4: INVASION OF PRIVACY

Objective: To communicate feelings evoked by sudden invasion of privacy.

Exercise: Students will empty out their pockets, purses, briefcases, or wallets onto a table in view of other students.

Discussion: (a) What specific response was elicited by this invasion of privacy (anger, pleasure, etc.)?

(b) What students would the students feel most comfortable doing this exercise with?

(c) Why would it be particularly important to respect an aging person's need for privacy?

MODULE 5: TERRITORIALITY

Objective: To acquaint students with the fact that each individual has his or her own personal space.

Exercise: Students pair up and, beginning from the outer boundaries of the classroom, approach each other gradually until they reach a degree of discomfort.

Discussion: (a) What differences can be noted in the distance between pairs?

(b) When was discomfort felt by students?

(c) How did the students react to this discomfort?

(d) How did students know when they were invading another student's personal space? What behavior cues were noted?

(e) How can this information be utilized when dealing with elderly residents?

SUMMARY

While there are many problems associated with residential care in a nursing home, the key factor in the care and treatment of residents is the recognition of each resident's need to return to a process of life and not to be treated in a stereotyped way. This implies that the nursing home and other like long-term care facilities utilize all available medical, psychological, and social knowledge in an attempt to carry forward programs that will meet the needs of their residents. Further, this implies that the home will conduct a full, careful assessment of needs during and after admission and a regular review in order to provide for changing needs and circumstances.

The specialist will have to develop skills in all areas associated with therapeutic recreation service. The specialist is concerned with helping the resident adjust to the nursing home and find a satisfying way of life there. Perhaps most important of all, the specialist must recognize the fact that no resident's needs will remain static; that solutions to problems should aim to deal not just with the present but should be concerned with seeking a pattern of successful care and treatment for each resident in a flexible way through varied group and individual recreative activity.

NOTES

1. Erving Goffman, *Asylums* (Garden City, N.Y.: Anchor Books, 1961).

2. U.S. Senate Special Committee on Aging, *Aging America: Trends and Projects* (Washington, D.C.: U.S. Government Printing Office, November 1983), p. 73.

3. Theodore H. Koff, *Long-Term Care* (Boston: Little, Brown & Co., 1982), p. 66.

4. Robert L. Kane and Rosalie A. Kane, *Values and Long-Term Care* (Lexington, Mass.: D.C. Heath & Co., 1982), p. 10.

5. U.S. Senate Special Committee on Aging.

6. Ibid., and Koff, *Long-Term Care.*

7. National Center for Health Statistics, *Health Status of Aged Medicare Beneficiaries,* series B, descriptive report no. 2, NMCUES (Washington, D.C.: U.S. Government Printing Office, September 1983), p. 9.

8. Veterans' Administration, *Caring for the Older Veteran* (U.S. Government Printing Office, July 1984), p. 72.

9. U.S. Department of Health, Education, and Welfare, Federal Council on Aging, *Public Policy and the Frail Elderly* (Washington, D.C.: U.S. Government Printing Office, December 1978), pp. 25–30.

10. Wesley Wiley Rogers, *General Administration in the Nursing Home,* 3rd ed. (Boston: CBI Publishing Co., 1980), p. 178.

11. Joan A. Koncelik, *Designing the Open Nursing Home* (Stroudsburg, Pa.: Dowden, Hutchinson, and Ross, 1976) pp. 36–42.

12. Cited by Richard Solomon, "Aging Individuals in Long Term Care Need Choice and Autonomy," *Generations* 5, no. 3 (Spring 1981), 32–38.

13. Elaine M. Brody, *Long-Term Care of Older People,* (New York: Human Sciences Press, 1977), p. 143.

14. Kane and Kane, *Values and Long-Term Care.*

15. Louis Lowy, *Social Policies and Programs on Aging* (Lexington, Mass.: D.C. Heath & Co., 1980), p. 101.

16. Brody, *Long-Term Care,* pp. 95–96.

17. Cited in Linda A. Byrne, "A Volunteer's Perspective," in *Working with the Elderly,* 2nd ed., ed., Irene Burnside (Monterey, Calif.: Wadsworth Health Sciences Division, 1984), pp. 442–43.

18. Lucille Taulbee and James Folsom, "Reality Orientation for Geriatric Patients," *Hospital and Community Psychiatry* 175, no. 8 (1966), 133.

19. Ibid., pp. 133–35.

20. A. M. Robinson, *Remotivation Techniques: A Manual for Use in Nursing Homes* (Philadelphia: American Psychiatric Association and Smith, Kline & French Laboratories, n.d.).

21. Burnside, *Working with the Elderly,* pp. 191–92.

22. A training program is offered at Philadelphia State Hospital and other centers by the National Remotivation Therapy Technique Organization with offices at Philadelphia State Hospital, 14000 Roosevelt Blvd., Philadelphia, Pa. 19114. Training aids can be obtained by writing the organization, and remotivation kits are available through the American Psychiatric Association, Publications Services Division, 1700 18th St., N.W., Washington, D.C. 20009. Kit no. 240 is for use in nursing homes.

23. Mary Ann Matterson, "Group Reminiscing for the Depressed Institutionalized Elderly," in *Working with the Elderly,* pp. 287–94.

24. Cited in Matterson, "Group Reminiscing," p. 289.

25. Ibid., p. 290.

26. Burnside, *Working with the Elderly,* p. 27.

27. Dulcy B. Miller, "Case Studies to Challenge the Nursing Home Activity Coordinator," *Therapeutic Recreation Journal* 13, no. 3 (1979), 22–32.

28. Nelida Ferrarri, "Assessment of Individuals in Groups of Older Adults," *Social Group Work with Older People* (New York: National Association of Social Work, 1963), p. 4.

29. Toba S. Kerson, *Understanding Chronic Illness* (New York: Free Press, 1985), pp. 18–19.

30. W. V. Bingham, "Introduction to the Effects of Music," in the *Effects of Music,* ed., M. Schoen (Freeport, N.Y.: Books for Libraries Press, 1968), p. 6.

31. H. L. Bonny and L. Savary, *Music and Your Mind: Listening with a New Consciousness* (N.Y.: Harper & Row, 1973), pp. 23–24; Mary Jane Hennessey, "Music and Group Work with the Aged," in *Nursing and the Aged,* ed., I. M. Burnside (N.Y.: McGraw-Hill Book Co., 1976), pp. 34–51; and J. Alvin, *Music Therapy* (N.Y.: Humanities Press, 1966), p. 132.

32. Kerson, *Chronic Illness,* p. 29.

33. Ibid., pp. 29, 32.

34. Florence Vickery, *Creative Programming for Older Adults* (New York: Association Press, 1972), p. 60.

35. The first figure is from Alzheimer's Disease and Related Dementias Association brochure (Mountain View, Calif.: the association, 1982); the second, from Mary A. Kiely, "Alzheimer's Disease: Making the Most of the Time That's Left," *RN* (March 1985), 38.

36. Kerson, *Understanding Chronic Illness,* p. 75.

37. Catherine Boardman, "Losing Control," *MCG Today* 15, no. 2 (1986), 14–17.

38. Kerson, *Understanding Chronic Illness,* p. 84.

39. Ibid., pp. 84–85; and U.S. Department of Health and Human Services Task Force on Alzheimer's Disease, *Alzheimer's Disease: A Scientific Guide for Health Practitioners* NIH publication no. 84–2251 (Washington, D.C.: U.S. Government Printing Office, May 1984).

40. Kerson, *Understanding Chronic Illness,* p. 92.

41. Ibid., pp. 96–99.

42. Ibid.

43. Ida M. Bean, "Alzheimer's Disease: Helping Families Survive," *American Journal of Nursing* 84, no. 2 (1984), 229–232.

SUGGESTED READINGS

AMERICAN HOSPITAL ASSOCIATION. *Coordinated Activity Programs for the Aged.* Chicago: the association, 1975.

ANDERSON, S. V., and E. BAUWENS. *Chronic Health Problems: Concepts and Applications.* St. Louis: C. V. Mosby, 1981.

BACHNER, J., and E. CORNELIUS. *Activities Coordinator's Guide.* Washington, D.C.: U.S. Government Printing Office, 1978.

BRACHT, NANCY F. "The Social Nature of Chronic Disease and Disability." *Social Work in Health Care* 12, no. 5 (1979), 129–44.

BRIGHT, RICHARD. *Music in Geriatric Care.* New York: St. Martin's Press, 1972.

BURNSIDE, IRENE. *Working with the Elderly* (2nd ed.). Monterey, Calif.: Wadsworth Health Sciences Division, 1984.

FAULKNER, ROZANNE W. *Therapeutic Recreation in Health Care Settings: A Practitioner's Viewpoint.* Greenville, N.C.: Leisure Enrichment Service, 1984, unit 12.

FERGUSON, DANIEL D. "Assessment Interviewing Techniques: A Useful Tool in Developing Individual Program Plans." *Therapeutic Recreation Journal* 17, no. 2 (1983), 16–22.

FOSTER, PHYLLIS. *Therapeutic Activities with the Impaired Elderly.* New York: Haworth Press, 1986.

GERSHOWITZ, S. Z. "Adding Life to Years: Remotivating Elderly People in Institutions." *Nursing and Health Care* 3, no. 3 (1982), 141–45.

GOODMAN, MARCENE. "'I Came Here to Die': A Look at the Function of Therapeutic Recreation in Nursing Homes." *Therapeutic Recreation Journal* 17, no. 3 (1983), 14–19.

GREENBLATT, FRED. *Therapeutic Recreation for Long-Term Care Facilities.* New York: Human Sciences Press, Inc., 1987.

HARRINGTON, CHARLENE, ROBERT J. NEWCOME, and CARROLL L. ESTES and ASSOCIATES. *Long Term Care of the Elderly: Public Policy Issues.* Beverly Hills, Calif.: Sage Publications, 1985.

HELGERSON, ELSBETH M., and SCOTT C. WILLIS. *Handbook of Group Activities for Impaired Older Adults.* New York: Haworth Press, 1987.

HISEK, DENNIS D. "Recreation Planning for a Nursing Home." *Therapeutic Recreation Journal* 12, no. 2 (1978), 26–29.

JANICKI, MATTHEW P., and ANN E. MACEACHRON. "Residential Health, and Social Service Needs of Elderly Developmentally Disabled Persons." *The Gerontologist* 24, no. 2 (1984), 128–37.

KANE, R. L., and R. KANE. *Assessing the Elderly.* Beverly Hills, Calif.: Sage Publications, 1982.

KERSON, TOBA S. *Understanding Chronic Illness.* New York: Free Press, 1985.

MILLER, DULCY B. "Case Studies to Challenge the Nursing Home Activity Coordinator." *Therapeutic Recreation Journal* 13, no. 3 (1979), 22–32.

———. "Suggested Methodologies for Auditing Activity Programs in Long Term Care Facilities." *Therapeutic Recreation Journal* 9, no. 3 (1975), 99–105.

ROGERS, WESLEY WILEY. *General Administration in the Nursing Home* (3rd ed.). Boston: CBI Publishing Co., 1980.

SCHOEN, M., ed. *The Effects of Music.* Freeport, N.Y.: Books for Libraries Press, 1968.

SOLOMON, RICHARD. "Aging Individuals in Long Term Care Need Choice and Autonomy," *Generations* 5, no. 3 (Spring 1981), 32–38.

STOLOV, W. S., and M. R. CLOWERS. *Handbook of Severe Disabilities.* Washington, D.C.: U.S. Government Printing Office, 1981.

TEAFF, JOSEPH D. *Leisure Services with the Elderly.* St. Louis: Times Mirror/Mosby College Publishing, 1985, pp. 121–70.

WOOD, JOAN B. *Meeting the Psychosocial Needs of the Elderly.* Burkeville, Va.: Piedmont Geriatric Institute, 1986.

9

Therapeutic Milieu Model

In recent years major changes have taken place in the provision of mental health care, in part because of the development of new psychotropic drugs and new administrative attitudes and in part because of the momentum of new ideologies, changing social values, new social policies, and the growth of a vigorous movement in support of the civil liberties of the mentally ill. These changes have also affected the delivery of therapeutic recreation services.

As we begin this chapter, it is useful to review and examine some of these changes. Even though this examination is lengthy, it is hoped that it will give the reader insight to where we are at present while at the same time helping to explain where we have been in the past two to three decades.

HISTORICAL BACKGROUND

It was not until the 1950s that significant changes took place in the care and treatment of the mentally ill. Prior to this time and for some decades before, the care and treatment of the majority of mentally ill was provided through state psychiatric hospitals, whose services were for the most part ineffective. According to many investigators, the ineffectiveness was the result of: (1) institutional overcrowding, which made adequate treatment impossible; (2) overworked staffs that were frequently untrained and ill paid; (3) a medical model that focused on finding organic causes for the various mental illnesses and using organic treatment procedures; and (4) too little money allocated by the states to their respective hospitals for care and treatment.[1] In 1950 the daily cost per patient in a state psychiatric hospital averaged less than $4.50 per patient while private psychiatric hospitals expended about $17 per patient per day, and the general medical hospital had a daily patient cost of more than $27 per day.[2]

Coupled with these problems was a new condition that appeared in patients with increasing frequency following their admission to psychiatric hospitals. This problem was in reality a number of symptoms that were thought to be brought about by the deficiencies just described above. The symptoms, grouped together under the term *so-*

cial breakdown syndrome, included severe withdrawal, loss of interest in social functioning and personal appearance, anger, aggressiveness, and personal dilapidation. The social breakdown syndrome was thought to be a socially determined disorder resulting from hospitalization, almost regardless of initial diagnosis. It appeared to be responsible for the increased chronic character of psychopathology. Further, since the syndrome was thought to be the result of deficiencies in psychiatric care, changes in the organization of that care would be required to bring the whole matter under control.[3] As a consequence of all these events, recovery rates decreased, and the hospitals filled up with chronic, virtually untreatable patients.[4]

CHANGES IN CARE AND TREATMENT

Starting in about 1950, four developments took place that set the stage for a major shift in psychiatric care and treatment by mental health professionals including therapeutic recreation specialists. Three of these developments had immediate impact upon patients in traditional psychiatric institutions. The other development was concerned with community mental health services and also incorporated two of the three developments associated with psychiatric institutions.

Psychopharmacology

The first of the three developments affecting psychiatric institutions was in the field of psychopharmacology. It was during this period that new tranquilizing and antidepressant drugs (also referred to as psychotropic, psychoactive, and antipsychotic) were developed (for example, reserpine and chlorpomazine for treating schizophrenia and mania). Although the organic therapies were still used, they no longer constituted the whole array of resources. In general, these drugs reduced anxiety, discomfort, and bizarre behavior in many patients; they altered the organization and content of the patient's thoughts and perception, thus

speeding discharge from the institution. Because these drugs modified the emotional components of psychiatric disorders without impairing intellectual capacities, they were far superior to the sedating drugs that had been used until this time. Not only was recovery accelerated, but many patients were able to avoid hospitalization entirely. Effective drug treatment stimulated the introduction of milieu therapy and the expansion of the "open-door" and "open-gate" policies as well as varied community mental health services.[5]

Decentralization or Regionalization

The second development focused on geographic decentralization or regionalization wherein patients were placed on wards according to their place of residence before hospitalization. Although there were a number of approaches, the most common method of decentralization was the unit system. The institution was divided into several autonomous units, each with a unit director, a program coordinator, and staff representing various disciplines. A twelve-hundred-bed institution might be divided into four three-hundred-bed units, each with its own staff, treatment program, and eating and sleeping facilities. Further, the decentralization concept minimized the traditional hierarchical and authoritarian professional roles found in psychiatric institutions.[6]

Patients of all degrees and types of psychopathology began to be housed according to their home communities, so that all patients from a particular city or geographic area might be placed on one ward. Admission services were abolished. Newly admitted patients were sent directly to their geographic unit. The unit became the mental hospital for the geographical area. Outpatient diagnostic and therapeutic services were also provided for the same population by the same unit. Follow-up observation and aftercare of the patients were carried out in the same manner. And finally, decision making about care and treatment came to be made at the ward or unit level rather than at higher administrative levels.

Some centralized services remained for those patients who required special services that would be impossible to duplicate in each unit, such as medical services. Separate treatment facilities were required for emotionally disturbed children and for those convicted of criminal acts, who were considered criminally insane. Most settings had a centralized activity building, which included the auditorium, gymnasium, and various activity or multipurpose rooms. Some settings had a facility that housed all the activity therapies and their activity areas. In fact, some facilities would make municipal recreation community centers look small by comparison.

Therapeutic Milieu

The third development has been variously referred to as milieu therapy, the therapeutic community, or the therapeutic milieu. While these labels are often used interchangeably, they were originally independent concepts. However, the emphasis of all three embraces a psychosocial approach to treatment.

In *milieu therapy* all aspects of the program—recreation, vocational, rehabilitation or therapy, patient government, patient-staff, and intrastaff interactions—were planned to promote the patient's recovery, including the attitudes that staff should assume in working with patients.[7] The *therapeutic community* differed only in that patients were explicitly called upon to exert a therapeutic influence upon each other, and decision making by staff-patients was more democratic. Thus, decisions regarding issues of daily living were reached democratically; communication was open and efficient; feedback and confrontation, with regard to staff as well as patients, was encouraged; and patients and staff shared responsibility

for assessing patient behavior and making recommendations for treatment planning. Lastly, patients had to justify their request for discharge or for changes in treatment status not only to staff but to their fellow patients.[8]

While the *therapeutic milieu* contained elements of the other two, there was never an agreed-upon comprehensive definition of the approach.[9] The approach, in addition to any one psychosocial theory, embraced the concept of allowing patients to assume personal responsibility for engaging in activities and improving their performance while at the same time interacting with others.[10] An important aspect of this approach was the support and encouragement patients received from staff while exposing themselves to a variety of new experiences.[11] In sum, the common goals of the therapeutic milieu consisted of facilitating patient responsibility, resumption (or learning) of appropriate problem-solving behavior, and the improvement of pathological behaviors, primarily through the use of group meetings, activities, and patient government.[12]

Community-Based Programs and Services

The fourth and last development was the expansion of community-based programs and services. As a result of the new tranquilizing drugs, geographic decentralization, and the therapeutic milieu, more individuals were being discharged into the community, and these same individuals were seeking community mental health services, which were limited. To meet this growing concern, Congress in 1955 enacted the Mental Health Study Act (PL94-182), which established a Joint Commission on Mental Illness and Health. The findings of this commission, which were published under the title *Action for Mental Health*, set the stage for federal support and emphasis on community mental health that marked the 1960s.[13] The response to the findings was the enactment of the Mental Retardation Facilities and Community Mental Health Construction Act (sometimes called the Community Mental Health Centers Act), based on the 1963 message to Congress by then President John F. Kennedy.

More recently President Jimmy Carter in 1977 created the President's Commission on Mental Health, whose recommendations concerning health care and needs were incorporated into the Mental Health Systems Act (PL96-398) in October 1980. In addition to authorizing funds to continue many of the provisions of the original community mental health centers programs and services, the act included provisions for grants specifically designed for the treatment of the chronically mentally ill, severely disturbed children and adolescents, and unserved or underserved populations as locally determined.[14]

Following the election of President Ronald Reagan, all the budgetary authorizations of the Mental Health Systems Act were repealed. Since that time, mental health services have been included in a block grant called the health services block. While some monies have been federally earmarked for specific services, funding for existing community mental health services are required to come from state authorizations. It is not clear after seven years what effect this has or will have on community-based programs and services.

The accomplishments of nearly three or more decades regarding the care and treatment of the mentally ill, whether in the traditional long-term psychiatric institutions or in the various community-based programs and services, have fallen short of what was anticipated in the opinion of many mental health experts.[15] It is clear, however, that mental health services from a community perspective are here to stay.

On the other hand, public psychiatric institutions continue to survive, even though in many situations their resources (funds, services, and even patients) have been redis-

tributed to community-based programs. An interesting aside regarding these factors: there was a concept that patients discharged from mental health centers would integrate quicker and better into the community than those discharged from public institutions. Another concept was that treating patients in the community was cheaper than institutional-based care. Neither concept was ever realized.[16]

The pattern of treatment or approach to treatment that was initiated in the public psychiatric institutions in the 1950s still exists today but in a less pronounced form. Other forms—such as behavior modification or operant conditioning, coping education, sensitivity training, and transcendental meditation, to name a few—exist along with the traditional medical or organic model, patient government, therapeutic milieu, and various psychotherapies and psychodynamic theories. Nevertheless, despite the confusion and ideological ferment of the past three decades, there is a growing recognition that social and community factors affect both the development and the course of various mental illnesses.[17] It is also beginning to be recognized that it may be possible to limit the magnitude of incapacity and disability of mental illness through manipulation of the social environment during and after treatment.[18]

Lastly, and of importance to therapeutic recreation specialists, is the emphasis on teaching patients skills within a therapeutic milieu that facilitates their social and personal adaptation or allows them to live more comfortably. The therapeutic milieu, according to one major study, aids patient movement and recovery, and a social therapeutic orientation is most effective in determining the course of treatment and the outcome. The rationale is that success in community life depends largely on the skills persons have in dealing effectively with others. Particularly important is the way the patient appears to others at work, at play, and at home as well as in the hospital.[19]

CHARACTERISTICS OF MENTAL HEALTH SERVICE

Therapeutic recreation specialists, like other professionals working in mental health settings, are expected to have some knowledge about matters other than those directly a part of their own service. These characteristics will include admission, patients' rights, rehabilitation or interdisciplinary team, release or discharge of patients, and quality assurance.

ADMISSION

There are two kinds of admission to psychiatric hospitals or units of general hospitals. The most desirable manner of obtaining treatment for mental illness is a voluntary admission. Voluntary admission is similar in procedure and legal consequences to admission to any other hospital. The individual simply signs an application and agrees to the treatment process and to abide by the rules of the hospital.

Unfortunately, many mentally ill persons lack insight concerning their behavior and will not seek hospitalization of their own volition. As a result, such an individual must be admitted involuntarily. Involuntary admission or civil commitment is a serious infringement of the patient's liberties and is not undertaken lightly or without due consideration of alternative approaches. While the laws are specific as to who may make application for hospitalization (spouse, relative, friend, guardian, physician, local government official, or the head of a general hospital), the grounds for involuntary admission vary from state to state. They all include some reference to judgment that the individual is dangerous to himself or others, is unable to care for physical needs, and needs care and treatment. In recent years, however, the involuntary commitment has been challenged as a result of the imprecision of the definition of mental illness, disability, and danger to himself or others, respectively.[20]

There are two other types of admission.

One is temporary involuntary admission, in which the period of time is designated by law for required observation, diagnosis, or short-term therapy. The other is emergency admission, which is provided for individuals considered to be dangerous to themselves or others.

The indications for admission to a psychiatric hospital or unit include the following:

1. Suicidal attempts, threats, or thoughts of suicide
2. Dangerous to others, overt attacks or threats of violence, brutal assaults on animals, or uncontrollable rage
3. Antisocial acts such as senseless desecration of a church, firesetting, or sexual crimes
4. Personality change, loss of control, disorganization, deterioration with a rapid downhill course, and failure to improve
5. Physical or neurological disease associated with mental symptoms that interfere with function
6. Transfer of an unmanageable patient with mental disorder from a medical ward in a general hospital
7. Pathological or noxious family that makes treatment impossible at home, necessitating removal to find a placement
8. Diagnosis, problem identification and evaluation, or time to ensure stabilization on drug therapy
9. Crisis or failure in outpatient treatment or when therapy cannot be safely started there, often because of distance from home
10. Withdrawal from drug or alcohol dependence[21]

PATIENTS' RIGHTS

The specialist needs to be aware of two matters that are important to care and treatment of the mentally ill: (1) the *right to treatment* and (2) the *right to refuse treatment*.

The right to treatment instead of custodial care in many long-term care facilities was affirmed in the Alabama case of *Wyatt v. Stickney* and *Lessard v. Schmidt* (right to due process), both in 1972. In the former litigation the federal district court judge agreed that the patient had a right to treatment that included certain standards of care. Subsequent court rulings have brought about additional changes. The trend in recent years has been toward restricting the grounds for civic commitment, reducing the length of time a person can be committed by physicians without judicial review, and requiring commitment through the courts with due process guarantees for longer-term commitments. In addition, the civil and personal rights of committed and voluntary patients have been given increased statutory recognition. Some of these rights, in addition to more humane care, are the right to communicate with persons outside the institution, to keep clothing and personal effects, to retain licenses, permits, or privileges established by law, and to enter into contracts.[22] In 1973 a legal suit, *Souder v. Brennan,* forced the provisions of the Fair Labor Standards Act of 1936 to be applied to the mentally ill and mentally retarded.

The right of committed patients to refuse treatment is not well recognized, even though there is evidence questioning the benefits and potential hazards of some of the treatment procedures—psychoactive drugs, ECT, behavior modification techniques, and psychosurgery. It is not surprising that few states have laws specifying the conditions under which various kinds of treatment or confinement (seclusion, use of restraints) may be employed. Where laws do exist, they vary considerably from state to state.[23]

REHABILITATION TEAM

A team approach to determining and providing care and treatment to patients is found in nearly all settings; this is especially so in relation to providing such services to the mentally ill. The team approach to treating mental illness evolved from the late-nineteenth-century belief that social influences could lead to mental illness. As therapists began to recognize the importance of the patient's complete social adjustment as a criterion of cure, the team concept in mental health emerged, with the addition of social workers to hospital psychiatric wards managed by psychiatrists and nurses.[24]

In the period between world wars the increased emphasis on specialization among mental health workers and a growing patient population contributed significantly to the expansion of interdisciplinary teams. And by the middle of the 1960s, in order to meet the needs of a variety of patient populations, the interdisciplinary team expanded to include a wide range of mental health workers, including paraprofessionals.[25]

As noted earlier, there are any number and kinds of teams that function in the various hospitals. In the recent psychiatric literature there is no general agreement as to who is included on the various interdisciplinary teams, but the psychiatrist, psychiatric nurse, psychologist, social worker, and various members of the activity or rehabilitation therapies, including therapeutic recreation specialists, usually are involved. Depending on the organizational structure of the hospital relative to care and treatment (unit plan, treatment plan, etc.), the therapeutic recreation specialist may assume leadership of the team or share in the leadership of the team and be a collaborator in the decision-making process.

An interdisciplinary team in mental health services, regardless of the kind of mental health setting, may be defined as a group of professionals and paraprofessionals from different disciplines who share the common goal of effective patient care and treatment. The team members utilize a single record and participate in any organized decision-making process regarding care and treatment, consciously utilizing the various approaches, skills, and knowledge of the different team members. Authority, decision making, and accountability for the services provided rest with each professional; ultimate responsibility for patient care and treatment remains with the team.[26]

It is important to recognize that each team member brings specific skills to the team; likewise there are shared skills. In addition, the interdisciplinary team also allows team members opportunities for growth and development, as each team member gains insights from others based on the sharing of treatment issues and the self-disclosure of personal doubts or areas of confusion. This overlap within the team is reflected in the petal model in Figure 9.1. Each petal represents the unique expertise of a particular discipline; the circular area in the center represents territory where expertise is shared.

Unfortunately, at times and in some situations biases may exist within the interdisciplinary team. Biases that are brought to the team by one profession toward another profession may affect teamwork. Social workers may preceive psychiatric nurses as effective treatment planners but question their skills as psychotherapists. Psychiatric nurses may perceive therapeutic recreation specialists as having the ability to establish rapport quickly, but the specialists' programs are centered around play, which is seen as having no mission in a hospital. Psychologists may preceive social workers as having skills in psychotherapy but want no part of them when it comes to research. Biases eventually work themselves out as members become more aware of the values, training, and customs of others on the team.

While no attempt is made here to stereotype the roles of the various professionals represented on the team, it might be interesting for the student to have some insight into the usual roles played by team members:

Psychiatrist. The role of the psychiatrist will vary with the setting; some will be in private practice and others employed by the hospital. Regardless of setting, they are involved with diagnostic evaluation, treatment planning, psychotherapy, medical services, and pharmacological matters.[27]

Social Worker. This team member provides information on environmental factors associated with a person's illness, col-

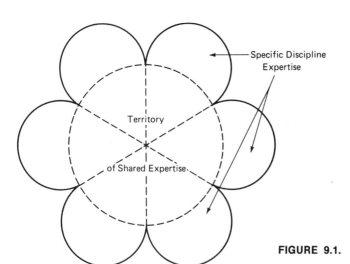

FIGURE 9.1. Interdisciplinary Sharing of Territory

laborates on the therapeutic design of the patient's stay, serves as a liaison between community, social, and rehabilitative service, does therapy with groups, and provides follow-up care.[28]

Psychologist. The role of the psychologist is as a collaborator in patient treatment planning as well as in treatment and as a data gatherer through psychodiagnostic testing. In some settings the psychologist takes the lead in research design and in data collection, analysis, and reporting.[29]

Psychiatric Nurse. This team member performs a broad range of duties depending on the setting. Most responsibilities are patient oriented: case-finding intake, goal setting and treatment planning, reporting and/or interpreting laboratory results, patient care, maintaining therapeutic milieu, psychotherapy, and reinforcement of desired behavior, to name just a few duties.[30]

Activity or Rehabilitation Therapists. This may include occupational therapists, art therapists, music therapists, therapeutic recreation specialists, etc., who use a variety of activities and modes of experience to further the goals of psychiatric treatment. They all assist in their respective roles and skills in problem identification, psychosocial/emotional development, and evaluation. (These therapists may be grouped together in a department or unit referred to as Activity Therapy or Rehabilitation Therapy. Moreover, any one of these therapists may represent all of the various therapists/disciplines at the team meeting, or each therapist may represent his or her own discipline; organizational structure and staffing patterns determine to a large degree the therapist/discipline representation. In recent years, the roles and responsibilities of the various therapists are less blurred than they were some years ago.)

In sum, the team model is a vehicle to enhance continuity of care and coordina-

tion of treatment. It promotes quality control, since team members work with, but are not subservient to, other interdisciplinary team members and are continually involved in describing and reformulating their approaches. In fact, the team itself can be a creative force in the development of approaches to treatment.

RELEASE OF PATIENT

As noted in a previous chapter, planning for release begins on admission and culminates when it appears the patient can continue convalescing at home. In the main, there are a number of ways a patient may be released from the hospital.

Patients who are admitted voluntarily may be released in one of two ways. Upon giving three days' notice (this may vary from state to state) the patient is free to leave the hospital with no other formality. A few years ago studies by Simmons and Freeman revealed that whenever two of the three participants—hospital (physician), patient, family—agreed on a release, then it occurred.[31] For the most part, those who discharge themselves usually have had a poor response to treatment or have found the close relationship on the ward too threatening.

The most frequently used method of discharge, whether it be a voluntary or involuntary admission, is that the ward or attending psychiatrist in a staff meeting makes a final examination of the case and recommends release. The patient may be discharged because of recovery or sufficient improvement to be treated through community resources. Unfortunately, once released, some patients do not carry out the recommendations of staff and are returned to the hospital for additional treatment or disappear into the community.

The above discharge process does not apply to those who are adjudged to be criminally insane. Such individuals are subject to the orders of a regular criminal court following the recommendation for release.

In preparation for release or discharge most states, at the discretion of the ward or attending psychiatrist, permit patients to return to their homes on a trial visit for a period of a few days, a few weeks, or even a year. This plan provides for a "trying-out" during which the patient can demonstrate the degree of recovery as measured by the ability to cope with normal social situations. The patient, however, remains under supervision of the hospital and must continue to visit regularly with the assigned psychiatrist or social worker. If the trial visit progresses satisfactorily, the patient may then be recommended for discharge.

QUALITY ASSURANCE

Quality assurance has evolved from being a voluntary, somewhat vague and implicit concept primarily used by inpatient mental health services to being an explicit practice mandated by federal laws, required by two important professional bodies—the Joint Commission on Accreditation of Hospitals (JCAH) and the Accreditation Council for Psychiatric Facilities, and expected by third-party insurance carriers.

By definition, quality assurance is the promise or guarantee made by mental health care providers (agencies, etc.) to funding sources, including third-party insurance carriers and consumers, that certain standards of excellence in mental health care are being met. It usually involves measuring the quality of care given to consumers in order to improve the appropriateness, adequacy, and effectiveness of care. In addition, a quality-assurance program is designed to detect deficiencies and errors in service and to control the cost of care.

An example of what is meant by quality assurance is found in the standards for patient treatment plans of the Accreditation Council for Psychiatric Facilities. Students may wish to consider these standards in relation to our case histories.

15.1 Each patient shall have an individualized, written treatment plan based on the assessments of that patient's fundamental needs.

15.1.1 The treatment plan shall be developed as soon after the patient's admission as possible.

15.1.2 Appropriate therapeutic efforts may begin before finalization of the treatment plan.

15.1.3 The treatment plan shall be a reflection of the program's philosophy of treatment and shall reflect appropriate multidisciplinary input by the staff.

15.1.4 The overall responsibility of the treatment plan shall be assigned to a member of the clinical staff.

15.1.5 The plan shall specify services required for meeting the patient's needs.

15.1.6 The plan shall include referral for needed services not provided directly by the program.

15.1.7 Speech, language, academic, and hearing services shall be available, when appropriate, either within the program or by written arrangement with a qualified clinician or facility, in order to meet the patient's needs.

15.1.8 The treatment shall include clinical consideration of the patient's fundamental needs.

15.1.9 Goals necessary for the patient to achieve, maintain, or reestablish emotional and/or physical health and maximum growth and adaptive capabilities shall be included in the treatment plan.

15.1.9.1 These goals shall be determined on the basis of the assessment of the patient and/or the patient's family.

15.1.9.2 Specific goals, with both long-term and short-term objectives, and the anticipated time expected to meet these goals shall be established.

15.1.9.3 Treatment plan goals shall be written in terms of measurable criteria.

15.1.10 The patient shall participate in the development of the treatment plan, and such participation shall be documented.

15.1.11 The treatment plan shall describe services, activities, programs, and anticipated patient actions and responses and shall specify the staff members assigned to work with the patient.

15.1.12 The treatment plan shall delineate the locations and frequency of treatment procedures.

15.1.13 The treatment plan shall designate the means for measuring the progress and/or outcome of treatment efforts.

15.1.14 The treatment plan shall delineate the specific criteria to be met for termination of treatment and aftercare services. Such criteria shall be a part of the initial treatment plan.

15.1.15 A specific plan for the involvement of the family or significant others shall be included in the treatment plan, when indicated.[32]

OUTPATIENT/INPATIENT SERVICE

As an introduction to therapeutic recreation service and the therapeutic recreation process in various settings, we should stop briefly and look at outpatient/inpatient service, which offers an interesting overview or perspective of such settings in general.

In the era before community mental health programs, the major form of patient care was inpatient. Today the primary setting for the treatment of mental disorders is the outpatient department found in the various public and private general medical hospitals and in community mental health centers.[33] These settings are followed by inpatient units of general hospitals, state and county psychiatric institutions, and private mental hospitals.[34]

The leading position of outpatient service settings is the result of a number of factors:

Consumer awareness of the importance of seeking help as quickly as possible

Positive change in the public's attitude about mental illness

Rise of psychotherapy

Provides help without disrupting the consumer's normal routine

Meets a need for assistance in a crisis, transient emotional symptoms, or milder forms of mental disorders

Services are accessible because they are close to the population and reachable with available transportation

Usually available when assistance is needed; seven days a week and twenty-four hours a day

Consumer awareness of the existence of the services

Entry into receiving services is uncomplicated

Emphasis on aftercare or service following release or discharge from inpatient service

Increase in insurance for outpatient services[35]

Even though these reasons are quite valid, problems still exist, which center around insufficient funds, programs and services for the population requesting or needing services.[36]

Although outpatient services are the primary setting for treating mental disorders, inpatient services still play a very important part for those who require more in-depth services because of the severity of the disorders (i.e., schizophrenia and affective disorders), pose a threat to themselves and others, or lack family or other resources to support their difficulties. Further, the move toward deinstitutionalization as related to state and private psychiatric institutions has been greatly slowed because (1) there is a lack of sufficient community services in already existing communities, (2) services are only of a standard nature, and (3) in many geographical areas no services exist.[37]

There is also no reason to believe, as society does, that inpatient service is associated with long-term hospitalization, especially in state and private psychiatric institutions. Long-term hospitalization is not the modal practice in inpatient facilities. The most recent figures available regarding length of stay show that the median length of stay in units of general hospitals and in private mental hospitals was in the range of seven to twenty-four days. State and county mental hospital patients stayed a median of forty-four days, with a discharge of 75 percent of admissions within three months and over 85 percent in six months.[38]

STATE MENTAL HOSPITALS

As we begin our discussion of the therapeutic recreation process in state mental hospitals, it is well to note that such hospitals have been and continue to be severely criticized for the quality of care and treatment they offer. On the other hand, a number of investigators have not agreed with that appraisal. In brief, these hospitals, according to one investigator, have within limitations promoted and reflected in their practices the state of scientific knowledge and the beliefs, attitudes, and values of society. Their achievements and failures are often the expression of social policy formulated outside the hospital and beyond its control.[39] Most significantly, what they have done well is shorten the length of stay and force the development of alternatives to hospitalization. In addition, they have provided a cost-effective alternative to expensive general hospital care for the patient who does not improve sufficiently to return home after three weeks of intensive care. And they continue to provide care and treatment for acute, severe and often recurrent mental illness, as well as providing continued care for those too sick and too disturbed for nursing home care.[40]

Purpose

In recent years the vast majority of state mental health services have reorganized under a human services umbrella. As a result, the major concept underlying human services, as related to treatment, is the dominance of social factors or stresses as the cause of mental disorders. This concept underplays the biological and intrapsychical factors as equal partners in a causative triad. This concept suggests a social goal of providing care and treatment to persons with mental illness so as to return them to the community relieved of symptoms in the shortest possible time. This goal fits well with the various secondary goals of safeguarding the public and protecting of individuals with self-destructive impulses, improvement and training in social skills to enhance socialization, rehabilitation of those with chronic disabilities, and the continuing care of the incurable.[41]

Organization

As we have commented earlier, the unit plan or system is the preferred organizational arrangement in most state mental hospitals. It objectives are to provide total care for a geographical area through linkages with community organizations, and a continuity of therapeutic effort with pre- and posthospital care, and with responsibility for decisions at the operating level. Advocates of this plan claim better total care, improved communication, and greater social responsibility result. As for therapeutic recreation specialists, they are usually assigned to a particular unit.

On the other hand, there are still some state mental hospitals that are organized around the concept of acute, intermediate, and continuous treatment programs, which was the primary arrangement prior to the unit plan. Acute or admission wards are usually those where stay is short and treatment intensive. Intermediate wards may keep patients up to six months; long-term wards (continuous treatment) house patients whose stay is over six months. Therapeutic recreation specialists in this kind of structure may be assigned to providing services to wards within a specific ward category or be assigned to provide services throughout the three categories.

The specialist needs to remember that the heart of any mental health inpatient setting is the ward. It is the setting where

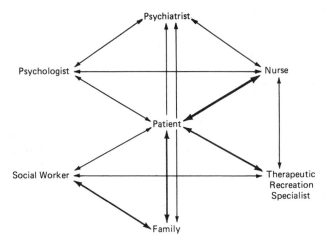

FIGURE 9.2. Ward Interaction
The thickness of the lines suggests the amount of interaction over a twenty-four-hour period.

nearly all treatment takes place. It is a specialized environment that facilitates the remission of symptoms, promotes social interaction, and encourages rehabilitation (see Figure 9.2). The psychiatric ward is unlike wards found in general medical and surgical hospitals where patients are usually in bed. Here patients are ambulatory. Things are not done to and for them but with them. Rooms provide privacy, but there is also space that fosters relationships and is used for socializing experiences and for activities. Ward size, staffing, and design differs from other medical units.

Therapeutic Recreation Service

Given the complex staffing arrangements and multiple therapeutic approaches to care and treatment in a state mental hospital, along with uncertainty in funding and position allocations and the need for accountability, it is extremely difficult, if not impossible, to outline the organizational structure, function, and approach to providing therapeutic recreation service. From a practical perspective, all of the above factors have led to a blurring of the professional identification and role of the therapeutic recreation specialist. No longer does the specialist lead only recreative activities. The specialist may lead activities that were traditionally the province of other activity-oriented thera-

pies, be responsible for leading various psychosocial intervention programs, serve as a group therapy leader or co-leader, or be the primary therapist for a number of patients.

These other responsibilities must usually fit into the organizational structure of the hospital in the delivery of therapeutic recreation service. There are today any number of organizational patterns. The unit plan, as discussed earlier, is one pattern wherein the specialist is assigned to a specific unit; where there is a shortage of staff the specialist may have two unit responsibilities. Another arrangement is the ward therapy team approach, wherein the specialist is assigned to various wards throughout the hospital. And still another is the treatment unit approach, wherein the specialist is assigned to a specific disorder unit—acute psychiatric unit, psychosocial treatment unit, geropsychiatric unit, children and adolescent unit, chemical dependency unit, and forensic unit. It is also quite possible that the specialist may function independently within the team with no home base (department) as such or return to a permanent base in his or her respective home department.

Programming

The opportunity to develop individual activity programs to meet specific individual needs is extremely limited in state mental hospitals. Patients are scheduled, according to their needs, for activity programs that have already been developed. Although a similar arrangement is found in nursing homes, programs in state mental hospitals tend to be more sophisticated as a result of the education and training of rehabilitation therapy staff, the organizational structure of the rehabilitation therapies, and the philosophy or mission of the hospital.

The activity program that has been initiated is usually based on the mission of the hospital and the goals that were developed to meet the mission statement. Thereafter, activities are implemented, based on objectives, to meet one or more of the goals that were developed earlier. Ideally, the total program will incorporate the professional services of therapy, leisure education, and participatory recreation as outlined by the

Philosophical Position Statement of the National Therapeutic Recreation Society (NTRS).[42] Further, in the delivery of service, the standards developed by NTRS will be followed: NTRS *Standards of Practice for Therapeutic Recreation Service* and *NTRS Guidelines for the Administration of Therapeutic Recreation Service in Clinical and Residential Facilities.*[43] It goes without saying that standards developed by the Joint Commission on Accreditation of Hospitals relative to activity therapies in a psychiatric setting will also be followed.

Although the variety of activities that can be offered in a state mental hospital is endless, much of the development will depend on the mission and size of the hospital, the size of the rehabilitation staff, and the resources available within and outside the hospital.

THERAPEUTIC RECREATION PROCESS

In our consideration of the therapeutic recreation process for a mental disorder, we will focus on an individual diagnosed as schizophrenic. It is one of the most common forms of mental disorder, as noted in an earlier chapter. Starting early in life, often during adolescence and still more often in the twenties, it can destroy a person's whole adult career and prevent the person from making any useful contribution to society. If spontaneous recovery does not occur, or if treatment is not successful, the patient may become a public charge for forty or fifty years.

Most investigators believe that schizophrenia has no single cause; rather, it is the result of a complex interaction of environmental and biological factors. The individual inherits a predisposition to schizophrenia, but the disorder is triggered by environmental stress.[44]

It is very difficult to address the complexity of schizophrenia and its treatment from a therapeutic recreation perspective since the disorder is a complex problem with a

range of human reactions not always understood by anyone. Almost any statement made about the disorder and its therapeutic recreation approach could rightly be accompanied by alternatives, exceptions, and multiple qualifications. Our hope is that we will describe a clear framework of the process in use with an individual diagnosed as schizophrenic.

Our approach is based on the psychosocial component of treatment, although we recognize that other therapy perspectives exist (medical, adaptational, and developmental modes).[45] This treatment focus is supported largely by the fact that many state mental hospitals approach care and treatment of this disorder from a psychosocial perspective.[46] The rationale, as related to this disorder, is that few individuals with this diagnosis respond successfully to psychotherapy.[47] Further, the patient has failed to acquire those psychological and social skills necessary for reasonable social adjustment; therefore, the need of the patient is to improve or develop new task and interpersonal skills that would enhance his or her chances of making a successful adjustment to community life.[48] At the same time the reader should not imagine that this approach will quickly enable the patient to function independently. A person diagnosed as schizophrenic becomes socially responsive, if at all, at a very slow pace.

Case History of George

George is a thirty-five-year-old man who has suffered two psychotic episodes since the age of twenty-one and is again returned to the hospital. Between hospitalizations he operates a grain-elevator business, which was left to him when his father died eight years ago. He is married and the father of two children. He was raised in an atmosphere of emotional confusion. Over the years the family isolated themselves and had few friends. Consequently, George had few friends.

His most recent episode is the result of a continued concern about finances. Two years ago he sold several acres of farm land which he inherited from his father. As a result, he and his wife were able to buy a larger house. Shortly thereafter George began to worry about finances. His worries were unfounded since the sale of the farm land produced a considerable profit. However, no amount of reassurance would help. He continued to worry and became so preoccupied with money that he sold the family car and the company truck and began walking to work. He lost his appetite, and his weight dropped some twenty pounds within a few weeks. He has not been to work for three weeks, refuses to talk to employees, and recently has withdrawn from any contact with his family. He no longer bathes and shaves. Three days ago he began reminiscing about playing in the high school band, his first date, and his first kiss. He spoke of these events as if occurring in the past week and in language more common to adolescents of his time.

George's axes according to the DSM-III-R multiaxial evaluation[49] might read as follows:

Axis I 295.64 schizophrenia, residual, chronic

Axis II 301.22 schizotypal personality (premorbid)

Axis III No diagnosis

Axis IV *Psychosocial stressors:* interpersonal problems with friends, associates, and employees; occupation; living circumstances

Severity: 4–5, severe to extreme (predominantly enduring circumstances)

Axis V Current GAF: 30
Highest GAF past year: 55

ASSESSMENT

As we have noted, the individual in need of hospitalization because of mental illness may be admitted through a voluntary or involuntary admission. In George's situation his admission is involuntary having been initiated by George's wife with a recommendation from the family physician. Since he is from Powell County, he is assigned to Unit B, which includes three counties and is a part of the unit plan structure found in Mosby State Hospital.

Within a day or two following admission, George is considered at a diagnostic staff meeting, which may be one and the same as the rehabilitation team meeting where the treatment plan is developed. Since George is a former patient, his previous file is reviewed. The file will usually consist of a psychiatric history, mental status examination, various psychosocial assessments, results of psychological tests, and in George's case, the former diagnosis. Added to this information will be the data collected since his most recent admission. Even though he has had two former commitments and there is a considerable amount of background material in addition to present information, the need for another assessment is essential and serves several purposes:

1. Identifying the condition (diagnosis) and problems

2. Identifying client motivations, strengths, and resources

3. Identifying forces that may hinder the therapeutic plan (forces both internal and external to the patient)

4. Identifying and determining goals and objectives

5. Determining appropriate intervention strategies

Before proceeding, a word about the information found in the file. Systems of collection and assessment vary among the various mental health agencies. As an example, the diagnosis may be made before, during, or after the team meeting. It is often seen as a function of the psychiatrist, although in some settings a tentative diagnosis will be made by the social worker. The psychiatric examination consists of the history and mental status examination, and in many situations psychological tests will be requested. These various examinations incorporate the following information:

Psychiatric history: Includes the complaint, present symptoms, previous hospitalizations and treatment, family background, personal history, and the individual's relationships with others, moods, feelings, interests, and leisure-time activities. This information may be given by the individual, but in some instances it is provided by others.

Mental status examination: Purpose is to gather data to be used in determining etiology, diagnosis, prognosis, and treatment. It seeks the following information: general behavior and appearance, characteristics of talk, emotional state, special preoccupations and experiences, orientation in terms of time, place, person, and self, memory, intellectual level, abstract thinking, and insight evaluation.[50]

Psychological testing: Includes intelligence tests and those tests concerned with the personality (sometimes called projective tests). A list and description of the more commonly used tests is found in Table 9.1.

TABLE 9.1. Common Psychological Tests in Clinical Use

Name of Test	Description	Method
Bender–Gestalt Test	A test of visual–motor coordination that is most useful with adults as a screening device to detect the presence of organic impairment. It may also be used to evaluate the level of maturation in the coordination of intellectual, muscular, and visual functions in children.	The client is asked to copy nine separate geometric designs onto plain white paper, one at a time. Sometimes the client is asked to draw the design from memory after an interval of forty-five to sixty seconds.
Blacky Test	A projective test used most frequently with children (although it is also designed for adults) to determine the level of psychosexual development.	The client is shown various cartoons about a dog (who may be identified as male or female) and the dog's family and is asked to make up a story about each cartoon.
Draw-a-Person Test	A projective test used with both adults and children to elicit information on the client's body image or perception of self and the client's relationship to the environment. It is also used as a	The client is asked first to draw a human figure and later to draw a person of the opposite sex. The test may be expanded by asking the client to draw a picture of a house and a tree as

TABLE 9.1. *(Continued)*

Name of Test	Description	Method
	screening device to detect the presence of organic impairment. With children it may be used to compare the age level of expression with the child's chronological age for a rough approximation of intelligence.	well (called the House-Tree-Person test), an animal, or a family.
Minnesota Multiphasic Personality Inventory (MMPI)	A self-administered objective (as opposed to projective) personality test designed to yield a broad examination of personality functioning that is amenable to statistical interpretation—such as self-attitudes, certain aspects of ego functioning, and profiles of symptoms or psychopathology.	The client responds to 550 statements, by indicating either "true," "false," or "cannot say." The client's personality profile is sketched in terms of: • Preoccupation with body diseases • Depression • Hysteria • Antisocial personality • Masculine or feminine features • Paranoid qualities • Anxiety, phobias, and psychogenic fatigue • Schizophrenic features • Manic features
Rorschach Test	A projective test that is the most highly developed of the personality tests. It reveals personality features and symptoms and is commonly used as a diagnostic tool.	The client responds to ten cards, one at a time, consisting of black and white or colored, standardized inkblots. Responses include the impressions, thoughts, and associations that come to mind while the client looks at the inkblot.
Sentence Completion Test	A projective test designed to elicit conscious associations to specific areas of functioning to illustrate the fears, preoccupations, ambitions, and idiosyncrasies of the client.	The client is asked to complete spontaneously sentences such as: "I feel guilty about . . . ," "Sex is . . . ," "My mother . . . ," "Sometimes I wish . . . ," Both mood and content are noted.
Stanford-Binet Intelligence Test	A general intelligence test based on an age-level concept from two years to about fifteen years. It is particularly useful to test children and to evaluate mental retardation.	The client is asked to do a graded series of tasks designed to correlate with the abilities of children of a particular age group. Each set is more difficult than the one before it.

(continued)

TABLE 9.1. (*Continued*)

Name of Test	Description	Method
Thematic Apperception Test (TAT)	A projective test offering a standardized set of stimuli for exploring the client's emotional life. Themes and interpersonal problems emerge in the client's responses.	The client is shown a series of ambiguous pictures of people in various emotionally significant situations and is asked to respond by describing what is happening in the picture and telling a story about it. Adaptations have been designed for use with children. In these, the central figure is a child or the pictures are cartoons of animals.
Wechsler Adult Intelligence Scale (WAIS)	A general intelligence test for persons sixteen years of age and older. It is the most widely used and best standardized intelligence test.	The client completes eleven subtests, which yield both verbal and performance scores as well as full-scale IQs. Subtest raw scores may also be compared to reveal variability in functioning. The subtests are: information, comprehension, arithmetic, similarities, memory for digits, vocabulary, digit symbol, picture completion, block design, picture arrangement, and object assembly.
Wechsler Intelligence Scale for Children (WISC)	A general intelligence test for children from five through fifteen years of age.	Similar to the Wechsler test for adults, this test asks the client to complete ten subtests, which yield separate verbal, performance, and full-scale scores.
Wechsler Memory Scale	A psychological test for immediate, short-term, and long-term memory.	The client is asked to do seven memory tests, including current information, orientation, mental control, logical memory, digits forward and backward, visual reproduction, and associate learning. A memory quotient (MQ) score is useful in the determination of organic mental syndrome.
Word Association Test	A projective test similar in form and organization to the Sentence Completion test. It is designed to elicit associations to areas of conflict.	The client is asked to respond spontaneously to a series of fifty or more words, presented one at a time. Words presumed to be related to the conflicts of the specific client are mixed with words that generally produce an emotional reaction.

SOURCE: Holly Skodol Wilson and Carol Ren Kneish, *Psychiatric Nursing*, 2nd ed. (Menlo Park, Calif.: Addison-Wesley Publishing Co., 1983), pp. 198–99.

Data Collection

We noted earlier that the collection of data comes from a variety of sources including but not limited to the patient's file, other staff, the patient's relatives, knowledge of the disorder, and the patient.

The patient's file, in this case George's file, reflects a history of symptoms associated with the disorder of schizophrenia since childhood coupled with stable-to-marginal adjustment. The psychiatric history notes an earlier failure of knowing "what is expected of me" from family and friends and the inability to manage relationships. Frequent reference is made to "feelings of anxiety" and "not fitting in." As a result of these feelings, George withdrew from relationships and social experiences; this in turn created anxiety and regression to simpler role relationships that had been fulfilled adequately in the past. However, as George grew older, expectations in social and work experiences made it impossible for him to sustain limited and confined role relationships. Ill-equipped, he was pushed into experiencing new situations, which eventually resulted in his initial hospitalization. With medication and psychotherapy, George weathered this crisis within a few days and returned home.

The second hospitalization occurred following the death of his father. Initially, anxiety appeared as a consequence of George's inability to handle the new situation of managing the grain elevator. Shortly thereafter, withdrawal from social contact was noted, along with George's spending an inordinate amount of time sleeping and daydreaming. Further, he began to give lengthy answers to questions that required only a yes or no answer. At other times, when asked a question, he appeared to be completely detached from the question, seemingly understanding it but not responding. Still later he began to think out loud and to arrange the pencils on his desk into various shapes or use a different pencil for each word or line. During his

second hospitalization his wife was involved in counseling. The therapeutic goals at this time were containment of social dysfunction and control of symptoms. The wife was asked to assume an increasing role in George's life.

While the psychiatric history and other records will provide considerable information about George, the therapeutic recreation specialist realizes that deterioration from a previous level of functioning frequently occurs in individuals having a schizophrenic disorder. This deterioration centers around work, self-care, and social situations. Further, schizophrenic patients present a veritable encyclopedia of disturbances associated with form of thought, perception, affect, language and communication, volition, sense of self, relationship to the external world, and psychomotor behavior.[51] However, these characteristics are not observed all together at one time in one person diagnosed as schizophrenic (nor are they seen only in schizophrenia).

The specialist knows that individuals who develop schizophrenia are usually reacting to a host of environmental stresses as well as to the disease itself. Many of the symptoms and behaviors of people with schizophrenia can be viewed as secondary: as stress responses, compensatory behaviors, and restitutive activities; as social responses to deviance; and as products of the interaction of the disease, the person, and the environment over long periods of time. A fundamental problem for individuals diagnosed as schizophrenic is a deficit in their ability to interpret or comprehend interpersonal relationships. They have difficulty forging and participating in social interactions; they are deficient in a large number of social skills and social behaviors. These characteristics are usually the result of several factors; namely, withdrawal and environmental deprivation.[52] Lastly, the specialist realizes that the treatment of the disorder is multidimensional and rehabilitation is a long-term process.

Interview

Prior to any further consideration of this case study, it is important to consider here the *therapeutic use of self* not only in relation to interviewing George and other psychotic patients, but in relation to all interactions with mentally ill patients. In many ways mentally ill patients may be the most challenging group of individuals the specialist ever works with. In a very real sense, the relationship can be one of the most important factors in the patient's therapeutic experience. However, many beginning specialists, like other therapists, frequently express concern about working with the mentally ill. These concerns include fear of bodily harm, fear of becoming mentally ill, fear of personal inadequacy, fear of loss of emotional control, and fear of rejection by patients. Most of these fears are experienced in varying degrees by almost everyone who works with mentally ill patients. They usually disappear as knowledge and understanding develop about the mentally ill. If the fears persist, one of the most helpful ways to reduce the feelings of fear is to share those feelings with others who are likely to have had similar experiences.

All therapeutic relationships possess common elements, although they are developed differently by each staff person depending on the characteristics of the individuals involved. If a relationship is to become therapeutic, it is necessary to recognize the patient, regardless of disorder, as a unique, important human being who experiences hopes, fears, joys, and sorrows as does everyone else. It is necessary to understand that the patient has a special set of problems and reactions to life. It is important for the therapeutic recreation specialist to develop a relationship with the patient so that he or she will understand, in a limited way at least, the emotional responses and probable meaning of the patient's behavior.

The basis of all therapeutic relationships is *acceptance*. Two other words that are of equal importance in the psychiatric setting are *consistency* and *nonjudgmental*. These three attitudes are basic to developing a therapeutic relationship with any patient. Acceptance implies that the specialist treats the patient as an important person and not as a diagnostic entity. It also implies that the specialist tries to understand the meaning the patient is conveying through various behaviors and through comments directed toward the specialist. One must remember that behavior—verbal or nonverbal—is an expression of the illness.

The word nonjudgmental is closely related to the concept of acceptance. A nonjudgmental attitude is neither condemning nor approving. Acceptance of patients and their behavior is often difficult to achieve, and almost everyone occasionally falls short of the ideal. The behavior of some patients is offensive at times. However, the specialist needs to realize that a patient's behavior will usually change as he or she gets better.

Consistency is another important element to be considered in the therapeutic relationship. The specialist maintains the same basic attitude toward the patient day after day so that the patient will learn what is expected. Such help lessens the patient's anxiety by simplifying decision making and by avoiding uncertainties.

Empathic listening is another important aspect of use of self therapeutically. There is probably no more important task than listening to a patient in a positive, dynamic, empathic way, without giving advice, stating opinions, or making suggestions. Empathic listening demands that the specialist be skillful in reflecting patient comments in such a manner that the patient will realize that the specialist is interested in the discussion and wants to hear as much as the patient needs to tell. It is not unusual for patients to pour out their problems and concerns more frequently to the specialist than to anyone else since they perceive the specialist as nonthreatening. However, the specialist is concerned with reality-oriented factors—the here and now—and leaves the problems of the unconscious to the psychiatrist or those trained to deal with such matters. By listening, the specialist may be able to provide an emotional experience that the patient has never been able to achieve.

Returning to George, it is no easy task to interview individuals with schizophrenia. They have a tendency to distance themselves from others because of their inability to handle or manage the exchange of information in a close relationship. If the relationship becomes too close, verbally or nonverbally, the patient may retreat, withdraw, become angry, or comment obliquely. Therefore, the staff needs to be sensitive to the patient, reflecting calmness and confidence.

In this particular situation, as in other assessment interviews, the interview will involve nonverbal, verbal, and environmental observations in addition to emotive, cognitive, and behavioral aspects. The specialist, in approaching George, restricts the interview to those matters that specifically focus on leisure and social functioning. To reduce any anxiety that George may have about the interview, the specialist introduces himself, invites George to be seated, and explains the context of the interview, including its purpose, in considerable detail. Thereafter, he explains how the information will be used in developing a treatment program and how George may benefit from participation in the program.

George responds to some questions concerning early recreative interest and experiences, but his responses to other questions and their relationship to him are rather inappropriate and far-fetched. Although interviews with other individuals diagnosed as schizophrenic and other psychotics can produce positive results, the specialist at this time will rely on George's past psychiatric history to develop a treatment plan. If time permits and an opportunity presents itself, the specialist will talk to other family members.

Team Meeting

The initial goal of George's treatment plan determined at the team meeting is to stabilize him. At the same time it is recognized that recovery is a process and a progression. Stabilizing means establishing a nonthreatening environment and treatment through medication; thereafter, psychotherapy and psychosocial interventions are introduced. It is anticipated that the interventions will improve basic social functioning (interpersonal communication, social skills, and behaviors) while decreasing abnormal subjective experiences, misperceptions, and bizarre behaviors. It is anticipated that George will gradually be moved into the milieu and social life of the unit so as to reduce social isolation and reestablish social patterns.

It is further anticipated that his symptoms will begin to subside quickly once proper medication is given since that is what occurred during the previous hospitalization. On the other hand, it is recognized that it might be several months before a significant remission of symptoms is noted. Antipsychotic medication differs from other psychotropic medication designed to relieve symptoms of anxiety and depression. Antipsychotic medication will directly alter the organization and content of George's thoughts and perceptions.

The team will also consider which member will be George's primary therapist and what psychotherapeutic approach will be taken to specific symptoms by the team as they interact with George. Consideration is also given to the degree of autonomy that George will be allowed on the unit. The latter two points are extremely important since they provide a structure that will tend to preserve self-respect and facilitate reality testing, rather than placing George in a confusing, unpredictable milieu. Lastly, consideration is given to continuing care and the management of the chronic illness. In this situation it is recommended that George's wife receive awareness counseling since she will be the primary support person following discharge.

As a result of the review of the psychiatric history, personal interview, and team meeting, the specialist has recorded the following information for consideration in planning George's treatment plan:

ACTIVITY INTEREST

Pet raising (4-H)
Square dancing
Fishing
Table games
Music playing—clarinet
Music listening

PROBLEMS

Withdrawal from social contact
Loss of self-esteem
Hallucinations
Detachment from surroundings
Blunt affect
Limited social skills
Thought disorder
Restrictive communication patterns
Bizarre preoccupations
Inappropriate responses
Illogical anxiety

PLANNING

There are many problems associated with George's schizophrenic state that could be considered in developing his treatment plan. In fact, the problem list is only partial. Medication will resolve some of the problems, assisted by a protective and pleasant environment and by psychotherapy and other psychosocial interventions. Other problems will require a more balanced approach involving all three intervention procedures.

From a therapeutic perspective, the specialist realizes that George has developed patterns of behavior that are ineffective in coping with the demands of daily life. However, the specialist also realizes that with a proper approach and attitude these faulty patterns of behavior can be unlearned and replaced by other, more effective and appropriate patterns to effect eventual integration into the social milieu of the unit. Thus, any goals must assist George to realize that reality can be bearable and even rewarding.

The specialist further recognizes that whatever goals are set forth, they will not be easily attainable since schizophrenic patients usually require special attention or assistance to begin their rehabilitation. Also, the specialist cannot forget that although George may appear to be out of touch with his surroundings, he should be told the goals of his treatment plan. Investigators have noted that while schizophrenic patients may not appear to be aware of their surroundings, a great number have reported later that they were well aware of their environment, of other patients, and of their therapists but could not communicate.[53]

Following consideration of those matters at the team meeting, the following initial goals were produced:

To promote self-identity
To promote self-esteem
To promote trust
To promote adult status
To promote socialization
To promote participation in activities

The rationale for these goals focuses primarily on the problems of withdrawal and limited social skills. The specialist initiates action to reverse further withdrawal from social contact, while at the same time reestablishing social skills and social interaction through participation in various activities. In this regard, the specialist may give consideration to the interactive process among individuals as outlined by Avedon and the type of group interaction skills the specialist wants George to obtain, as delineated by Mosey.[54] These interactive processes and interaction skills are appropriate regardless of special population and setting. In addition, when George participates in activities, a feedback mechanism operates wherein he begins to observe himself facing reality, and that promotes his self-identity. With success in activities comes self-esteem; likewise, trust in others is initiated.

Increasingly in recent years the approach of therapy with schizophrenic patients has been directed toward the adult rather than the infantile aspects of the personality. Therefore, within the activity the specialist will allow George choices and decision-making opportunities, albeit limited, which will promote not only adult status but also George's sense of his own identity and self-esteem.

Mosby State Hospital provides an extensive number and range of activities. Activities are primarily of a group nature with few, if any, one-on-one activities. Further, the size of the group may vary from small to large, from four or five patients to fifty or sixty, depending upon the type of activity. Some activities are conducted on the ward or unit, while others are scheduled in the centralized activity building, which is similar in nature to the traditional public recreation community center. Then too, depending upon the patient's treatment plan, activities are scheduled in community resources.

George will be assigned to two activity groups. One is the arts and crafts group number two, which is for lower-functioning patients. It meets three times a week. The second activity is the music appreciation class, which meets twice a week. Both activities are conducted in the activity center. In addition, George will have the opportunity to attend the weekly dance and movie and have access to the recreation room in the activity building. This room is adjacent to the canteen and offers the opportunity for patients to socialize through playing pool, ping-pong, cards, and other table games and just conversing.

The members of the arts and crafts group that George is assigned to are concerned with learning about their needs and emotions. Although the completion of a project is important, it is secondary to the group goal. The goal of the group is to develop basic skills or facets of the private and public self. In this low-functioning group the specialist decides initially what projects might be the most appropriate for patients to work on, but eventually allows patients to make their own choices. The specialist will also determine the kinds of behavior to encourage and the focus of discussion. Overall, the specialist determines or controls the dynamics and process of the group. This particular group helps patients develop a greater understanding of who they are and what they are. It is used to help patients take the first step toward developing living skills necessary for independent functioning following discharge.

In addition to allowing George to make choices which will assist him in feeling like an adult, the group will help George reestablish interaction patterns and participation skills. Although a completed project is secondary, it does assist in organizing orderly thinking and brings a feeling of personal worth and respect, which is extremely valuable to George. It is anticipated that this activity will provide the opportunity to bring satisfaction in accomplishment, in personal endeavor, and in success.

The music-listening group has a number of group goals: to provide an aesthetic experience, to influence behavior, to change mood, to stimulate various bodily processes, and to maintain contact with reality, to name a few. Scheduling George for the music-listening group places him in an activity that is nonthreatening and noncontroversial but at the same time has socializing effects. The activity lends itself to resolving feelings of fear and mistrust, thus providing a feeling of order and well-being. Further, as George improves, the therapist can involve George more and more in the discussion of the music being played since directed music listening with discussion is better than undirected listening, which may stimulate loss of contact with reality.

Having determined the goals and activities for George, it now becomes necessary for the specialist to develop terminal expectations. They are as follows:

Goal: To promote self-identity
Activity: Arts and crafts class and music-listening class
Behavioral Objective: After sixty days George will verbally express his feelings about his present and future behavior.

Goal: To promote self-esteem
Activity: Arts and crafts class and music-listening class
Behavioral Objective: After sixty days George will have:
completed two simple craft projects
selected one song to be played and discussed in the music-listening class

Goal: To promote trust
Activity: Arts and crafts class and music-listening class
Behavioral Objective: After sixty days George will show a heightened confiding relation with both the arts specialist and the music specialist, as determined by them.

Goal: To promote adult status
Activity: Arts and crafts class and music listening class
Behavioral Objective: After 60 days George will have:
chosen a specific craft project
selected a specific song to be played and discussed

Goal: To promote socialization
Activity: Arts and crafts class and music-listening class
Behavioral Objective: After sixty days George will voluntarily engage verbally with one or more of the other patients during the activity.

Goal: To promote participation
Activity: Arts and crafts class and music-listening class
Behavioral Objective: After sixty days George will engage in:
a group arts and crafts project as selected by the therapist
the selection of songs to be played and discussed in the music-listening class

In addition to these behavioral objectives, George will be monitored by all staff as he does or does not participate in other social activities—dances, movies, and visits to the canteen and recreation room.

The plan now becomes a part of the record on file. Since treatment is a process and a progression, these goals will change as George progresses and additional problems are identified.

IMPLEMENTATION

In implementing the plan, the specialist needs to be scrupulously honest in all dealings with George. Few things are more destructive to a therapeutic relationship than deliberate deception. However, the obligation to be truthful does not imply that the specialist must be brutally honest. A *tactful* concern for the patient's sensitivities and anxieties is an equally important dimension in a mutually trusting relationship. It is not unusual, for example, for a patient to ask the specialist directly about a diagnosis. Patients with schizophrenic disorders usually ask about their diagnosis because the term is particularly frightening. The most favorable response is to suggest that they ask their psychiatrist or primary therapist.

Another matter encountered with psychotic patients, including George, is medication side effects. When neuroleptic medication is used in full antipsychotic doses, the incidence of undesirable side effects is high. Sedation is perhaps the most common problem noted, with patients having difficulty staying awake. As psychotic agitation decreases, the sedative effects of the medication may remain. In some instances patients may fall asleep or become drowsy during the activity, and the specialist should not assume that the activity is a failure. Although tolerance often develops to this side effect with the passage of time, gradual reduction of the dosage is often necessary before the problem improves.

Other common side effects of neuroleptic drugs include dry mouth, blurred vision, constipation, and postural hypotension. Of special concern to the specialist are heat intolerance and photosensitivity reactions to exposure to sunlight. Patients need to be advised to use a sunscreen preparation and avoid excessive heat during summer months. (The various kinds of neuroleptic medication and side effects are found in Appendix B.)

Returning to George and his involvement in activities, it is important that the specialist recognize that recovery is usually characterized by slow, uneven progress. Excessive rules and unreasonable regulations in activities cause problems, if not flight. In such an atmosphere George, who is struggling to reorganize, grow, and regain some sense of dignity, independence, and autonomy, would not fare well. On the other hand, a laissez-faire or confused structure will promote disorganization and hinder his progress. A balance must be found that will support rehabilitation goals, promote health, and facilitate reality testing and avoid a confusing, unpredictable milieu for George.

The specialist's direction of activities is clear, simple, and explained in a dignified fashion. Further, the approach must be consistent from activity to activity. Consistency means that the specialist in his interaction with George means what he says and says what he means, rather than saying one thing and doing the opposite. Such an approach improves rehabilitation efforts and promotes George's healthy functioning. If he is to turn toward reality, he must be convinced that reality is safer and more desirable than the refuge he has chosen.

EVALUATION

We have noted elsewhere that evaluation is the final phase of the therapeutic recreation process, although in practice some form of evaluation is an ongoing process. Therefore, it is imperative that the specialist review the assessment of the patient's problem and the plan for helping the patient as well as the actual outcome of the program developed for the patient. The focus of evaluation is on the result of the planned intervention—the achievement of the goals of the treatment plan.

The recording of George's progress follows the same procedures that have been used in other settings. The evaluation findings may be written and recorded in the chart or verbally reported in a team meeting and recorded in the chart later. What is recorded should be written simply, accurately, and straightforwardly and should avoid psychiatric jargon and labels.

In preparing George's evaluation, the specialist is cautious about overestimating George's level of skill competence or social functioning, or that of any schizophrenic patient for that matter, since his social skills may appear to be better within the safe hospital environment than they would be in a less structured environment. An evaluation of George at the end of sixty days might read as follows:

A reestablishment of social patterns has been noted, accompanied by control of symptoms. He is attempting to establish a level of stability by less acting out. Consistently coming to activities and participating is noted. Has completed three projects in his group and interacts at times in music activity. Interaction with other patients at the weekly dance appears to be stressful. When encouraged to dance responds with "I can't," although patient can dance. [There are many interpretations that can be offered for "I can't." The specialist will bring the matter to the attention of the team at the next meeting.] Trust seems to be developing and specialist will begin to increase warmth and informality.

In conclusion, the future for George is difficult to predict. Estimates of the outcome of schizophrenia are influenced by three factors: consistency of treatment programs, social and cultural context (familial, social, and cultural realities influence the course of schizophrenia), and resources and economics. Some patients attain a high level of independent functioning and do not require even periodic care. At the other end of the spectrum are those who, in spite of hospitalization, medication, psychotherapy, and social-vocational rehabilitation programs, are barely able to function in the community. These people may require, and usually do, continuing professional support.

PRIVATE PSYCHIATRIC HOSPITALS

Private psychiatric hospitals occupy a very important and frequently unrecognized position in the treatment of psychiatric patients. Such hospitals are active treatment institutions that admit patients with a wide range of psychiatric disorders including alcoholism and drug dependence, provide continuous twenty-four-hour service, and have organized psychiatric staffs. The hospital may serve only adults, or only children and adolescents, or a combination of the two. The hospital usually provides care as a part of a delivery system in which the patient is in treatment with a physician or psychiatrist in private practice. Hospitalization is by referral, but occasionally the family or the patient comes to the hospital seeking care. The most recent statistics indicate that two-thirds are operated by corporations, individuals, or partnerships, or on a for-profit basis; only one-third are not for profit.[55]

The private mental hospital services the private system in much the same fashion as the public mental health hospital services the public delivery system. It has nearly the same indications for use and for change and almost the same problems. Its reason for being is to provide a specialized environment for those who can pay for their services.

The advantages of private psychiatric hospitals over public hospitals might be as follows: (1) the greater acceptability to patients because of greater privacy and less stigma; (2) to be with others from similar backgrounds and common interests; (3) better intensive treatment, better patient-staff ratio, quality staff, and pleasant surroundings, as opposed to the austerity found in some psychiatric units of general hospitals and public psychiatric hospitals; (4) protective privacy for the well known and socially prominent; and (5) the fact that referring

psychiatrists may continue care of their patients during hospitalization and following discharge so that there is no break in the patient-doctor relationship. We would anticipate that some of these reasons could be challenged by some public psychiatric hospitals.

The organizational structure of the private psychiatric hospital will vary with the purpose of the hospital, services provided, disorders treated, and kinds of individuals being treated—adults, children, or adolescents. Naturally, the therapeutic recreation service will be organized around the mission, goals, and objectives of the hospital. In such hospitals therapeutic recreation service may be a separate service or department or be part of an activity therapy department. The therapeutic recreation specialist may provide services to wards within specific treatment units (admission, acute), to specialized units (children, adolescents, geriatric), or to wards throughout the hospital regardless of kind of treatment or unit specialization.

The care and treatment procedure found in private psychiatric hospitals is similar to what is found in public psychiatric hospitals. The patient is admitted, diagnosed, and considered in a team meeting. The therapeutic recreation specialist assesses the patient, formulates goals, writes a treatment plan, implements the plan, evaluates periodically, alters goals and the treatment process as the patient progresses or regresses, and prepares the patient for eventual discharge. Patients are assigned to group activities based on their needs, which correspond with the goals and objectives of the activities. However, there is usually more opportunity in private hospitals to initiate an activity to meet individual needs. Also, more commercial community resources are used as part of the program of services.

Aside from being members of treatment teams and conducting activities, therapeutic recreation specialists are largely restricted to the performance of their responsibilities in a more traditional manner. The opportunity to be a primary therapist or direct a basic psychosocial group (reality orientation), as might be done in a state psychiatric hospital, is limited. This is not unusual. In the 1960s and well into the 1970s, the trend was to blur roles as much as possible. Today the trend has swung back toward capitalizing on the uniqueness of each of the activity-oriented professions. Whether or not a clear trend is really noted, there has always been a separation of responsibilities by discipline because of the nature of the setting, third-party payment, necessity for assurance of uniformity and quality of performance in association with accreditation, and the fact that referring or attending physicians have full responsibility for the total care and treatment of the patient; the last is a legal-administrative concern.

GENERAL MEDICAL HOSPITALS— PSYCHIATRIC UNITS

The psychiatric unit of a general medical hospital may provide a variety of care services or just two or three services. The following services are typically found in the psychiatric unit of larger general hospitals: inpatient care, day care, outpatient care, emergency care, consultation to other non-psychiatric wards in the hospital, and detoxification of substance abusers. For our purpose, we will focus on inpatient care.

The number of general medical hospitals with separate psychiatric inpatient service has increased dramatically since World War II, and the number of individuals treated nearly tripled between the midfifties and the late seventies. According to one source, about half of all patients requiring admission for a mental disorder are now going to a general hospital.[56] The increase in units or wards and individuals using them is the result of increased insurance coverage, construction of psychiatric beds because of legislative funding, increased training of mental health workers, treatment closer to home, and relationship with various outpatient services.

The inpatient unit or ward varies in size and complexity depending upon the site and needs of the hospital and community. Because the number of beds available is limited, the hospital cannot afford to allocate them for custodial use. Therefore, the hospital concentrates on admitting those acutely ill patients who are most amenable to short-term intensive care. This usually means that the unit functions as a private delivery system with initial treatment of the patient by the psychiatrist in community practice, who then attends the patient in the hospital and provides continuing management after release. The unit also functions as a component in the public delivery system by receiving and returning patients to the community mental health center. Admission, for the most part, is voluntary.

The treatment process in most psychiatric units is directed toward the immediate resolution of the problem, with activities being tailored to those appropriate after the patient leaves the hospital. The principal modalities of treatment employed include the therapeutic community approach, token economy, behavior modification, drug therapies, and individual and group psychotherapies within a milieu therapy environment.[57] A full range of professional disciplines provide the service with a high patient-staff ratio.

Therapeutic Recreation Service

Therapeutic recreation service is a viable service within a psychiatric unit of a general medical hospital. If it is not provided, that is usually the result of problems associated with third-party payment (payment by an insurance carrier to a person or agency for services rendered to an individual, for example, Blue Cross-Blue Shield, Medicare, Medicaid). Therapeutic recreation service may be represented by one, two, or more specialists depending upon the size of the unit. The specialist may function independently within a therapeutic recreation service or department or within a rehabilitation or activity therapy department or occupational therapy department. The last is found in some settings so as to comply with reimbursement regulations. The services provided by the specialist may incorporate all three services recommended by the NTRS position statement or just one or two. Again, the philosophy of the unit will determine the approach. Because of the short-term nature of total inpatient service and the physical structure of such units therapeutic recreation resources may be limited. However, considerable use may be made of community resources including community recreation centers. If the opportunity is presented, specialists will develop a leisure-counseling program with a referral system to a community recreation agency or in conjunction with the unit's referral approach to community aftercare.

Although patients will be assigned to groups of two, three, four, or more, it is not unusual for the specialist to arrange frequent one-on-one programs. Much depends upon the goals and functioning level of the patient as to the approach taken as well as the anticipated length of stay.

Case History of Joan Ann

Joan Ann is a forty-six-year-old mother of two children who was admitted on the referral of the family physician. For the past three to six months she had had crying spells, severe headaches, felt depressed, had little appetite, had not slept well, and had lost interest in family and social matters. Her husband found her with a butcher knife in her hand when he came home from work, which he felt she intended to use on herself since she recently had been talking about suicide.

On admission she looked wan and pale and had an anxious face. At the mention of her children she began to cry. The oldest boy is seventeen, and she feels she has failed him because he just gets by in high school although he is popular and plays sports. The youngest is thirteen, is mentally retarded, and has been in an institution for five years.

She gave a history of a thyroidectomy in 1957, surgery for tubal pregnancy in 1969, and a hysterectomy in 1972. In addition, she was hospitalized as a teenager for a "nervous breakdown." Socially, she had friends as a child and teenager but developed few outside activities. School was difficult, and the family was poor and money in short supply.

There was no history of neurological disorder, but she stated that she has had frequent headaches most of her life. Her lab and X-ray were normal. She has no insight into her problems, as indicated by a psychological test, and no evidence of thought disorder. Intelligence is average. She smokes nervously and shows a fine tremor of hands and head.

Diagnosis (according to DSM-III-R[58]) although an arbitrary one, might read as follows:

Axis I	300.40 dysthymic disorder (depressive neurosis)
Axis II	301.87 atypical personality disorder
Axis III	No diagnosis
Axis IV	*Psychosocial stressors:* parenting, living circumstances, and possible interpersonal problems
	Severity: 3–4 moderate (predominantly acute events)
Axis V	Current GAF: 48
	Highest GAF past year: 67

THERAPEUTIC RECREATION PROCESS

Our discussion of the therapeutic recreation process with Joan Ann will be limited because of space considerations and the knowledge the specialist should have about diagnosis, Axis I, and Axis II. The instructor and students may wish to consider these items as a classroom learning experience.

ASSESSMENT

To make an intelligent therapeutic care plan for Joan Ann, the specialist realizes he needs to understand the nature of the patient's conflict and the meaning of her symptoms. This can be obtained only through good data collection and eventual discussion and collaboration in a team meeting.

The specialist knows that depressive neurosis usually occurs in relation to the loss of an important source of satisfaction—person, possession, or position. The patient represses the resulting feeling of hostility and turns it inward upon herself by the use of *introjection:* it is better to feel sad than to feel angry. The specialist also knows that the symptoms of this disorder—despondency, guilt, and despair—serve two purposes: (1) it punishes Joan Ann for her "bad" feelings, and (2) it punishes others around her for disappointing her. No kind of behavior, in reality, is more hostile or punishing than that of depression, the specialist recalls.

Because of Joan Ann's overwhelming feelings of guilt and ideas of self-depreciation, the specialist does not greet her in the interview with "How do you feel?" since this will produce a flood of verbal complaints and cause more guilt. Nor does the specialist end the interview with "Let's see you smile," since this will add to feelings of guilt and thus more sadness.

The interview with the patient produced the following:

PROBLEMS

Depression
Guilt
Anxiety
Slow speech
Gloominess
Headaches

ACTIVITY INTEREST

Cooking

PLANNING

The first step in the treatment process for Joan Ann consists of relief of her distress as well as the relief of the symptoms of her illness, since the symptoms are based upon her emotional distress rather than the other

way around. In response to these factors, the attending psychiatrist has already initiated the administration of a minor tranquilizer and an antidepressant drug.

During the team meeting it is determined that the psychological treatment of choice will be psychotherapy supported by as many psychosocial approaches as possible to widen Joan Ann's perspective of herself and the world she lives in. The overall approach will be to help Joan Ann increase her acceptance of herself, lessen her repression, increase her satisfaction, and in general find better ways of satisfying her needs. As many positive reinforcing experiences and new avenues of expression as she can tolerate are recommended. Lastly, structured recreational activities will be more therapeutic and have greater value than unstructured activities in decreasing the level of depression.[59]

The psychosocial approach has been determined by the treatment team, which includes the therapeutic recreation specialist. If you were the specialist, what would you consider to be the goals, the activities to match those goals, and the behavioral objectives? You need to give a rationale for the goals developed and the activities used.

In developing the treatment plan, keep in mind that Joan Ann is in a twenty-five bed psychiatric unit, which includes a multipurpose room, a lounge room, and a self-contained kitchen area. Community resources are used when opportunities are presented. Supplies and equipment are limited to table games, arts and craft materials, pool table, ping-pong table, and a shuffleboard layout in one corridor. One therapeutic recreation specialist and an occupational therapist are employed.

IMPLEMENTATION

Regardless of the treatment plan developed, the specialist realizes that attempting to change Joan Ann's mood through logical suggestions during activity encounters early in the treatment process is fruitless and should be avoided. In fact, the specialist will avoid as much as possible any reinforcement of Joan Ann's distorted picture of herself as unworthy, inadequate, and inferior and of her pattern of failure, rejection, hostility, guilt, and self-punishment. In addition, the specialist will attempt to assist Joan Ann to direct her hostility outward. The process of self-punishment must be relieved before further injury to self.

As the specialist begins to interact with Joan Ann and others in the group activity, the attitude of acceptance and reassurance is reflected. The specialist does not reassure her by telling her that she need not worry or that she is going to be all right, especially when her convictions tell her differently, but she is reassured when the specialist treats her with concern, respect, knowledge, and a sense of responsibility.

Since Joan Ann has reflected suicidal tendencies, care must be exercised regarding her physical safety in those activities that require materials or tools that she could use to hurt herself. In such activities the use of equipment must be restricted. In many hospitals the file of a patient who is a suicidal risk is marked by a color code to indicate self-destructive tendencies. With Joan Ann the specialist will be alert to such tendencies, since patients usually provide cues to their feelings and to their intended behavior.

With these brief comments about interacting with Joan Ann during the implementation of her therapeutic recreation treatment plan, we might now ask you, the specialist/student, "How would you interact with Joan Ann or the group in implemented activities?"

EVALUATION

Any treatment plan, to be effective, must be aimed at meeting the needs of the patient for whom it is intended. Those needs include physical, emotional, and social needs, so the program must include physical, emotional, and social treatment. The plan is aimed at the whole person, Joan Ann in this case, not parts of her, and not Joan Ann in isolation, but Joan Ann as a member of a group. Successful and comprehensive treatment has as its goal helping patients return to optimum functioning in a community setting.

The effectiveness of the treatment plan is determined by the resolution of the problems on the problems list and disappearance of symptoms present on admission. Also valued are interaction with other patients, participation in treatment, ability to manage one's self, and the depth of relationships.

Subjective reports by Joan Ann are determinants of progress under treatment. The lifting of depression, disappearance of headaches, diminution of anxiety, and even generalization of "feeling better" are markers on the road to recovery. In addition to these reports, objective measures of the effectiveness of treatment may be employed with Joan Ann. The specialist may want to use any one of a number of tests to assess improvements that were mentioned in Chapter 5 or may depend upon those that may have been developed in the unit. As a specialist/student, what would you consider as markers to the improvement or effectiveness of treatment? Did the intervention accomplish the behavioral objectives? Does a review of the progress notes indicate improvement?

The discharge plan for Joan Ann was tailored to her needs, with emphasis on periodic counseling on an outpatient basis, group association, use of leisure time with others, and employment. Studies have shown that the last three factors play an important part in reducing rehospitalization rates.[60] Joan Ann was encouraged to learn to drive so that she would not be confined to the house. She was urged to explore volunteer assignments. Full-time employment was also discussed, which might help with financial problems. The problem with her mentally retarded son was discussed, and she was encouraged to accept her mixed feelings as being those that most parents would experience in similar circumstances.

COMMUNITY MENTAL HEALTH CENTERS (DAY TREATMENT)

As we noted in an earlier chapter, the community mental health center (CMHC) with its affiliated general hospital and state mental hospital is a primary-care facility in the public mental health service delivery system chiefly providing outpatient services for children, adolescents, adults, the elderly, and the alcoholic and drug dependent. CMHCs vary in size, in organizational structure, in facilities being used community-wide, and in the distribution of services throughout its catchment area. Services may run from initial contact or early therapeutic intervention, to inpatient, to providing a transitional facility for patients being discharged from inpatient services who require continuing therapy, to rehabilitating or maintaining long-term chronic patients on a drug maintenance program.[61]

Rehabilitation and aftercare include those activities (including recreation) and therapies geared toward enhancing a patient's capacities to integrate or reintegrate into a community. Such services are usually found within a day treatment facility. Day treatment patients spend most of the day at the facility in structured activities but return home in the evening. Most day treatment programs provide opportunity to enhance coping skills with everyday experiences. An important aspect of this service is that it is moving patients away from a hospital focus for their care and treatment. The total effort of day treatment is one of habilitation and rehabilitation: the process by which patients are progressed to their fullest physical, psychological, social, vocational, and economic capabilities.[62]

Therapeutic Recreation Service

Therapeutic recreation service in a CMHC day treatment program may incorporate all three therapeutic recreation services—therapy, education, and participation—or just one or two. The approach is dictated by such things as philosophy, funds, policies, personnel, resources, and facility size.

Most programs focus heavily on helping individuals fill their leisure time with newly learned activities that they can do with other individuals. Some of these activities are done at the day treatment center, especially for those patients too fearful or too ill to go out into the community, while others are purposely chosen to use the community's existing recreational facilities and programs to move those patients who can do so into the recreational mainstream. Such patients appreciate the exposure to activities in a structured leisure-counseling group program because this lessens their initial fears of finding out when the activity is being offered, finding the location, and actually going and participating with others.

In some communities a social club of former patients may be established, with a therapeutic recreation specialist assigned as director or staff member of the club in addition to having CHMC or day treatment responsibilities. In other communities the specialist's sole responsibility may be the club. Social clubs focus on here-and-now problems, develop social skills, and utilize the membership for mutual aid. In still other communities the specialist may be employed in a halfway house, which not only provides housing for former patients but a varied social and recreational program to enhance self-esteem and social skills and develop leisure habits.

THERAPEUTIC RECREATION PROCESS

We will consider here the case of a young woman living at home with her mother who is referred to a CMHC and eventually to a day treatment program associated with a CMHC.

Case History of Diane

For the past six months Diane, an eighteen-year-old single female, has had the recurrent idea that she should kill her mother. This thought has upset her so much that she has become increasingly anxious, tense, and preoccupied with washing her hands.

Patient is younger of two children, with a brother two years older who does not live at home. Father died several years ago of a heart attack. Mother is an aggressive, matronly woman who dominates Diane, making most of her decisions, choosing her clothes, and even talking for her.

Diane completed high school with average grades. She participated in few activities and had a few close girlfriends. When it came time to date, she usually went with a group rather than a particular boy. She states she never had a boyfriend. Mother has discouraged her in dating and has become even more possessive since father's death.

In the past few weeks Diane has gotten steadily worse so that her mother has had to stay home from work to care for her. Diane spends considerable time in the bathroom washing and wiping her hands. She has difficulty thinking, eating, and sleeping.

The family physician suggested to the mother that Diane be taken to the CMHC after a physical examination revealed no evidence of physical illness.

Diane's assessment at the CMHC would include not only an in-depth interview regarding her problem, but a detailed family social history, a psychosocial developmental history, a mental health status examination, and other significant contacts and tests deemed appropriate. In addition, her mother would be interviewed to determine her emotional and functioning level, since children and adolescents are affected by a variety of elements including level of family functioning. (A side point here is that children and adolescents from female-headed families are admitted to outpatient facilities at four times the rate of such individuals from two-parent families. The difference in admission rate is believed due to the higher family stresses associated with single parenthood.[63])

Not only is a thorough diagnostic evaluation necessary to formulate treatment goals and objectives for Diane and her mother, but an inaccurate assessment can lead to poor treatment and waste of time and money, which is usually in short supply in CMHCs. Also, more time is needed in working with children and adolescents than with adults, since staff members need time on a daily basis to review the patient's progress, to discuss any relevant changes in the family, to adjust individual treatment plans, and to coordinate, if need be, with other relevant community professionals. Likewise, time is needed to work with parents since they need special information, knowledge, and skills to care adequately for their emotionally disturbed child as well as time to better understand and resolve their own emotional problems.

The diagnostic evaluation team decides that Diane and her mother need initially to be involved in individual outpatient psychotherapy; thereafter, both are to be involved together in counseling sessions. It is further recommended that because of her limited social experiences Diane be referred to the day treatment program to expand psychosocial skills and develop new leisure outlets. The referral consists of scheduling Diane for day treatment three days per week and three hours per day.

The diagnostic categories associated with Diane as determined by the team might read as follows:

Axis I	300.30 obsessive compulsive disorder
Axis II	301.60 dependent personality disorder
Axis III	None
Axis IV	*Psychosocial stressors:* persistent parental discipline, limited and inadequate peer relationships, lack of self-confidence
	Severity: 3—4 severe (predominantly acute events)
Axis V	Current GAF: 32
	Highest GAF past year: 55[64]

In addition to the above factors, the following stressful factors or problems associated with Diane are noted by the team and included in the referral to the therapeutic recreation specialist in the day treatment program:

Anxiety   Lingering loss of a significant person
Fear   Parent working out of the home
Loneliness   Allowing others to assume responsibility

ASSESSMENT

The therapeutic recreation assessment of Diane will follow the general principles and procedures used in other settings. The specialist may be involved in the initial diagnostic evaluation or, following the referral, to the day treatment center. In our situation the interview takes place following the referral.

In the interview process the specialist will be aware that establishing rapport with Diane may be more difficult than with adults since adolescents may see the specialist as authoritarian, "square," or in collusion with the patient's parents. Then too, some adolescents like to test or challenge the specialist by acting out, or refusing to give answers to questions in the interview, or even verbally assaulting the specialist. As long as the specialist can remain objective and avoid personalizing verbal assaults, this experience can be a valuable one for the patient as he or she learns that anger and disagreements do not inevitably destroy relationships or people, and that people who have different beliefs and frames of references can genuinely care about each other. It should be remembered that for the disturbed adolescent rebelling against staff is immeasurably safer than rebelling against or disagreeing with parents. On the other hand, the specialist needs to respect the adolescent as a person with a problem and with rights and treat the person as such.

Naturally, the specialist will have knowledge about the problems associated with Diane's diagnosis as well as general knowledge about the physical, emotional, and social growth and development of any adolescent. Adolescence is the period of transition from the expectations and competencies of childhood to a whole new set of expectations and competencies of adulthood. The changes that occur in the physical, emotional, and social spheres of development, as the specialist knows, are simultaneous or in a series. They are interrelated and affect one another. Diane will emerge from this period as the kind of person she will be as an adult. Erikson describes the overwhelming stress in adjustment at this time: "In no other stage of the life cycle are the promise of finding oneself and the threat of losing oneself so closely allied."[65]

After the interview the specialist, in addition to confirming factors associated with the diagnosis and information provided in the referral, notes the following leisure interests of Diane:

Watching TV—soap operas
Listening to music
Looking at clothes in magazines
Attending school social functions with girlfriends
Driving around town with girlfriends
Talking on the telephone to girlfriends
Going to movies with girlfriends

While some of these activities appear to indicate that Diane is involved with her peer group, the specialist noted that the activities involving girlfriends were restricted primarily to high school years. Also, during the interview Diane commented that she had only a few dates while in high school and none since graduation. Throughout the whole interview Diane appeared anxious, hardly moved in her chair, and spoke very softly. She was doll-like in appearance, with long red hair and large green eyes. She appeared neat and gave the impression of being fragile enough to break easily.

PLANNING

Before considering and developing the therapeutic recreation treatment plan for Diane, consideration needs to be given briefly to the day treatment center in action.

Day Treatment Center in Action

Our hypothetical day treatment center operates from 9:30 A.M. to 5:30 P.M., Monday through Friday, but schedules are adjusted to the individual patient. The center is self-contained. A large lounge room is divided into a number of smaller areas: a place to sit, read, or talk; an activity area for social interaction; and a kitchen area. Card tables, games, a piano, a sewing machine, and a radio and television are in frequent use. Adjacent to the large activity lounge are a number of smaller rooms, which include the arts and crafts room, a music room for quiet listening and reading, a small library, offices for staff, various therapy rooms, and a nursing office. A bulletin board on one wall contains not only official notices but also a random collection of articles and cartoons about mental health. Behind the facility are a patio and space for outdoor activities. (The regional mental health board is giving thought to initiating a vocational counseling office in the center and adding a sheltered workshop in the vacant adjunct building.) The physical arrangement of the facility is geared to encouraging group interaction or socialization during periods when the individual or groups are not involved in treatment programs.

Although the atmosphere throughout the day is informal, staff members are attuned to the interaction between staff and patients for evidence of feelings and motivations and clues to problems and behavior. In this calculatedly open environment, with no one arbitrarily dictating behavior, the staff assumes—and makes clear in one way or another to children, adolescents, and adults—that they are expected to act like responsible human beings. Realistic standards are set in matters of general behavior, dress, feeding, and toileting.

An individualized, goal-oriented program is planned for each patient per referral from the CMHC. Some patients may initially be assigned to an individualized program while others are scheduled for a group activity. Much depends on the individual and/or group goals, behavior, age, and symptoms of the patient. Some individual and group activities meet once a week, while others meet as much as three, four, or even five times a week.

Diane's Treatment Plan

The treatment plan will focus on Diane's current problems. As a result of the therapeutic recreation specialist's interview and the referral from the diagnostic evaluation team, the following initial treatment plan was designed for Diane. (The plan is far from complete, but it does provide a general approach to some of the areas of concern.)

Need:	To improve functioning level
Goal:	To decrease anxiety
Activity:	Activity area
Behavioral Objective:	After two sessions Diane will reflect a decrease in anxiousness, as judged by the specialist.
Need:	To improve functioning level
Goal:	To improve self-identity
Activity:	Personal-charm class
Behavioral Objective:	After two sessions Diane will verbalize to the specialist and other staff an interest in changing her makeup, jewelry, dress, and hair style.
Need:	To become a more integrated person
Goal:	To increase socialization skills
Activity:	Activity area
Behavioral Objective:	After two sessions Diane will freely interact with male and female peers, as judged by the specialist.
Need:	To increase leisure experiences
Goal:	To develop awareness of varied leisure activities

Activity: Leisure counseling
Behavioral After two sessions Diane will iden-
Objective: tify twelve leisure activities of interest to her, as judged by the specialist.

The limited number of goals and associated activities is not unusual in light of the
potential daily changes in patient schedules.
This is Diane's first treatment plan, and it
will change as she becomes more involved
in her psychotherapy sessions and as psychotherapeutic drugs take effect. The concern from an overall program perspective is
to introduce Diane slowly into the day treatment program, while attempting to dispel
the anxiety that accompanies obsessive-
compulsive reactions and initiate socialization, improve self-concept, and develop new
leisure experiences.

A major concern initially will be with Diane's compulsive behavior of washing her
hands, which borders on the ritualistic. The
dynamics behind the decision to deal first
with the handwashing is that Diane needs
an orderly climate in which she can function
to her own satisfaction without being over-
whelmed by her repressed anxieties. A compulsion is an overpowering repetitive, unwanted act and is a way of alleviating,
controlling, or disguising the anxiety that
comes from underlying emotional conflict.
In Diane's case she is trying to make up for
her "bad" thoughts and actions directed
toward her mother. Handwashing is a very
typical symbolic behavior of obsessive-
compulsive disorders. As a result of the concern with Diane's handwashing, a strict time
limit is put on her bathroom use.

IMPLEMENTATION

During the following weeks Diane continues to improve; she becomes less tense,
more able to concentrate and care for herself. In psychotherapy she begins to recognize and talk about some of her feelings
toward her mother. She also becomes increasingly aware of the fact that she has
other problems besides her feelings about

her mother, and she begins to explore her
inner conflicts regarding her identity. Her
mother, in psychotherapy, begins to see her
part in her daughter's illness.

In day treatment, Diane's treatment plan
is frequently revised and updated. She participates in the assertiveness training session
conducted by the specialist, learns to feel
comfortable voicing her opinions even
though other patients disagree, and learns to
recognize when she is beginning to feel anxious, while at the same time learning constructive ways to keep from becoming depressed and isolated through involving
herself in activities and social situations in
which she feels confident. She also begins
to interact more frequently with male peers
as her personal appearance changes, and
prior to her discharge is spending considerable time with another male adolescent patient who is shy and retiring.

Her leisure awareness has expanded and
her use of community recreation resources
increased as a result of participation in leisure counseling. Diane has been encouraged to invite friends or fellow day treatment attendees to go with her to various
leisure resources and to use the staff as informational resources. As many positive reinforcing experiences and new avenues of
expression as Diane can tolerate are helpful
in her situation.

EVALUATION

The final phase of the therapeutic recreation process, as we have frequently noted, is
the evaluation of care and treatment. It
bears repeating that evaluation is the process of determining the degree of success in
achieving a predetermined objective. It also
serves as a guide to improvement of the procedure to reach the objective or goal. Evaluation of a patient's treatment plan begins
with the formulation of an objective that is
practical, followed by the development of
criteria to be applied in measuring achievement and in answering the question, "Was
the objective reached?"

In Diane's situation it would appear that the objectives were reached, even though the objectives continued to change on a somewhat continuous basis. Such revisions in a treatment plan are not that unusual in day treatment centers. However, in working with chronic patients, revision of treatment plans is less frequent.

Diane was discharged after six weeks. Although there were some problems about her bathroom activities, she did not have a recurrence of her upsetting thoughts. Medication was discontinued, and it was recommended that both she and her mother continue psychotherapy on an outpatient basis.

SUMMARY

Mental health care has come a long way in the past seventy-five years. Public psychiatric hospitals and private care have been supplemented by outpatient clinics, psychiatric units in general hospitals, day-care programs, halfway houses, and a federally mandated network of community mental health centers. A short stay in a state mental hospital or in a general hosptial's psychiatric unit may begin treatment to be continued in an aftercare clinic or day treatment center. Moreover, many effective new treatment procedures have been discovered. Likewise, many new professionals, including therapeutic recreation specialists, have become members of the mental health delivery service team. In fact, according to one source several years ago, more therapeutic recreation specialists worked in mental health settings than in any other setting.[66] Despite the progress that has been made, much still needs to be done. Adequate insurance coverage of mental disorders, legal rights of patients, legal duties of care-giving institutions, and third-party payment for therapeutic recreation service remains unresolved issues. It is hoped that these problems will resolve themselves in the closing decade of the twentieth century.

NOTES

1. J. Sanbourne Bockoven, *Moral Treatment in American Psychiatry* (New York: Springer Publishing Co. 1963), pp. 23–25; Albert S. Norris, Anthony E. Rayes, and Robert L. Kelley, "Mental Hospitals," in *Handbook of Psychiatry*, 2nd ed., ed. Philip Solomon and Vernon D. Patch (Los Altos, Calif.: Lange Medical Publication, 1971), pp. 143–51; and Bernard L. Bloom, *Community Mental Health* (Belmont, Calif.: Brooks/Cole Publishing Co., 1977), pp. 8–10.

2. Martin J. Witken, *Provisional Patient Movement and Selective Administrative Data, State and County Mental Hospitals, Inpatient Services by State: United States 1976*, statistical note 156 (Washington, D.C.: U.S. Government Printing Office, 1979).

3. Cited in Bloom, *Community Mental Health*, p. 10.

4. E. M. Gruenberg, "Mental Disorders," in *Maxey-Rosenau Public Health and Preventive Medicine*, 11th ed., ed. J. M. Last (New York: Appleton-Century-Crofts, 1980).

5. Jack Meislen, "Rehabilitation Medicine in Contemporary Psychiatry," in *Rehabilitation Medicine and Psychiatry*, ed. Jack Meislen (Springfield, Ill.: Charles C Thomas, Publishers, 1976), pp. 22–28; and Frederick H. Meyers and Philip Solomon, "Drug Therapy," in *Handbook in Psychiatry*, 2nd ed., ed. Philip Solomon and Vernon D. Patch (Los Altos, Calif.: Lange Medical Publication, 1971), pp. 354–89.

6. Norris, Royes, and Kelley, "Mental Hospitals," pp. 143–51.

7. E. T. Carlson and Norman Dain, "The Psychotherapy That Was Not Moral Treatment," *American Journal of Psychiatry* 117, no. 52 (1960), 519–24.

8. Maxwell Jones, *Social Psychiatry: The Idea of a Therapeutic Community* (New York: Penguin Books, 1968).

9. J. J. Rossi and William J. Filstead, eds., *The Therapeutic Community* (New York: Behavioral Publications, 1973).

10. Jerry S. Visher and Martha O'Sullivan, "Nurses and Patient Responses to a Study of Milieu Therapy," *American Journal of Psychiatry*, 127, no. 34 (1970), 451–56.

11. M. I. Herz, H. Wilensky, and A. Earle, "Problems of Role Definition in the Therapeutic Community," *Archives of General Psychiatry* 4, no. 11 (1966), 270–76.

12. J. Cumming and E. Cumming, *Ego and Milieu* (New York: Atherton Press, 1962).

13. Joint Commission on Mental Illness and Health, *Action for Mental Health* (New York: Science Editions, 1961).

14. U.S. Congress, *P.L. 96-398—Mental Health Systems Act* (Washington, D.C.: U.S. Government Printing Office, 1980).

15. Cited in Bloom, *Community Mental Health*, p. 51.

16. S. A. Kirk and M. E. Therrin, "Community Mental Health Myths and the Fate of Former Hospitalized Patients," *Psychiatry* 38, no. 12 (1975), 209–17; and H. H. Robbins, "Social Implications of Deinstitutionalization," *Journal of Community Psychology* 10, no. 9 (1982), 82–83.

17. Walter E. Barton and Gail M. Barton, *Mental Health Administration*, vol. 2 (New York: Human Sciences Press, 1983), p. 603.

18. Leonard I. Stein and Mary Ann Test, "From the Hospital to the Community: A Shift in the Primary Locus of Care," in *Alternatives to Acute Hospitalization*, vol. 1, ed. H. Richard Lamb (San Francisco: Jossey-Bass, Publishers, 1979), pp. 15–32.

19. Charles G. Smith and James A. King, *Mental Hospitals*. (Lexington, Mass.: Lexington Books, 1975), pp. 162–189.

20. Richard A. Weatherley, "Mental Health Policy and Patients' Rights," in *Handbook on Mental Health Administration*, pp. 66–86.

21. Barton and Barton, *Mental Health Administration*, vol. 2, p. 538.

22. Lorrin M. Koran, "Mental Health Services," in *Health Care Delivery in the United States*, 2nd ed., ed. Steven Jonas (New York: Springer Publishing Co., 1981), pp. 262–64; and L. H. Roth, "A Commitment Law for Patients, Doctors, and Lawyers," *American Journal of Psychiatry* 136, no. 11 (1979), 1121–27.

23. Weatherley, "Mental Health Policy and Patients' Rights," pp. 68–76.

24. N. I. Brill, *Team Work: Working Together in Human Services* (Philadelphia: W. B. Saunders, 1976), p. 312.

25. Kermit B. Nash, "Managing Interdisciplinary Teams," in *Handbook on Mental Health Administration* pp. 166–67.

26. Brill, *Team Work*.

27. American Psychiatric Association, *What Is a Psychiatrist?* Task Force Report (Washington, D.C.: the association, 1975).

28. *Profile* (Washington, D.C.: National Association of Social Workers, n.d.).

29. Richard R. Bootzin and Joan Ross Acocella, *Abnormal Psychology*, 4th ed. (New York: Random House, 1984), pp. 641–42.

30. Holly Skodol Wilson and Carol Ren Kneisl, *Psychiatric Nursing*, 2nd ed. (Menlo Park, Calif.: Addison-Wesley Publishing Co., 1983), pp. 16–39.

31. O. G. Simmons and H. E. Freeman, *The Mental Patient Comes Home* (New York: John Wiley & Co., 1965).

32. Joint Commission on Accreditation of Hospitals, *Principles of Accreditation of Community Mental Health Service Programs* (Chicago: the commission, Accreditation Council for Psychiatric Facilities, 1979), p. 78.

33. Koran, "Mental Health Services," p. 242; and Barton and Barton, *Mental Health Administration*, vol. 1, p. 359.

34. Barton and Barton, *Mental Health Administration*, vol. 1, p. 360.

35. Koran, "Mental Health Services," p. 248; and National Institute of Mental Health, *Provisional Data on Patient Care Episodes in Mental Health Facilities—1975*, statistical note 139 (Washington, D.C.: U.S. Government Printing Office, 1977).

36. Michael J. Austin and William E. Hershey, "Issues in Management Practice," *Handbook on Mental Health Administration*, ed. Michael J. Austin and William E. Hershey (San Francisco: Jossey-Bass, Publishers, 1982), pp. 2–3.

37. Bootzin and Acocella, *Abnormal Psychology*, pp. 641–42.

38. Barton and Barton, *Mental Health Administration*, vol. 1, p. 365.

39. Ibid., pp. 366–71.

40. Ibid., pp. 366–68.

41. Ibid., pp. 62–75.

42. National Therapeutic Recreation Society, "Philosophical Position Statement of the National Therapeutic Recreation Society." Adopted May 1982.

43. Book published by the National Therapeutic Recreation Society (Alexandria, Va.: 1980).

44. David F. L. Dawson, Heather M. Blum, and Giampiero Bartolucci, *Schizophrenia in Focus* (New York: Human Sciences Press, 1983), pp. 13–48; and Bootzin and Acocella, *Abnormal Psychology*, p. 381.

45. Dawson, Blum, and Bartolucci, *Schizophrenia in Focus*, pp. 51–63.

46. Ibid., p. 72.

47. Bootzin and Acocella, *Abnormal Psychology*, p. 363.

48. Charles J. Wallace, et. al., "A Review and Critique of Social Skills Training with Schizophrenic Patients," *Schizophrenia Bulletin* 6, no. 2 (1980), 64–69.

49. American Psychiatric Association, *Diagnostic and Statistical Manual of Mental Disorder*, 3rd ed. (Washington, D.C.: the association, 1980), pp. 17, 28–31, 192.

50. S. M. Small, *Outline for Psychiatric Evaluation* (Parsippany, N.J.: Sandoz Pharmaceuticals, 1980).

51. American Psychiatric Association, *DSM-III-R*, pp. 181–93.

52. Ibid.

53. M. E. Pattison and M. L. Pattison, "Analysis of a Schizophrenic Psychosocial Network," *Schizophrenia Bulletin* 7, no. 6 (1981), 135–44.

54. Elliott M. Avedon, *Therapeutic Recreation Service: An Applied Behavioral Science Approach* (Englewood Cliffs, N.J.: Prentice-Hall, 1974), pp. 612–72; and Anne Cronin Mosey, *Activities Therapy* (New York: Raven Press Publishers, 1973), pp. 8–9, 120–35.

55. Barton and Barton, *Mental Health Administration*, vol. 1, p. 371.

56. Ibid., p. 372.

57. Ibid.

58. American Psychiatric Association, *DSM-III-R*, pp. 18–19, 220–22, and 329–30.

59. Katharine B. Wassman and Seppo E. Iso-Ahola, "The Relationship between Recreation Participation and Depression in Psychiatric Patients," *Therapeutic Recreation Journal* 19, no. 3 (1985), 63–70.

60. Leonard J. Stein, Mary Ann Test, and Mary J. Jarz, "Alternative to the Hospital: A Control Study," *American Journal of Psychiatry* 132, no. 7 (1975), 517–22.

61. Jonas, *Health Care Delivery*, p. 251.

62. Barton and Barton, *Mental Health Administration*, vol. II, p. 602.

63. Peter J. Pecora and Maureen A. Conroyd, "Child and Adolescent Mental Health Services," in *Handbook on Mental Health Administration*, pp. 558–59.

64. American Psychiatric Association, *DSM-III-R*, pp. 18–19, 234–35, and 324–25.

65. Erik Erikson, *Identity: Youth and Crisis* (New York: Norton Publishing Co., 1968), p. 244.

66. Gerald S. Fain, Lynn Champion, and Daniel G. Scully, "Employment Status Study of Therapeutic Recreation Personnel" (unpublished study, Boston University, Department of Movement, Health, and Leisure, n.d.).

SUGGESTED READINGS

AMERICAN PSYCHIATRIC ASSOCIATION. *The Diagnostic and Statistical Manual of Mental Disorders* (DSM-III-R). Washington, D.C.: A.P.A. 1987.

ANDERSON, STEPHEN C., DEBRA B. WOLF, and VICTOR C. PAPPAS. "On Becoming Interdisciplinary: Implications for Therapeutic Recreation." In *Expanding Horizons in Therapeutic Recreation XII*, Gerald Hitzhusen, ed. Columbia, Mo.: Department of Recreation and Park Administration, University of Missouri, (1984), 104–117.

BARTON, WALTER E., and CARL J. SANBORN, eds. *An Assessment of the Community Mental Health Movement*. Lexington, Mass.: Lexington Books, 1977.

BEAN, PHILIP. *Mental Illness: Changes and Trends*. New York: John Wiley & Sons, 1983.

CARTER, MARCIA., GLEN E. VAN ANDEL, and GARY M. ROBB. *Therapeutic Recreation: A Practical Approach*. St. Louis: Times Mirror/Mosby College Publishing, 1985, pp. 197–242.

DUNN, JULIA KENNOW. "Leisure Education: Meeting the Challenge of Increasing Independence of Residents in Psychiatric Facilities." *Therapeutic Recreation Journal* 15, no. 4 (1981), 17–23.

GREENFIELD, DAVID. *The Psychotic Patient: Medication and Psychotherapy*. New York: Free Press, 1985.

HERZ, M. I. "Short Term Hospitalization and the Medical Model." *Hospital and Community Psychiatry* 30 (1979), 117–21.

KRAUS, RICHARD. *Therapeutic Recreation Service: Principles and Practices* (3rd ed.). Philadelphia: Sanders College Publishing, 1983, pp. 181–227.

LAMB, H. RICHARD, and VICTOR GOERTZEL. *Social Rehabilitation in Rehabilitation in Community Mental Health*. San Francisco: Jossey-Bass, Publishers 1971.

MASSERMAN, J., ed. *Current Psychiatric Therapies*. New York: Grune & Stratton, 1975.

MECHANIC, DAVID. *Mental Health and Social Policy*. Englewood Cliffs, N.J.: Prentice-Hall, 1980.

MEYER, ROBERT G., and YVONNE H. OSBORNE. *Case Studies in Abnormal Psychology*. Newton, Mass.: Allyn & Bacon, 1981.

MOSEY, ANNE CRONIC. *Activities Therapy*. New York: Raven Press, Publishers, 1973.

PAKES, DEBORAH L., and GARY E. PAKES. "Anti-Psychotic Drug Side Effects and Therapeutic Recreation Program Considerations." *Therapeutic Recreation Journal* 16, no. 1 (1982), 12–19.

PETERSON, CAROL ANN, and SCOUT LEE GUNN. *Therapeutic Recreation Program Design: Principles and Procedures* (2nd ed.). Englewood Cliffs, N. J.: Prentice-Hall, 1984.

SHIVERS, JAY S., and HOLLIS F. FAIT. *Special Recreational Services: Therapeutic and Adapted*. Philadelphia: Lea & Febiger, 1985, pp. 172–91.

TALBOTT, JOHN, ed. *The Chronic Mentally Ill: Treatment, Program Systems*. Port Washington, N.Y.: Human Science Press, 1981.

VALE, WALLACE H., and SYLVESTER R. MLOTT. "An Assessment of Treatment Enjoyment and Effectiveness in Psychiatric Hospitalization." *Therapeutic Recreation Journal* 17, no. 1 (1983), 26–32.

10

Education and Training Model

The education and training model of service is used extensively in the field of therapeutic recreation. In fact, as noted in Chapter 6, it transcends all settings, residential and nonresidential. The model is employed in special schools and training centers for mentally retarded persons, in settings that provide health services to those with sensory and neurological impairments, and in correctional facilities for juvenile and adult offenders. It is also applied in sheltered workshop facilities and can be utilized on a temporary or permanent basis with homebound individuals.

The model focuses on three major areas of human service:

1. Formal or informal academic educational programs
2. Prevocational and/or vocational preparation and work adjustment
3. Leisure skill/socialization development

There is a strong belief among human service personnel that this comprehensive approach is most valuable in the rehabilitation process. Heynes makes this point strongly when considering the application of this model in correctional settings:

It is obvious, however, that if we are to aid the inmate in preparing for satisfactory social living, we must be concerned with all aspects of normal living: the ethical and moral, the economic and industrial, mental and physical health, satisfactory relationships . . . and the wise use of leisure.[1]

Likewise, Capobianco reflects upon the merits of a holistic education and training paradigm when serving mentally retarded persons:

Vocational habilation must provide comprehensive service to people with handicapping conditions. A total person approach is suggested. Merely instructing a person to perform a specific job, and neglecting his or her social needs is counterproductive. Treating the person as only a worker, and not taking into account his/her recreational needs is also dysfunctional. Professionals must serve the total individual, not segments of the person. Handicapped people have the right to adequate treatment—they also have the right to enjoy themselves through appropriate leisure outlets. If we as professionals do not include instructions on how to use unobligated time constructively, we are wasting our efforts toward the development of an independent person.[2]

Smith and Reynolds have also extolled the virtues of combining educational, vocational, and leisure services within an outpatient psychological-counseling clinic. The desirable features of this approach may be summarized as follows:

1. *Comprehensiveness:* The major areas of service complement each other and result in improved patterns of behavior in *each* of the spheres.
2. *Availability of Support:* All members of the staff are free to work with the client on social skills required for leisure participation.
3. *Interchange and Pooling of Knowledge:* Psychological-counseling staff assisted therapeutic recreation specialists in refining their counseling techniques. Similarly, therapeutic recreation personnel assisted clinical staff in locating community resources.

4. *Potential for Follow-Up:* Because clients received other services after visits to the clinic ceased, it was possible to track their progress in meeting various educational, vocational, and recreational goals.[3]

The actual services provided by the therapeutic recreation specialist in this model are influenced strongly by the setting in which the model is found. Specifically, these services will be affected by the other disciplines present, the philosophy of the agency, and various administrative considerations. However, as the previously cited literature indicates, emphasis will be placed upon the use of recreative experiences to improve patients' self-concept, social and activity skills (which can be used in leisure pursuits following completion of the program), and leisure education to examine their values, attitudes and patterns of leisure participation.

IMPLEMENTATION OF THE MODEL

This chapter illustrates the application of this model by providing current examples of instruments, processes, and programmatic techniques that are used by therapeutic recreation specialists in the four phases of assessment, planning, implementation, and evaluation. Case-study examples will again be employed to highlight the application of the model. Additionally, several contemporary examples of this approach will be described in the final section of the chapter.

ASSESSMENT

Because the education and training model focuses on three broad areas of human service (education, vocation, and leisure) and is employed in a wide range of settings, the application of this approach requires a comprehensive client assessment process. It would be impossible to provide here all available instruments and techniques that

could be used to obtain such information. Table 10.1, however, details the major types of data that might be gathered in implementing a multidisciplinary program of education and training. It also specifies when and how this information would be obtained and the individuals who would be responsible for its acquisition.

The therapeutic recreation specialist working within the education and training model has a variety of standardized assessment instruments available to establish a baseline measurement of the client's ability level at the onset of instruction. These tools determine both the functional level (how well the client performs in activity settings) and the client's leisure-skill repertoire (how many leisure interests the client has). The instruments vary greatly in the specificity of the behaviors they evaluate. Also, some measure only specific skills, while others provide an index of overall leisure function-

TABLE 10.1. Categorical Elements for Multidimensional Assessment

Client Attributes	Assessment Techniques	Evaluator	Setting	Data Collected
Socialization	Written tests Performance tests	Therapeutic recreation specialists	Formally (in agency)	Preprogram
Self-concept	Questionnaires Medical records	Occupational therapists	Home	At beginning of program
Mental status	Recommendations and referrals	Rehabilitation counselors	School	At regular intervals during program
Daily living skills	Observations	Social workers	Job site	Randomly throughout program
Vocational skills	Role playing	Doctors		Postprogram (follow-up)
Physical abilities	Inductive comments	Teachers		
	Diary/records	Parents		
Activity skills	Nonverbal demonstrations	Referring agents Clients (self-reports)		
Feelings, attitudes, and understandings concerning leisure	Leisure Valuing exercises	Volunteers		

SOURCE: Adapted from Lynn D. Saslow, "Multidimensional Approach to Camper Assessment," *Therapeutic Recreation Journal* 12, no. 4(1978), p. 32.

ing. Some tools are designed for group administration; others rely on input from those who are in daily contact with the client, namely, parents and staff. Table 10.2 lists some of the more popular instruments that may be used in the education and training model and their respective target populations.

CASE STUDIES

At this point it is useful to present two individual case studies to illustrate the process of this model. It should be noted that these case studies are designed to provide the reader with a feel for the application of the education and training model. They are not intended to illustrate the full range of services that would be provided to individuals over an extended period of time.

Client One: Tom R.

Tom R., a juvenile offender, enters a learning center operated by the Youth Services Division of the State Department of Corrections. For the first three weeks following his admission Tom receives the services of a reception and diagnostic center. At this facility he is examined by a physician, who takes a complete medical history, determines his current state of health, notes special conditions such as heart murmurs, and records any medication that could affect Tom's performance by producing side effects. A psychologist also administers a series of diagnostic tests that provide insights into Tom's verbal and mathematical aptitude, self-concept, and other psychological attributes. Specific tests designed to assess academic performance, such as reading comprehension, are then administered by an educational specialist. At this point, if indicated, separate testing may be performed to detect possible learning disabilities and suggest remedial learning activities. The client may also spend consider-

TABLE 10.2. Sample Leisure Assessment Tools

Leisure Assessment Instruments	Target Population	Leisure Assessment Instruments	Target Population
1. Avocational Activities Inventory (Overs 1974)	EMR	13. Leisure Skills Curriculum Assessment Inventory (LSCDD) (Wehman and Schleien 1979)	Developmentally Disabled
2. Bogan's Group Assessment (Bogan 1974)	All	14. Minimum Objective System (MOS) (Williams & Fox 1977)	Severely Handicapped
3. Comprehension Evaluation in Recreational Therapy Scale (CERT) (Parker 1975)	Short-term Psychiatric	15. Mirenda Leisure Interest Finder (Wilson 1975)	Normal Intelligence
4. Constructive Leisure Activity Survey (CLAS) (Edwards 1975)	Normal	16. Recreation Therapy Assessment (Cousins, Brown 1977)	Nonambulatory Adult
5. I Can (Wessel 1976)	TMR-Children	17. Self-Leisure Interest Profile (SLIP) (Hubert 1969)	Normal Intelligence
6. Davis' Recreational Directors' Observational Report (Davis 1957)	Psychiatric	18. Sonoma County Organization for the Retarded Assessment System (SCOR) (Westaway, Apolloni 1977)	Developmentally Disabled
7. Iowa Leisure Education Program Assessment form (Maddy 1977)	Hospitalized	19. State of Ohio Curriculum Guide for Moderately Mentally Retarded Learners (1977)	TMR
8. Joswiak's Leisure Counseling Assessment Instruments (Joswiak 1975)	Developmentally Disabled	20. Toward Competency: A Guide for Individualized Instruction (Oregon Dept. of Ed. 1974)	All special populations
9. Knox, Hurff & Takata Deaf-Blind Assessment (Takata 1974)	Deaf-Blind Birth–Adolescence	21. Vineland Social Maturity Scale (Doll 1965)	All
10. Leisure Activities Blank (LAB) (McKechnie 1975)	Normal		
11. Leisure Interest Inventory (LII)	Normal		
12. Linear Model for Individual Treatment in Recreation (LMIT) (Compton 1975)	Developmentally Disabled		

SOURCE: P. Wehman and S. Schleien, "Relevant Assessment in Leisure Skill Training Programs," *Therapeutic Recreation Journal* 14, no. 4(1980), 14–15.

able time with other professionals, including speech therapists, audio pathologists, and optometrists. Several evaluations are then performed by an occupational therapist. These include a variety of perceptual-motor tasks designed to detect any deficits Tom might have in his overall motor performance.

As an integral part of these admissions procedures, a therapeutic recreation specialist reviews Tom's classification records for the purpose of determining past and current leisure pursuits and interests. Specifically, educational reports are reviewed, with particular attention paid to performance in physical education classes, team sports, and intramural activities and comments from teachers, athletic staff, and others. Tom and members of his family are interviewed concerning his current recreation interests and future goals, peer activities, family recreational patterns and interests, affiliation with clubs, church groups, and other organizations, as well as transportation and financial resources available for recreation. Additionally, Tom is asked to complete a simple leisure-interest finder, which determines past and current involvement in such areas as active games and sports, social activities, musical pursuits, arts and crafts, drama, dancing, nature and outings, and hobbies. Other staff members, such as cottage personnel, are also asked to provide information concerning Tom's expressed attitudes toward recreational participation, ability to use free time constructively, motivational level in respect to leisure, ability to conform to rules, and impulse control during competition.

Client Two: Ms. T.

Ms. T. is a thirty-year-old mentally retarded woman who has been discharged from a large residential facility and placed in a community-based group home for adults. She currently attends a sheltered workshop where she receives vocational training. Prior to her placement in the group home, a social worker from the residential facility met with staff members of the home and reviewed Ms. T.'s records. In addition to basic demographic and family-related information, her relevant educational and daily living (self-help) skills were reviewed. Data concerning vocational interests, skills, and training were forwarded to rehabilitation counselors affiliated with the vocational training center. Similarly, information concerning her recreational skills and interests was provided to the therapeutic recreation specialist employed by the group home. After a two-week period in which Ms. T. was welcomed to the facility and introduced to the recreational resources available in the home and nearby community, the therapeutic recreation specialist administered a questionnaire designed to assess both her knowledge of the concept of leisure and her ability to identify recreational resources. Ms. T.'s responses to this

interview/questionnaire are shown in Figure 10.1.

PLANNING

As previously stated, the development of goals for individual clients within the education and training model is an interdisciplinary process involving the client and those responsible for educational, vocational, and leisure/social skill development. This procedure ensures that each discipline may use its respective medium to work toward the same ultimate end. The planning process within the education and training model as related to our two clients is illustrated below.

Client One: Tom R.

At the learning center an interdisciplinary meeting takes place involving the cottage staff, academic instructors, therapeutic recreation specialists, and occupational therapy personnel who will have daily contact with Tom. At this point a team coordinator is designated to overview the specific plan that will be developed. After a review of the medical, psychological, and educational evaluations that have been performed, and after Tom's family history and scores on motor skill and fitness tests and recreational assessments have been noted, several trends emerge. Tom appears to be of average intelligence, an underachiever in school, deficient in motor skills, and below national fitness norms. Furthermore, his family, teachers, and cottage staff categorize him as a "loner." Tom expresses little knowledge or interest in recreational activities other than television, video games, and antisocial pursuits. Using this information, the team determines that Tom would benefit from participation in new activities, particularly those available in his immediate neighborhood. The center's leisure-education class appears to be an ideal vehicle to work toward this general goal. As in the previously described models of therapeutic recreation service, it is now necessary for the specialist to develop terminal expectations.

Tom's objectives are as follows:

Goal: To increase involvement in leisure pursuits available in Tom's immediate neighborhood

FIGURE 10.1.   Objective Assessment Sheet

Name: Ms. T.

X = attained
O = failed to attain

1. Awareness of the meaning of play and leisure.
　　　　　　　 1A: Awareness of the concept of play. (Identifies five out of six "play" photographs and five out of six "work" photographs.)
　　　 ___ Number of "play" photographs correctly identified.
　　　 ___ Number of "work" photographs correctly identified.
　　 X 　　 1B: Knowledge of the concept of free time. (Identifies one of the following points.)
　　　 X 　a. " . . . free from doing things that we have to do."
　　　 ___ b. " . . . free to do whatever we want as long as it doesn't break the law or hurt anybody."
　　　 X 　c. " . . . time when we have fun."
　　 X 　　 1C: Knowledge of when personal free time occurs. (Identifies 85 percent of the following appropriate blocks of time.)
　　　　　　 During the week:
　　　 X 　In the mornings.
　　　 X 　In the afternoons.
　　　 X 　After work/school.
　　　 X 　After supper.
　　　　　　 Saturday:
　　　 X 　Morning after waking up.
　　　 X 　Afternoon.
　　　 X 　Evening after supper.
　　　　　　 Sunday:
　　　 X 　Morning after waking up.
　　　 X 　Afternoon.
　　　 X 　Evening after supper.
　　 O 　　 1D: Knowledge of the beneficial effects of play. (Identifies two of the following points.)
　　　 O 　a. " . . . a chance for exercise or physical activity."
　　　 O 　b. " . . . a chance to be with and talk to people."
　　　 O 　c. " . . . a chance for learning."
　　　 O 　d. " . . . lets us have fun," or " . . . it makes us feel good."
　　 O 　　 1E: Knowledge of the potential relationship of leisure activities and mood alteration. (Identifies all of the following points.)
　　　 O 　a. Identifies a period of time (if appropriate).
　　　 O 　b. Describes the mood.
　　　 O 　c. Selects an appropriate activity.
　　　 O 　d. Presents an appropriate rationale.
　　 O 　　 1F: Ability to select and engage in a leisure activity for the purpose of mood alteration. (Describes and discusses the activity and the mood.) Record below the activity and the mood.
2. Awareness of leisure resources in the home.
　　 X 　　 2A: Knowledge of personal leisure resources. (Identifies and describes a minimum of three personal leisure resources.)
　　　 X 　Provide the number of resources identified.
　　　　　　 Record below those resources identified.
　　　　　　　 Client's paint set.
　　　　　　　 Client's cassette recorder.
　　　　　　　 Client's domino game.

_____ 2B: Ability to use one's personal leisure resources. (Utilizes two different resources in two different activities.)

___ Provide the number of resources identified.

Record below those resources identified.

Uses cassette tapes in dance activities.

Engages in domino games with other residents.

___X___ 2C: Knowledge of leisure resources owned by the facility. (Identifies and describes four resources.)

X__ Provide the number of resources identified.

Record below those resources identified.

Billiard table.

Stereo.

Pets.

Kitchen.

___X___ 2D: Ability to use leisure resources owned by the facility. (Utilizes one resource in a leisure activity.)

Grooms pets.

Bakes cookies.

___O___ 2E: Knowledge of appropriate procedure for borrowing leisure resources. (Identifies all of the following points.)

O__ a. " . . . ask the owner for permission."

O__ b. " . . . use the way it is supposed to be used."

O__ c. " . . . tell the owner if it is broken or lost," or " . . . offering to pay for it."

O__ d. " . . . returning it when done with it."

___O___ 2F: Knowledge of leisure resources owned by peers willing to share. (Identifies three resources and their owners.)

O__ Provide the number of resources identified.

Record below those resources (and the owners) identified.

___O___ 2G: Ability to borrow resources from peers. (Engages in two different activities using two different resources borrowed from peers, in the manner described below.)

O__ a. Request for permission.

O__ b. Use in accordance with rules, norms, etc.

O__ c. Notification of the owner if broken or lost, or offer to pay for it.

O__ d. Return of the resources when done.

Record those resources (and their owners) utilized.

3. Awareness of leisure resources in the community.

___O___ 3A: Knowledge of leisure resources within walking distance. (Identifies and describes four resources.)

O__ Provide the number of resources identified.

Record below those resources identified.

___O___ 3B: Ability to use a leisure resource within walking distance. (Utilizes one resource.)

Record below the resource(s) utilized.

___O___ 3C: Knowledge of leisure resources accessible primarily by car or bus. (Identifies four resources.)

O__ Provide the number of resources identified.

Record below those resources identified.

___O___ 3D: Ability to use a leisure resource accessible primarily by car or bus. (Utilizes one resource.)

Record the resource(s) utilized, below.

(continued)

FIGURE 10.1. Objective Assessment Sheet (*Continued*)

___X___ 3E: Knowledge of information sources. (Identifies four of the following sources.)
    X a. Radio.
    X b. Television.
    X c. Asking friends or staff at work/school.
    ___ d. Observing different places when traveling around town.
    X e. Using the telephone to call appropriate places.
    ___ f. Entertainment, advertisement, and "What's Happening around Town?" sections of the newspaper.
    ___ g. Billboards and posters around town.
    ___ h. Magazines and publications dealing with "things to do" in town.
    ___ i. Yellow Pages.
    ___ j. City or state map.
    ___ k. (If unable to read) Requesting literate acquaintances to refer to appropriate sources, e.g., Yellow Pages.
    ___ l. Any other appropriate source identified by the client.

___X___ 3F: Ability to utilize an information source. (Identifies and describes the appropriate process for utilizing one of the information sources listed in EO 5.)
    Record below the process identified.
        Switches television to public broadcast channel.

Comments:

SOURCE: Adapted from K. F. Joswiak, *Leisure Counseling Program Materials for the Developmentally Disabled* (Washington, D.C.: Hawkins and Associates, 1978), pp. 127–31.

Activity:	Biweekly cottage leisure-education session
Behavioral Objectives:	Upon being asked, "What are the things you can walk to from home that will help you to have fun?" Tom will identify a minimum of four leisure resources within walking distance of his home.

Upon being asked, "What are the things you can get to by car or bus that will help you to have fun?" Tom will identify a minimum of four leisure resources that are accessible primarily by car or bus.

Upon being asked, "What are the ways that we can find out about places to go for fun or things happening in town?" Tom will identify a minimum of four of the following information sources:

Radio
Television
Asking friends
Observing places when traveling around town
Entertainment sections of the newspaper
Billboards and posters
Magazines and publications
Yellow pages
City map[4]

Client Two: Ms. T.

In reviewing Ms. T.'s records from her former residence, the group home staff and therapeutic recreation specialist note that she avoids activities requiring cooperative interaction with staff and other residents. This observation is confirmed by rehabilitation specialists at the sheltered workshop and by responses on items 2E, 2F, and 2G on the objective assessment sheet. Also, her self-help skills are found to be deficient, particularly in the areas of grooming and food preparation. Finally, the interview based on the *objective assessment tool* reveals a lack of understanding of the concept of leisure and its role in her life and an inability to identify leisure resources beyond her immediate environment.

From this assessment, the team feels that Ms. T. could benefit from activities of a group nature that would also assist her in activities of daily living. A cooking class at the group home has the potential to meet both these overall goals.

Ms. T.'s specific objectives are as follows:

Goals: To increase cooperative responding in structured group activities
To improve food-preparation skills

Activity: Cooking class

Behavioral Objectives: In a group discussion concerning the flavor and type of cake to be made, Ms. T. will express an opinion, yet willingly abide by the group concensus expressed in a majority vote.
After a demonstration by the therapeutic recreation specialist, Ms. T. will correctly measure the following amounts of ingredients:
    2 cups flour
    1 cup milk
    1/2 teaspoon salt
    1/2 cup shortening
After receiving verbal instructions from the therapist, Ms. T. will share responsibility for mixing the cake's ingredients with one other client. They will each take at least one turn at mixing during the session.

IMPLEMENTATION

In implementing the education and training model, the therapeutic recreation specialist must now design specific learning experiences that will help each client meet the previously outlined objectives. At this point other professionals on the team will also undertake this process, utilizing their own media. For example, it is likely (and desirable) that several disciplines will be working on the previously identified goals. Coordination among disciplines is therefore essential. The implementation phase may extend over a period of weeks and months and involve several separate but related educational or training sessions. In this fashion the therapeutic recreation specialist plans a systematic intervention or curriculum which will ultimately meet all objectives that have been developed in the goal-determination phase.

Conducting the Individual Educational Session

While a variety of formats exist for implementing specific education or training sessions, most plans include the following steps:

1. Choosing an activity designed to meet selected objectives
2. Stating the specific behavioral objectives that may be achieved by participation in this activity
3. Developing a strategy or guidelines for conducting the activity
4. Determining the success of the session in terms of its effectiveness in meeting the objectives identified in step 2.

To illustrate this process, it may be helpful to describe how a therapeutic recreation specialist might plan and conduct an activity session for both of our hypothetical clients. Let us begin with Tom R. Before conducting the leisure-counseling session, the therapeutic recreation specialist developed the following special strategies:

The therapeutic recreation specialist will judge the appropriateness of the response.

Antisocial responses will not be considered acceptable.

Clients will take turns or raise hands before answering questions.

If clients exhibit difficulty in answering questions, the therapeutic recreation specialist will provide an example of a correct response.

Clients will be encouraged to share the content of the discussions with their families.

The therapeutic recreation specialist would keep a narrative report of the major events of the session, particularly as they relate to the three performance measures developed for Tom. For example:

Session began at 7:05 P.M. shortly after cleaning up for dinner. After the group settled down, the therapeutic recreation specialist initiated a warm-up exercise in which the group members were asked to talk about any enjoyable activities they had engaged in since the last session. Tom reported that he had enjoyed a special trip to a baseball game and an ice cream party planned by the cottage. Other responses from the group included "working in the garden," "pool," and "horseshoes." Most members of the group were able to identify four recreational opportunities within walking distance of their homes. Tom's answers included "a park," "a movie theater," "a video arcade," and "a shopping mall." The client, however, exhibited a minimal knowledge of resources in the community. Other than mentioning "a stadium a long ways away," he could not identify any leisure opportunities. When asked to list four information sources, the client responded "Ask other people," "Look in the phone book," "T.V." and "Listen to the radio," thus meeting performance measure number 3. Throughout the session the client was cooperative and listened attentively to the reactions of the other group members. Upon discharge, the therapeutic recreation specialist will suggest that Tom's case worker initiate an activity exploration session by accompanying him on public transportation to several resources in the community. As an assignment for the next meeting, the group members were asked to make a list of things that they could do in their communities that would cost less than two dollars. The session ended at 7:50 P.M.

A similar implementation approach is used with Ms. T. Noting that several residents of the group home have upcoming birthdays, the therapeutic recreation specialist enlists the help of four residents (including Ms. T.) in planning a special party. Capitalizing on an interest Ms. T. has expressed in baking, the therapeutic recreation specialist schedules a cake-baking session in the home's kitchen. In anticipating this activity, the therapeutic recreation specialist develops the following strategies or guidelines:

Select other group home members who are known and liked by Ms. T.

Provide mixing utensils with large handles.

Use tape to mark proper levels of ingredients on measuring cups.

Provide appropriate verbal reinforcement to Ms. T. throughout the session.

Rotate responsibilities among group members if more than one cake is to be baked.

At the conclusion of this session, the therapeutic recreation specialist would record Ms. T.'s progress in meeting the performance measures, note any deviations from the planned routine, and make suggestions for future activity sessions. An evaluation of the hypothetical session might read as follows:

The activity took place in the home's kitchen from 2:00–3:45 P.M. In attendance were Ms. T., Mr. R., Ms. L., and Mr. H., all of whom appeared excited at the prospect of baking cakes. Following a brief discussion of the type of cake to be baked, the therapeutic recreation specialist asked for a vote on the two cakes that were suggested—chocolate bundt and lemon chiffon. Ms. T. cast the sole vote for the chocolate cake but said, "Oh, OK" without prompting from the therapeutic recreation specialist, who immediately praised Ms. T. for following the group's decision. The therapeutic recreation specialist then reviewed the basic steps in baking the cake and emphasized that it would require a team effort, with each individual performing certain required tasks. At this point Ms. T. attempted to measure the four ingredients specified. She accurately poured the salt and shortening but could not manage the larger flour and milk containers. In the future it will be necessary to provide smaller, intermediate containers and to instruct Ms. T. in their use. Ms. T. completed behavioral objective number 3 successfully by alternating turns twice with Mr. R. after verbal prompting by the therapist. In the future such prompting will gradually be phased out. Other recommendations include reducing the size of the baking group from four to three because of the size of the kitchen area and baking several smaller cakes to provide more practice on the various tasks involved.

A technique that has proven to be most effective in the education and training model is termed *task analysis*. This procedure involves breaking down a complex activity into its more basic steps and teaching these steps to a client or clients in a sequential fashion. To illustrate, if Ms. T. had been less adept at the cake-baking task, the therapeutic recreation specialist might have taught the activity over several sessions in the following progression:

1. Selecting utensils (mixing bowls, spoons, measuring instruments, egg beaters, baking pans)
2. Selecting ingredients (eggs, milk, flour, extracts, sugar, flavoring)
3. Measuring ingredients
4. Mixing ingredients
5. Preparing stove (setting temperature, preheating, setting timer)
6. Removing cake
7. Frosting cake (repeating steps 1–4)

This application of the education and training model relied heavily upon a leisure-counseling or leisure-education approach. While this text cannot fully describe the various orientations in the delivery of leisure counseling and/or leisure education, most models would fall under one or more of the following headings as described by Allen and Hamilton:

Leisure Resource Guidance. This orientation focuses on information sharing where the therapeutic recreation specialist matches the interests of the client with existing leisure resources. Many of the efforts of the therapeutic recreation specialist were directed toward this goal in Tom's case study.

Skill Development. This approach analyzes an individual client's strengths and weaknesses in the areas of socialization, social interaction, reasoning, or physical skills and then structures experiences that will enhance the client's functioning in these areas. Elements of this orientation were evident in the case study of Ms. T., where an activity was used for the purpose of increasing interaction and reasoning skills.

Lifestyle Awareness. This third orientation focuses upon clarifying leisure values and attitudes and promoting an understanding of forces in the external environment that can affect the individual's perception of leisure.

Leisure-Related Behavioral Problems. This remedial approach goes beyond the exploration of values and attitudes in the previous orientation. Specifically, feelings of boredom, guilt, anxiety, and nervousness must be dealt with directly in the counseling process.

Counseling through Activity Involvement. This medium is used when an individual client's problems transcend his or her leisure. It is similar to traditional forms of counseling or psychotherapy. As such, it would be employed in conjunction with the efforts of other disciplines in the team approach described earlier in this chapter.[5]

EVALUATION

At this point it may be apparent to the reader that this highly structured approach to the delivery of therapeutic recreation service has a built-in evaluative mechanism that functions in two ways. First, short-term progress may be gauged by the client's performance on each of the highly specific behavioral objectives that appear in the activity plan. The plan's narrative provides evidence of this progress *and* suggestions for new teaching strategies to achieve these goals. Second, by periodically noting which goals have been met, the therapeutic recreation specialist can obtain a global index of client progress over weeks or possibly months.

Before concluding the case-study section of this chapter, the authors wish to alert readers to certain limitations inherent in presenting hypothetical examples. First, due to space considerations, only a limited number of goals and behavioral objectives could be dealt with. In reality, the therapeutic recreation specialist employing this model would structure several different educational sessions designed to meet these ex-

tensive goals. The reader may also be curious about the choice of activities—baking and discussion groups. The authors chose these media because they were based on the interests of the clients, were appropriate to the hypothetical settings, and would directly illustrate the incorporation of certain educational goals into a leisure activity. Many other activities would have served an identical function. Space limitations also prevent describing in detail the efforts of other disciplines in meeting client objectives. However, the reader can easily envision a vocational instructor working on Ms. T.'s measuring skills in a carpentry project and a cottage supervisor verbally reinforcing Tom's participation in a new group activity. Finally, the reader may feel a bit uncomfortable when contemplating the large number of goals that can be developed for an individual client. There are, however, certain considerations that will limit the number of goals and establish their priority. Client interest and motivation to work on certain objectives is an obvious factor. Likewise, the therapeutic recreation specialist will have to consider the overall importance of each possible objective in contributing to the independence of the client. Skills and abilities should be selected that are likely to *transfer* to other settings and that *complement* the efforts of other disciplines. Available staff, facility, equipment, and transportation resources will also have to be considered.

THE MODEL IN PRACTICE

So far in this chapter we have provided a conceptual overview of the education and training model and described each of its four major processes by utilizing two case studies as illustrations. The remaining section of this chapter contains descriptions of several contemporary programs that portray the application of this model in a range of settings and activity media with a variety of clients.

PROGRAM ONE: LEISURE EDUCATION

An excellent example of the education and training model is Project SELF (Special Education for Leisure Fulfillment) as described by authors Schnorr and Bender.[6] This particular intervention features the use of leisure education as an integral part of a public and nonpublic school-based program for handicapped children and youth, grades K–12. The curriculum consists of eight leisure domains. These classifications and samples of specific activities are as follows:

1. *Play and games:* tetherball, croquet, shuffleboard, Old Maid, Simon Says
2. *Sports and physical development:* bicycling, ice-skating, swimming, canoeing, cross-country skiing, sauna
3. *Camping and outdoor activities:* catching live bait, backyard barbecues, chopping wood
4. *Nature study, appreciation, and development:* observing wildlife, beachcombing, birds
5. *Hobby activities:* finger painting, model airplanes, bottle collecting
6. *Craft activities:* drying food, candle making, leather work, wood refinishing
7. *Art activities:* photography, sketching, ceramics, creative rhythms
8. *Educational entertainment and cultural activities:* viewing sports events, dining out, traveling

Here is an illustration of how this curriculum was infused into a program. A profile was presented of a fourteen-year-old moderately mentally retarded student who was in a self-contained classroom. This student functioned at a first-grade level but had somewhat higher interpersonal skills. Other handicaps included an inability to speak clearly and problems in gross motor coordination. The general goal statements of his Individualized Educational Plan (IEP) were:

1. To improve his reading from a 1.3 to a 2.5 grade level
2. To improve his arithmetic skills from a 1.8 to a 2.5 grade level
3. To improve his skills of daily living
4. To improve his hand-eye coordination
5. To promote his participation in a variety of leisure activities

The specific objectives from his IEP included:

1. To be able to write the numbers 0–100
2. To be able to add math facts (11–18)
3. To be able to subtract math facts (11–18)
4. To recognize coin values of 1, 5, 10, 25, 50¢
5. To count change under $1
6. To add one- and two-digit numbers to 100[7]

To achieve these goals, shuffleboard was first introduced to develop a specific motor-sequence pattern and teach the rules of the game and its scoring procedure. In this fashion both social and academic skills could be reinforced. Following the mastery of shuffleboard, the client was introduced to Jarts, a game with a similar movement pattern but a new release dimension. The scoring procedure was again practiced to enhance mathematics skills. Bowling was then undertaken to reinforce cross-lateral extension and meet such objectives as writing and adding numbers, recognizing coins and change necessary to pay for the cost of bowling, and using speech in daily activities and in skills like reading the phone book and bus schedules. A final activity, supervised barbecueing, was then implemented to provide practice in reading labels on products, counting money, and listing the names of items to be purchased.

PROGRAM TWO: DEVELOPMENTAL ACTIVITIES

Using a similar but broader approach, Martin and Ovans found evidence that the education and training model could result in significant improvement in the gross motor, language, auditory, manipulative, and cognitive skills of pre- and primary-school children with a variety of developmental disabilities.[8] Specifically, small-group instruction two hours per day, five days per week for five weeks was given stressing total body movement as a learning modality. A partial list of developmental activities modules included:

Gross motor coordination: crawling, climbing, walking, skipping, balancing and free-style tumbling, etc.

Fine motor coordination: building with blocks and logs, playing with tools, molding clay, buckling and buttoning buckles and buttons, attaching geometric figures to a cube, drawing, painting, etc.

Language development: reading and telling stories, singing, programming puppet shows, identifying letter and number symbols, geometric shapes, etc.

Social adjustment: engaging in group play and rhythms, participating in associative play, etc.

Self-image: learning to identify body components by means of a moving clown, etc.

PROGRAM THREE: PERCEPTUAL-MOTOR TRAINING

Mosher has also developed a perceptual-motor training program for autistic children based on the specific needs and characteristics of this disability group.[9] His curriculum is designed around eight specific stations which have distinct rationales. Children do not spend the same amount of time at, or even visit, each and every station. Rather, they attend those areas that meet their developmental needs. A brief description of the eight stations that make up this training system follows:

Station 1, Sequential skills 1: This station is designed to ameliorate the immature movement patterns prevalent in autistic children. It includes a progression of creeping, crawling, walking, hopping, skipping and jumping activities.

Station 2, Sequential skills 2: The emphasis here is on the development of more advanced skills such as catching, throwing, kicking, and striking. These skills are required for peer interaction, which will lead to improved self-concept and in turn to a higher level of socialization.

Station 3, Body-image development: These activities are designed to correct a major deficit exhibited by autistic children—the ability to interpret the position of the body and its relationship to objects in the environment. Sample training exercises include identification of specific body parts, touching body parts with eyes closed, identifying the movement of body parts when prone or supine and drawing shapes with arms and legs.

Station 4, Fine motor skills-manual dexterity: Here activities involving designs, puzzles, block assemblies, and peg boards are used. These manipulative tasks are related to the right hemisphere of the brain, which is generally less affected in autistic children. Hence, these activities are interesting, enjoyable, and relatively easily mastered.

Station 5, Vestibular stimulation: This cluster of activities is designed to provide appropriate stimulation to the vestibular (sensorimotor) system. Trampoline exercises, spinning net hammocks, tumbling stunts, and scooter boards are among the activity offerings at this station.

Station 6, Swimming: Water activities promote socialization, body image, self-concept development, and general fun. Peer and family interaction is also a by-product of these activities. Normal swimming instructional sequences are followed, with extensive use made of floats, rubber balls, and inner tubes.

Station 7, Cognitive skills: The station is used to provide appropriate cognitive stimulation and prevent regression when the child is not receiving formal academic training. Sample activities include the use of number and word concepts (high-low etc.) in relay and stunt situations.

Station 8, Arts and crafts: Activities such as cutting, pasting, papier mâché, and puppets are used to promote motor coordination and serve as a break from large-muscle movements.

PROGRAM FOUR: FORM PERCEPTION

There have also been several interventions reported in the literature that use specific media or specialized techniques in an education and training mode. MacNeil suggests an interesting application of this model in discussing form-perception training for children who are visually or auditorially impaired or mentally retarded.[10] This system of training is based on the assumption that the ability to discriminate between basic objects in the environment is essential for intellectual performance. A brief overview of the three key elements in the form-perception matrix proposed by this author follows:

Component 1, Form recognition: These activities are designed to assist children to differentiate specific forms from global masses. The therapeutic recreation specialist starts with relatively simple exercises, such as having the child differentiate between blocks of sharply contrasting shapes, sizes, or colors. Gradually, objects can be made more similar, or additional objects can be added. Ultimately, objects can be replaced by drawings or pictures.

Component 2, Matching activities: These exercises build upon the previous recognition training and can include sorting objects of the same size, shape, and color and then grouping objects, such as foods or furniture, by function. Eventually, the therapeutic recreation specialist can progress to having the child match objects by their component parts, for instance, objects with wheels or objects with faces.

Component 3, Constructive-form activities: This final phase of perception training involves the transformation of previously identified objects into new forms. In this component, the therapeutic recreation specialist will ask the client to combine materials such as form boards, puzzles, clay, dough, and Lincoln Logs into recognizable objects.

PROGRAM FIVE: AQUATICS

Aquatics has traditionally been a popular medium for use in the education and training paradigm. Priest provides a sample curriculum, which can be implemented to remediate academic deficiencies and promote motor learning in a variety of disabled clients. The following are some sample learning areas:

Arithmetic concepts

    Retrieving and counting objects
    Identification of geometric shapes of retrieved objects

Auditory discrimination

    Games that use a sound signal such as "go" on whistle, "stop" on bell

Creativity and self-expression

    Exercises that encourage listening to auditory cues and moving the way the sound "makes you feel"

Coordination

    Retrieving objects such as ping-pong balls
    Throwing objects such as sponges
    Catching objects such as Frisbees
    Hitting objects such as beach balls

Sequential thinking

    Water relays
    Retrieving objects of a particular nature from the bottom of a pool[11]

PROGRAM SIX: MUSIC

Music has also been shown to be a powerful medium for use within the education and training model. Birkenshaw outlines several major areas where music can help developmentally disabled children.

1. *Motor-sensory*: Running, skipping, and jumping to a drum beating out songs in a rhythm-and-movement pattern can develop laterality and directionality. Performing actions to a song creates body awareness. Freezing the body in various shapes assists in developing body image.

2. *Rhythmic training*: Echoing rhythms clapped by another person and playing instruments can develop inner rhythmic abilities.

3. *Auditory awareness*: This area uses movement to focus on listening. For example, children can vary their pace to the sound of a drum. The sounds of several instruments can also be used to guide children in several different directions.

4. *Speech training*: Children can clap to the syllables of several contrasting words or move to the sounds of words and poems.

5. *Indirect learning*: The alphabet song can be used to learn letters. Poems and songs encourage children to read words. Spelling in rhythm can be taught.[12]

PROGRAM SEVEN: PLAY ENVIRONMENT

Therapeutic recreation specialists have also employed specific training techniques in the play environments of handicapped children to improve language skills and increase verbal interactions. Lewko and Erickson suggest the following measures for achieving these goals:

Technique 1, Verbalizing an action while performing it: For example, subject-verb utterances, such as "ball roll," may be readily acquired when paired with the direct action of rolling a ball in front of a child.

Technique 2, Parallel talk: This technique is a basic description of action currently taking place, such as "Jimmy is pulling the wagon." It can also be followed immediately by the therapist's modeling the

behavior and stating, "I'm pulling the wagon."

Technique 3, Echo expansion: Here the therapeutic recreation specialist uses the child's verbalization as a base and tries to expand its duration. For example, the child's statement, "That is a slide," would be followed by the therapist's statement, "Yes, that is a big slide."[13]

PROGRAM EIGHT: OUTDOOR EDUCATION/CAMPING

Outdoor education and camping experiences have proven to be most popular backdrops for the application of the model. Havens and Witman provide a strong rationale for using outdoor programming to achieve the goals of the individualized educational plans for severely disabled children.[14] Their model includes the modules shown on p. 277.

PROGRAM NINE: OUTDOOR EDUCATION/ACTIVITIES

A similar outdoor education program has been designed by Stoudenmire to meet the educational and perceptual-motor needs of emotionally disturbed children. His curriculum is outlined in Table 10.3.

PROGRAM TEN: OUTDOOR EDUCATION

Rawson found that behavior-modification methodologies applied in an outdoor education setting could significantly improve the self-concept, academic and interpersonal skills, and attitudes toward school of behaviorally disordered children.[15] Reinforcers such as verbal praise, physical gestures of approval, awards of tokens, and recognition in public ceremonies were used in a variety of camp activities. As in previously described programs, mathematical skills were taught in water games. Geography and spelling were integrated into nature activities, and language skills such as sentence struc-

PROCESS CONSIDERATIONS	CONTENT CONSIDERATIONS
1. Rationale for outdoor programming	1. Communication skills
2. Basic outdoor skills, knowledge and attitudes	2. Independent living skills
3. Activity analysis, selection, and adaptation	3. Learning skills
4. Planning and implementation considerations	4. Motor skills
5. Evaluation	5. Social skills

A sample of their active and challenging curriculum is outlined below.

IEP OBJECTIVES	OUTDOOR ACTIVITIES
1. A ropes-and-obstacles adventure course: 1A. To roll independently	1A. Gradually reduced prompts on rolling portion of course
1B. To demonstrate increased balance	1B. Walking forward, backwards, catching an object on a natural balance beam
1C. To demonstrate increased endurance	1C. Jogging at the outdoor center
2. Outdoor cookery: 2A. To plan a menu	2A. Each student plans own Dutch treat
2B. To follow a simple recipe	2B. Follows recipe at campfire
2C. To pour from pitcher to cup	2C. Practice during meals plus a water-pour relay
3. Initiative tasks: 3A. To help others	3A. Student leads other student in blind trust walk
3B. To participate with others in group activity	3B. Stump stand
3C. To contribute to and accept group decisions	3C. Group process in deciding how to move the entire group over the "wall"
4. Hiking and orienteering: 4A. To demonstrate improved short-term memory	4A. Remembers instructions (at red marker, turn right) on adapted orienteering course
4B. To distinguish colors	4B. Finds natural objects to match all the colors on a Color Lotto card
4C. To develop a hobby interest	4C. Photographs variety of natural objects
5. Acclimatization activities: 5A. To precede nouns with adjectives	5A. Sensory-description exercise (big, green, slimy rock)
5B. To discriminate by touch	5B. Touchy-feelly box (match items in box with models outside)
5C. To tolerate and adapt to new activities	5C. Swamp walk

ture, punctuation, and grammar rules were taught through campcrafts. Unit participation "learning modules" emphasizing long-term, cooperative activities were also stressed. These projects were centered around tasks that would benefit an entire group of campers, such as clearing a site for an evening campout.

PROGRAM ELEVEN: TEACHING OUTDOOR EDUCATION

Albert outlines a curricular approach to teaching outdoor education to educable and trainable mentally retarded adults living in a residential facility.[16] He recommends the following one-week units:

TABLE 10.3. Camp Activities Having Both Educational and Emotional Objectives

Activity	Educational Objective	Emotional Objective
Motor area		
Calisthenics	Gross motor body control	Improved body image and body awareness
Pantomime	Knowledge of body parts	Social perceptiveness
Sports (swimming, softball, etc.)	Fine and gross motor body control, visual alertness	Social skill refinement (e.g., teamwork), self-acceptance of abilities and limitations
Arts and crafts (painting, modeling clay, etc.)	Fine motor control, visual-perceptual skills	Emotional catharsis
Perception area		
Card games and dominos	Mastery of shapes, numbers, colors	Socialization
Learning sounds heard on hikes (e.g., birds, wind, cars, water, etc.)	Knowledge of sounds, auditory perceptiveness	Ego-enhancement through knowledge of results and knowledge acquisition
Memory area		
Recalling sounds or events occurring on hikes	Memory training	Self-pride for memory acquisition
Issue directions for camper to follow (e.g., "Take your ball glove to the field." "Get the equipment from the shed.")	Memory training	Self-pride for accomplishment, some socialization
Language area		
Recall and discuss the new names being learned at camp (e.g., trees, birds, camp equipment, activities, emotions, ideas)	Language development and vocabulary enlargement	Self-confidence in discussion-group settings
Letter writing	Increase letter writing knowledge, improve spelling ability, reinforce camper's memory of his address	Maintenance or improvement in intrafamily communication
Signlettering (lettering signs for cabin door, foot lockers, camp zoo exhibits)	Increase spelling ability, fine motor control	Personal-organization skills, self-identity, socialization (where lettering was a group project)
Numbers area		
Activities calling on the camper to count ("We need four groups of people, with five people in each group." "This lean-to needs two more boards, each six feet long with three nails in each end and two in the middle.")	Increase number skills of counting, measuring, etc.	Self-pride for accomplishment, some socialization enhancement where group projects are involved

SOURCE: John Stoudenmire, "Including Educational and Perceptual Training in a Therapeutic Camp for Emotionally Disturbed Children," *Therapeutic Recreation Journal* 11, no 1(1977), 14. Reprinted by permission of National Therapeutic Recreation Society/National Recreation and Park Association.

1. Plants
2. Seeds
3. Trees and leaves
4. Insects
5. Higher animals—reptiles, birds, mammals
6. Water life
7. Rocks, minerals, and soil

Each unit is approached through four subject areas: science, art, language development, and social studies. Lesson plans consisted of the following:

1. Behavioral objectives
2. Concepts
3. Materials
4. Vocabulary and definitions
5. Procedures and activities
6. Evaluation

An evaluation revealed that as a group residents were more able to recognize objects in the outdoors and explain their use to humans, understand simple science concepts, and note color, shape, and composition of wilderness features after participation in this program.

PROGRAM TWELVE: LEISURE COUNSELING/EDUCATION

As stated earlier in this chapter, leisure counseling/education has been a common technique used within this paradigm. Aikens reports on a progressive leisure-counseling/education program for young persons with traumatic spinal cord injuries in a rehabilitation center in Canada.[17] In keeping with the comprehensive nature of the education and training model, this program focuses on specific problems in the areas of leisure awareness, social skills, and planning skills and interests. After an initial assessment, the following ten-step process is implemented:

Step 1. The client is encouraged to review the potential problem areas identified by the therapeutic recreation specialist, comment and set goals based on this information.
Step 2. The client identifies his or her attitudes and values toward leisure.
Step 3. The client explores his or her leisure needs.
Step 4. Leisure interests are explored.
Step 5. Barriers to leisure participation are examined.
Step 6. Feasible leisure activities are identified.
Step 7. Community resources within the client's discharge area are identified.
Step 8. Specific barriers to participation, such as transportation and architectural accessibility, are dealt with.
Step 9. The client participates in an exploratory activity and evaluates this experience.
Step 10. Follow-up is undertaken to determine the client's level of satisfaction with his or her leisure.

PROGRAM THIRTEEN: LEISURE COUNSELING/EXPERIENTIAL LEISURE

There have also been creative, albeit limited, efforts to incorporate the teaching of human sexuality in education and training programs that feature leisure counseling and the provision of experiential leisure opportunities. Stensrud has outlined several innovative techniques for meeting the sociosexual needs of mentally retarded adults.[18] Her model education and training approach concentrates on these major practices:

1. *Sociosexual leisure-competency evaluations:* observations, interviews, specific tests, and leisure counseling.
2. *Formal education:* small-group rap sessions utilizing books, magazines, films, and visual aids to reach each participant on his or her own level, covering the following:
   a. *Body awareness:* body-part identification and purpose, differences between

males and females, feelings about our own body and about others' bodies.

b. *Puberty:* early sexual behavior, menstruation, masturbation, nocturnal emissions, adolescent anxieties, role changes, attitudes, and problems.

c. *Social relationships and activities:* developing socialization skills, conversation, large-group activities and dating.

d. *Sexual activity-sexual intercourse:* biological, social, and emotional considerations, sexual options, experimentation and adaptations.

e. *Sexual consequences:* basic information and comparison of various birth control methods, premarital sex, genetic counseling, exploration of self-esteem and attitudes.

f. *Marriage, parenthood, and alternatives:* responsibilities, social attitudes, changing trends and values.

g. *Considerations and problems:* institutional and community attitudes, moral and ethical implications, legal restrictions.

3. *Experimental opportunities:* controlled and sequentially planned activities for each individual such as:

a. *Integrative social activities:* for example, folk dancing, where many types of people come together, or to provide opportunities to touch, talk, dance, and to be in couples and to have fun in a normal adult recreational event.

b. *Normalization club:* one staff member trained in sociosexual skills will go out on a planned date with a special group individual and help that person learn the skills that he or she needs.

c. *Small parties:* held in homes, providing individuals with the opportunity to integrate and experience normal adult leisure and to help them acquire the ability to choose friends and develop relationships and to become more independent.

4. *Leisure counseling:* playing an important part in helping the special individual understand his or her abilities and potential as a social-sexual being. This type of leisure counseling may have to go far beyond the usual matching of resources that leisure counseling in the past has provided. Leisure education and even leisure stimulation may be included. Individuals who have been made to believe that they have no sexual potential may need to be turned on to their potential through the use of films, books, and activities before they are interested in developing their skills in this area. Counseling techniques can be employed to help individuals identify their needs, assess their ability, understand problems, and find solutions to these problems.

5. *Parent education:* constant communication, involvement, counseling and education for parents, helping them to cope with their child's sexuality.

SUMMARY

The education and training model is widely used in the field of therapeutic recreation. It is highly structured in its approach to client assessment, goal determination, implementation, and evaluation. The model relies heavily upon objectives that are measurable and observable. As such, it can be applied to the teaching of specific recreational skills or, more broadly, to helping individuals acquire knowledge about their leisure lifestyles. A cooperative approach is a most common pattern of service delivery in facilities employing this model. Therefore, the therapeutic recreation specialist must be prepared to function as an active member of an interdisciplinary team whose efforts are aimed toward the development of client independence.

NOTES

1. G. Heynes, "Penal Institutions," *Annals of the American Academy of Political Science* 313 (September 1957), 73.

2. John J. Capobianco, "Continued Socialization," *Leisurability* 4, no. 1 (1977), 6.

3. Debby A. Smith and Ronald P. Reynolds, "Integrating Leisure Counseling and Psychological Services," *Therapeutic Recreation Journal* 12, no. 3 (1978), 29.

4. Adapted from K. F. Joswiak, *Leisure Counseling Program Materials for the Developmentally Disabled* (Washington, D.C.: Hawkins and Associates, 1978), 66–69.

5. Lawrence R. Allen and Edward J. Hamilton, "Leisure Counseling: A Continuum of Services," *Therapeutic Recreation Journal* 14, no. 1 (1980), 18–20.

6. Janice M. Schnorr and Michael Bender, "Project SELF: Special Education for Leisure Fulfillment," *Therapeutic Recreation Journal* 16, no. 3 (1982), 9–16.

7. IEP is the terminology used for writing an educational plan for a student with a disability who is in the school system, as required by PL 94-142.

8. Margaret Mary Martin and Phyllis M. Ovans, "Learning Games Are Pathways to Cognizance for Young Handicapped Children in Therapeutic Recreation," *Therapeutic Recreation Journal* 6, no. 4 (1972), 153–57, 171.

9. Richard Mosher, "Perceptual-Motor Training and the Autistic Child," *Leisurability* 2, no. 3 (1975), 29–35.

10. Richard D. MacNeil, "Form Perception Training: Implications for the Recreation Therapist," *Therapeutic Recreation Journal* 12, no. 1 (1978), 28–32.

11. E. Louise Priest, "Academic Remediation in Aquatics," *Therapeutic Recreation Journal* 10, no. 2 (1976), 35–37.

12. Lois Birkenshaw, "Music for the Handicapped Child," *Leisurability* 2, no. 2 (1975), 3–9.

13. John H. Lewko and Joan Good Erickson, "Language Development in the Play Environment," *Leisurability* 5, no. 2 (1978), 16–20.

14. Mark Havens and Jeff Witman, "From Frill to Necessity: Outdoor Programming as a Component of Individual Education Programs and Treatment," in *Expanding Horizons in Therapeutic Recreation VII*, ed. Gerald Hitzhusen, Julie Elliott, David J. Szymanski, and M. Gary Thompson (Columbia: Curators, University of Missouri, (1979), pp. 61–68.

15. Harve E. Rawson, "Short-Term Residential Therapeutic Camping for Behaviorally Disordered Children Aged 6–12: An Academic Remediation and Behavior Modification Approach," *Therapeutic Recreation Journal* 12, no. 4 (1978), 17–23.

16. Russell Albert, "A Concentrated Program of Outdoor Education for Educable and Trainable Retarded," *Therapeutic Recreation Journal* 3, no. 3 (1969), 25–28.

17. Ann Aikens, "An Institutional Perspective: Recreation and Leisure Services in Spinal Cord Rehabilitation," *Leisurability* 9, no. 2 (1982), 27–31.

18. Carol Stensrud, "Recreation's Role in Meeting the Socio-Sexual Needs of Special Populations," *Therapeutic Recreation Journal*, 10, no. 3 (1976), pp. 94–98.

SUGGESTED READINGS

HAWKINS, D. E. A *Systems Model for Developing a Leisure Education Program for Handicapped Children and Youth, (K-12)*. Washington, D.C.: Hawkins and Associates, 1976.

JOSWIAK, K. *Leisure Counseling Program Materials for the Developmentally Disabled*. Washington, D.C.: Hawkins and Associates, 1975.

Kangaroo Kit. Alexandria, Va.: National Recreation and Park Association, 1977.

KELLEY, JERRY D., ed. *Recreation Programming for Visually Impaired*. New York: American Foundation for the Blind, 1982.

MCDONALD, JESSYNA M. "Special Adaptive Recreation as Intervention in Vocational and Transitional Services for Handicapped Youth." *Therapeutic Recreation Journal* 19, no. 3 (1985), 17–27.

OVERS, R., E. O'CONNOR, and B. DEMARCO. *Avocational Activities for the Handicapped*. Springfield, Ill.: Charles C Thomas, Publisher, 1974.

RAWSON, HARVE E. "Short-Term Residential Therapeutic Camping for Behaviorally Disordered Children Aged 6–12: An Academic Remediation and Behavior Modification Approach." *Therapeutic Recreation Journal* 12, no. 4 (1978), 17–23.

REYNOLDS, R. P., and M. H. ARTHUR. "Effects of Peer Modeling and Cognitive Self Guidance on the Social Play of Emotionally Disturbed Children." *Therapeutic Recreation Journal* 16, no. 1 (1982), 33–40.

SESSOMS, H. DOUGLAS. "Organized Camping and Its Effects on the Self-Concept of Physically Handicapped Children." *Therapeutic Recreation Journal* 13, no. 1 (1979), 39–43.

SCHLEIEN, STUART, RANDY PORTER, and PAUL WEHMAN. "An Assessment of the Leisure Skill Needs of Developmentally Disabled Individuals." *Therapeutic Recreation Journal* 13, no. 3 (1979), 16–21.

SCHNORR, JANICE, and MICHAEL BENDER. "Project SELF: Special Education for Leisure Fulfillment."

Therapeutic Recreation Journal 16, no. 3 (1982), 9–16.

VOELTZ, LUANNA M., and BONNIE BIEL WUERCH. "A Comprehensive Approach to Leisure Education and Leisure Counseling for the Severely Handicapped." *Therapeutic Recreation Journal* 15, no. 4 (1981), 24–35.

WEHMAN, P., and S. SCHLEIEN. *Leisure and Handicapped Individuals: Adaptations, Techniques, and Curriculum.* Baltimore: University Park Press, 1981.

WUERCH, B. B., and L. M., VOELTZ. *The Ho'Onanea Program: A Leisure Curriculum Component for Severely Handicapped Children and Youth.* Honolulu: University of Hawaii, Department of Special Education, 1981.

11

The Community Model

Community-based programming represents a new and most challenging dimension of therapeutic recreation service. Although the number of therapeutic recreation specialists employed in residential facilities has traditionally greatly outnumbered those working in the community, there are several trends that will most likely cause a shift in this distribution. Such factors as legislative measures promoting physical and programmatic access to recreational opportunities, shortened hospital stays, trends toward deinstitutionalization, and a growing recognition that the vast majority of persons with disabilities do reside in the community at large all underscore a growing need for community-based services. This chapter provides a brief overview of some examples of interest in the community-based therapeutic model that have been an outgrowth of these trends and then illustrates the application of this model in the four phases that have served as the organizational basis for the preceding chapters.

The Assessment section stresses the necessity to examine both the individual's needs and interests and the external factors in the environment that may impede his or her recreational participation. It then provides concrete procedures and instruments for conducting the assessment process on both of these levels. In keeping with this dual approach to needs determination or goal development, the Planning section centers on a behavioral approach to operationalizing client information into program plans and translating environmental assessments into procedures designed to remove barriers. As in the initial phase, current examples are given to illustrate each of these measures. The Implementation section contains three related topics. First, the concept of recreation integration is discussed to emphasize the continuum of leisure services in the community model and to highlight the ultimate goals of the specialist working in this setting. Attention is then given to the unique roles community therapeutic recreation personnel must perform in achieving these objectives. The section concludes with a description of five major types of service that might be provided in a municipal recreation department and an example of a progressive municipal therapeutic recreation program. The chapter concludes with a brief discussion of how the resources described in the assessment and goal-determination phases can be used as evaluative tools.

COMMUNITY INTEREST: AN OVERVIEW

One general indication of the surge of interest in community-based programming for disabled individuals has been the large number of "state-of-the-art" reports that have been published in the therapeutic recreation literature. Early evidence of sporadic interest in determining the status of services for the mentally retarded came as early as 1967, when municipal recreation departments in 166 major cities in the United States were polled about their offerings for this client group.[1] In 1977 community recreation services for disabled persons became a major concern of the White House Conference on Handicapped Individuals. Proceedings from this symposium included a state-of-the-art overview and survey of current programs meeting the recreational needs of the disabled.[2] In the twelve-year period from 1971 to 1983, the *Therapeutic Recreation Journal* and *Leisurability* contained a plethora of reports summarizing the numbers and characteristics of disabled persons using community-based recreation services. In the United States municipal departments were surveyed in Iowa, Texas, Oregon, Indiana, and Minnesota.[3] Canadian departments were surveyed nationally and separately in the case of Ontario.[4] Interest in this topic also surfaced in England where the city of Manchester was surveyed about its recreational opportunities.[5] In addition to these state-of-the-art investigations, articles on the provision of therapeutic recreation in the community began to appear in professional journals. A sampling of these topics includes: "Community Recreation for the Mentally Retarded," "National Therapeutic Recreation Society and the American Park and Recreation Society Liaison Report" "Environmental Barriers to Persons with Physical Disabilities," and "Recreation in

Community Mental Health."[6] Interestingly, articles instructing recreation directors in how to interact with parents of disabled children also began to emerge.[7] Similarly, guides for parents describing where to find recreational services for their disabled child were also published.[8] During this time therapeutic recreation specialists in the community continually addressed such topics as the removal of architectural barriers, modification of areas and facilities, activity planning, and leadership with respect to disabled persons.[9]

Today interest, involvement, and commitment to providing community leisure opportunities have greatly transcended the parameters of municipal recreation departments. The following paradigms, identified by the National Institute of New Models, are illustrative of the varied approaches to community leisure services for disabled persons in operation today.

Leisure consumer models: programs organized and conducted by people who are handicapped (Wheelchair Athletic Association)

Consumer leisure-competency models: programs that help the handicapped become aware of recreation and leisure opportunities (educational and counseling programs)

Leisure for handicapped advocacy-group models: organizations that advocate handicapped rights with respect to leisure needs of the handicapped (National Therapeutic Recreation Society)

Special recreation for handicapped facility and service models: recreation programs and facilities specifically designed for use by the handicapped (San Francisco Recreation Center for the Handicapped)

Commercial recreation for handicapped models: travel agencies, equipment manufacturers, private facilities (theaters, bowling establishments, and the like), and transportation agencies that serve the handicapped

Community service and civic organization models: (Toastmaster, Chamber of Commerce, PTA, political parties)

Creative and performing arts models: organizations and clubs that offer programs in the area of dance, music, art, and the like at both a spectator and participation level (Theater of the Deaf)

Education and school models: preschool through postsecondary education

Park and recreation departments: full range of leisure services to the handicapped at all levels (national, state, local, urban, and rural)

Rehabilitation, health, social, and welfare models: federal, state, and some private funding for specific services to the physically, emotionally, socially, and mentally handicapped

Support-service models: services of consultation, planning, in-service training, information research, which are provided by national or state organizations to both participants and practitioners (National Consortium on Physical Education and Recreation for the Handicapped; U.S. Bureau of Education for the Handicapped; Information and Research Utilization Center in Physical Education and Recreation for the Handicapped (IRUC); Cooperative Extension Service in Therapeutic Recreation)

Voluntary health agency models: agencies serving specific impairments or disabilities

Youth service models: (Boy Scouts, Girl Scouts, 4-H, YMCA)[10]

In response to the broad areas of leisure service inherent in these models, the term *recreation integration,* referring to the involvement of disabled persons in community leisure opportunities, became commonplace in the therapeutic recreation literature of the 1980s. One source identified twenty-one research articles alone on the subject that appeared over a nine-year time span.[11]

A quick perusal of the literature indicates that service clubs, day camps, preschool daycare centers, community mental health agencies, and municipal park and recreation departments were popular sites for these integrative efforts.

It is apparent from even this brief review that in certain instances it is hard to distinguish therapeutic recreation service from the general recreation that may be provided to persons with disabilities in a community setting. Kennedy, Austin, and Smith have summarized this dilemma as follows:

> Within the field of therapeutic recreation two philosophical points of view have emerged. One defines therapeutic recreation primarily as the provision of leisure services for those people who have some type of limitations. This position has been adopted by the National Therapeutic Recreation Society, a branch of the National Recreation and Park Association. The other view holds that therapeutic recreation should restrict itself to the application of purposeful interventions employing the therapeutic recreation process, and should, therefore, relinquish the provision of community recreation for special populations to community recreation personnel.[12]

The polarity that at times has existed between therapeutic and special recreation has been studied empirically. Following a comparison of the relationship between therapeutic and community recreators, one researcher noted:

> The results of this study indicate that significant changes have occurred in the attitudes of community recreators toward therapeutic recreators within eight years. Even though there exists a variety of changes, community recreators and therapeutic recreators have a long way to go to mutual understanding of roles and mutual acceptance of the other for even better services for the handicapped populations. We need to hope for a continual increase in the employment of therapeutic recreation specialists in community settings and more interaction among members of community recreation and therapeutic recreation.

We need to encourage the development of sufficient recreation programs in the community for the variety of handicapped populations that exist and utilize trained personnel for the development of these programs.[13]

The authors feel that several events that have taken place since these words were written in 1978 have decreased the polarity between therapeutic recreators and those who provide special recreation service. One such event has been the sharp increase in the number of trained therapeutic recreation specialists employed in settings such as those outlined above in the New Models study. Another development has been the adoption of the 1982 Philosophical Position Statement of the National Therapeutic Recreation Society. This document substantiated the need for therapeutic recreation specialists to provide therapy, leisure education, and general recreation to disabled persons, when appropriate, regardless of setting. A final trend has been the erosion of the notion that services in clinical, medical, or rehabilitation settings are synonomous with prescriptive, interventionist, treatment, or individualized therapies, while community programs are diversional in nature. Today many community-based therapeutic recreation programs serve a developmental purpose. Many trained therapeutic recreation specialists employed in the community conduct individual client assessments, develop goals, and implement plans designed to achieve specific client objectives.

In view of this discussion, the reader is asked to keep these points in mind concerning the material that follows:

1. The information is designed for persons being trained as therapeutic recreation specialists. Nevertheless, it is expected and hoped that these practitioners will work closely with community recreation personnel and persons from outside the recreation profession when implementing this model of service.

2. The following process is applicable not only to therapeutic recreation specialists employed in municipal recreation departments, but also to those who will seek employment in other areas such as advocate associations, group homes, outpatient clinics, and schools.

3. Some overlap with the practices presented in the preceding four chapters is both natural and desirable. In many cases these chapters can be viewed as a continuum of services designed to help clients realize their fullest potential.

IMPLEMENTATION OF THE MODEL

ASSESSMENT

Assessment in the community model of therapeutic recreation service uses a unique two-pronged approach. As in the preceding models, assessment must include a thorough analysis of the functional abilities, leisure needs, and past, present, and future recreational interests of the *individual*. Additionally, however, a comprehensive evaluation must be made of factors in the *environment* that could impede a client's progress in participating successfully in leisure opportunities. The therapeutic recreation specialist working within the community model must be well versed in both processes. Some of the most successful techniques and instruments that have been developed for the assessment of individual and environmental factors in the community model are described below.

Individual Assessment

Stanley has suggested several guidelines for conducting an initial functional assessment of an individual in a community-based recreation setting. The following represents a summary of the areas that should be considered by the therapeutic recreation specialist:

1. *Placement:* Where the applicant is placed in school (a regular public school classroom, a resource room in the public school, a self-contained special education classroom, a special education regionalized school or district) or at work (a rehabilitation workshop, an adult activity center, regular employment).

2. *Family situation:* Is it supportive or nonsupportive? Are there appropriate models in the home for the applicant to emulate? Is there anyone in the family who takes an interest in the individual's leisure pursuits or who recreates with the individual?

3. *Social skills:* How does the applicant get along with others? (withdrawn/outgoing? friendly/hostile? submissive/aggressive?)

4. *Learning skills:* What is the individual's attention span? Rate of learning and retention? What motivational factors need to be considered?

5. *Emotional factors:* How does the applicant feel about himself or herself? Is self-concept healthy? Are any behaviors such as anger, fear, frustration exhibited in an overt manner?

6. *Physical skills:* At what development level are the gross motor skills? Fine motor skills? Physical fitness aspects? Hand-eye/foot-eye coordination?

7. *Self-help skills:* Can the applicant attend to personal needs (toileting, feeding, clothing, dressing, cleaning, grooming)?

8. *Interests and skills:* What does the applicant like to do? In what recreational areas does he or she exhibit proficiency? What has he or she expressed an interest in doing? What does he or she actually do during leisure time?[14]

This information can be obtained from many sources, including:

Interest surveys: involving the client's family members

Interviews: including filling out applications, touring the facility, administering leisure-interest forms

Registration forms: providing information relative to the disability, medicines, mechanical aids, self-help skills, and previous recreational interests

Health history and physical examination forms: describing the disability, related limitations, and special considerations

Consultation: with other persons who have knowledge of the participant including parents, school personnel, vocational rehabilitation personnel; or for those recently discharged from a residential facility, recreation, occupational, and/or physical therapists[15]

An extremely comprehensive client-assessment process for developmentally disabled adults, which is directly applicable to the community-based model of therapeutic recreation service, has been developed by Congdon, Conley, and Duecker. Described in their book, *A Part, Not Apart: A Systematic Approach to Integrated Recreation and Leisure*, this system centers around evaluation of the following three areas:

1. *Client characteristics:* The client is rated on abilities related to expressive and receptive communication, general intelligence, cognitive abilities, creativity, mobility, fine and gross motor coordination, mannerisms and personality, appearance, socialization and interpersonal skills, values, and academic performance.

2. *Home environment:* An extensive thirty-four-question form is used to assess the client's home situation. Major areas of inquiry concern the client's transportation needs, social involvement, spectator interests, time utilization, responsibilities, and recreational involvement.

3. *Client assessment:* This process is divided into three parts:

a. An open-ended interview, which determines the client's general leisure competency and knowledge.
b. A slide presentation designed to measure the client's identification, participation, enjoyment, and interest in six major activity areas.
c. A determination (again through the use of slides) of patterns of recreational interest.[16]

The extensive nature of information gathered in the assessment process obviously requires that appropriate recording procedures be developed. Because participants' age ranges, disabilities, and functional levels will vary widely in community settings, forms should be designed that will readily record basic demographic, health, perceptual-motor, and recreational data while being flexible enough to accommodate intraindividual differences. Additionally, the information contained on the form should be readily interpretable to nontherapeutic recreation personnel who may have contact with the client. Figure 11.1 represents one data collection instrument found to be useful in community-based therapeutic recreation assessment.

Environmental Assessment

To date there has been much general discussion concerning environmental barriers, yet relatively little systematic assessment of these factors. One promising instrument that has been developed for this purpose is called the AEBLE (Assessment of Environmental Barriers to Leisure Experiences Scale).[17] Although developed for use with orthopedically disabled children, it is a promising prototype for other ages and disability groups. The questionnaire analyzes six major factors that can pose serious barriers to an individual's recreational participation. Individuals are asked to respond to several questions concerning each of these factors by answering "usually," "sometimes," or "not a problem." Figure 11.2 represents a brief description of the six potential problem areas and two sample questions related to each factor.

After the questionnaire is completed, a composite profile is developed yielding an overall picture of critical constraints that prevent leisure participation.

In communities where little groundwork has been done about identifying disabled persons, determining their leisure interests, and identifying leisure opportunities, the therapeutic recreation specialist may be faced with a much more fundamental assessment task. Witt outlines the type of information that may be obtained in a preliminary community survey.

1. *Determining number and location of individuals with various disabilities:* gaining estimates of numbers of disabled persons from advocate associations, local governmental agencies, or other sources.

2. *Determining leisure needs and interests of disabled persons:* holding meetings with representatives of advocate associations, parent groups, and/or individual citizens, and visiting local workshops, day centers, and schools to determine perceived barriers to leisure involvement.

3. *Evaluating the number, type, location, and level of leisure services currently available:* surveying institutions, advocate associations, service clubs, municipal departments, and agencies that serve youth. Topics of the survey should include philosophy of service, goals, major objectives, groups served, type and location of services, fees, and future service plans.[18]

Once the survey is completed, the therapeutic recreation specialist will have to make a determination concerning the status of recreational services based upon two factors—*availability* and *quality* of local leisure opportunities. Lyons and Reynolds offer the following guidelines for evaluating these two dimensions.

FIGURE 11.1. **Participant Assessment**

Demographic Data:

Name _____ _____ _____ Age _____

      (Last)   (First)   (Middle)

Address _____

Phone: Home _____ Work _____ Emergency _____

Weight _____ Name of person filling out form

Height _____ _____

Sex _____ Relationship to participant _____

Most recent school attended _____ Teacher _____

Do you have your own transportation? Yes _____ No _____

Classification:
Please check one

Trainably mentally retarded _____

Educably mentally retarded _____

Severely mentally retarded _____

Multiply handicapped _____

Orthopedically impaired _____

Hearing impaired _____

Visually impaired _____

Emotionally disturbed _____

Other _____

Cause of handicap _____

Current medications _____

Drug reactions _____

At what intervals does medicine have to be taken?

Medicine _____ Dosage _____ Time _____

_____ _____ _____

(*continued*)

FIGURE 11.1. (*Continued*)

Allergies:

Food _____ Other _____

Seizures:

Type _____ Frequency _____ Duration _____
                              (how often)   (how long)

Management _____

Health or behavior habits (biting, running, must not become overheated, etc.):

Type _____ Management _____

Please rate: (1) Never observed   (2) Never   (3) Sometimes   (4) Most of the time   (5) All of the time

Fine Motor Skills:

1. Grasping _____

2. Touching _____

3. Building _____

4. Pouring _____

5. Stringing _____

6. Drawing _____

7. Cutting _____

8. Hammering _____

9. Zipping _____

10. Buttoning _____

Gross Motor Skills:

1. Body awareness _____

2. Balance _____

   a. static _____

   b. dynamic _____

3. Creeping/crawling _____

4. Walking _____

5. Rolling _____

6. Pushing/pulling _____

7. Lifting _____

8. Throwing _____

9. Catching _____

10. Striking _____

11. Climbing _____

12. Running _____

13. Hopping _____

14. Skipping _____

15. Jumping _____

Socialization Skills:

1. Communicates with adults _____

2. Communicates with peers _____

3. Plays independently _____

4. Small group participation _____

5. Large group participation _____

6. Responds to instructions _____

7. Completes activity _____

8. Other _____

Behavioral Skills:

1. Participant will attempt new activities _____

   Comment _____

2. Participant easily attempts new situations and/or changes in routine _____

   Comment _____

3. Participant interacts with others in group situations _____

   Comment _____

4. Participant understands directions _____

   Comment _____

5. Participant can follow directions _____

   Comment _____

6. Participant persists in completing a task _____

   Comment _____

7. How well does the participant communicate? _____

   Comment _____

8. How does the participant react to a structured situation? _____

   Comment _____

9. How does the participant react to an unstructured situation? _____

   Comment _____

(continued)

FIGURE 11.1. (*Continued*)

Please comment:

1. What behavior management techniques are utilized? _____

_____

2. Please list any activities the participant particularly enjoys. _____

_____

3. What specific goals and behavioral objectives outlined in the participant's activity program would you like to see continued and enhanced in our program? _____

_____

_____

Recreation Skills:
Please rate as follows: (1) Never observed   (2) Never   (3) Sometimes   (4) Most of the time   (5) All of the time

Arts and Crafts:

1. Ceramics _____

2. Cut and paste _____

3. Drawing _____

4. Handiwork _____

5. Other _____

Music and Dance:

1. Singing _____

2. Dancing _____

3. Rhythm instruments _____

4. Musical games _____

5. Other _____

Nature and Wildlife:

1. Camping _____

2. Hiking _____

3. Horticulture _____

Sports and Games:

1. Table games _____

2. Active sports _____

3. Quiet games _____

4. Low-organized games _____

5. High-organized games _____

6. Other _____

Drama and Puppetry:

1. Imaginary play _____

2. Plays with puppets _____

3. Costume play _____

4. Drama games _____

5. Story time _____

6. Other _____

4. Outdoor experiences _____

5. Field trips (list, if any) _____

_____

_____

_____

6. Other _____

Other staff observations:

SOURCE: Developed as part of a class project for a course in Program Development in Therapeutic Recreation at Virginia Commonwealth University by Ronald Reynolds, Veronica Davis, B. J. Mines, and Andrew Wilds.

FIGURE 11.2.   Assessment of Environmental Barriers to Leisure Experiences Scale

Factor 1: Community Resources
(Refers to the presence or absence of programs that meet the needs of the client)
Sample Questions:
I don't go to recreation centers because they don't offer activities I can join.
Comments:

I don't go to the park because it's too hard to move around on the grass or rough ground.
Comments:

Factor 2: Architectural Barriers
(Both manmade and naturally occurring obstacles that are inherent in the design and construction of a facility)
Sample Questions:
Narrow doors and stairways make it hard for me to get around a building.
Comments:

It's hard for me to join in any outdoor activities unless they are done on a hard surface.
Comments:

FIGURE 11.2.   *(Continued)*

Factor 3: Family Support
(Members of the child's family providing forms of emotional, physical, psychological, and financial support)
Sample Questions:
My parents don't take me to local recreation activities.
Comments:

My brothers or sisters don't encourage me to get involved in recreational activities.
Comments:

Factor 4: Community Support
(Programs designed to supplement existing available recreation programs)
Sample Questions:
There aren't any recreation programs for me at school.
Comments:

There aren't any recreation programs offered by any of the neighborhood service groups like the Y.
Comments:

Factor 5: Care-Giver Support
(Includes efforts on the part of parents, guardians, relatives, teachers, therapists, and recreation leaders)
Sample Questions:
When I'm at a recreation activity, the leader doesn't try to get me involved.
Comments:

My teacher doesn't encourage me to join in recreation activities.
Comments:

Factor 6: Accessible and Available Transportation
(Involves public transit, private transportation enterprises, and family automobiles)
Sample Questions:
My parents or other family members are unable to drive me to recreation activities.
Comments:

There is a lack of accessible buses and taxis to get me to community recreation facilities.
Comments:

SOURCE: Division of Recreation and Leisure Studies, *Manual for Utilization of the Assessment of Environmental Barriers to Leisure Experiences* (Denton, Texas: North Texas State University, 1982).

CONCERNING THE AVAILABILITY
OF SERVICE:

1. Are facilities and programs interspersed throughout the given locale, thus allowing maximum access for all disabled people?

2. Are facilities conveniently reached by public transportation?

3. Are programs offered during time periods which are convenient for disabled persons?

4. Can disabled people afford program admission and participation fees?

5. Are facilities physically accessible to disabled persons?

6. Are disabled persons informed of existing leisure opportunities by the mass media and individual agencies?

7. Are the types of information concerning programs available in a variety of forms including braille, cassette tapes, large print, etc.?

8. Are programs advertised in a dignified way that indicates that they are available to disabled persons?

9. Are the opportunities offered appropriate and available to all age groups?

CONCERNING THE QUALITY OF SERVICE:

1. Are the types of activities and experiences offered and the locales of programs appropriate to the age of the client?

2. Is the program offered in such a manner that the client can proceed at his or her own rate?

3. Are instructors and leaders comfortable with disabled participants? Do they have the skills and abilities to adapt or modify programs if necessary?

4. Are participants given the opportunity to help in the planning of programs and experiences?

5. Is the leader/participant ratio small enough to insure individual instruction of disabled persons?

6. Do program staff regularly evaluate the progress of the client and the satisfaction of the client with the program?

7. Are a variety of programs, services, and experiences offered within a given community? For example, are there programs requiring different skill levels for participation? Are there individual and group experiences? Is there a variety of social, cultural, dramatic, craft, and spectator activities offered?

8. Do the majority of leisure services offered involve the opportunity for disabled and nondisabled people to interact with each other?

9. Are leisure opportunities provided by a variety of agencies and organizations? For example, does a large cross section of public, private, commercial, and voluntary leisure services exist, or is the provision of recreational opportunities chiefly the function of the municipal recreation department?[19]

PLANNING

Once the process of assessment is complete, the therapeutic recreation specialist is faced with three related tasks within the goal-development phase. These may be viewed as (1) translating client-assessment information into behavioral goals, (2) translating environmental assessments into goals related to the removal of barriers, and (3) developing programs or interventions designed to meet the objectives established in tasks 1 and 2. The following sections provide an overview of procedures relative to this process and give examples to illustrate each facet of the planning phase.

Individual Goal Determination

The importance of the individual goal-development process in the community-based model has been highlighted by Stanley:

Regardless of whether the individual is to be mainstreamed totally or in part (or to be placed in a specialized/segregated setting) a *goal setting procedure* is undertaken for each of the applicants. This process helps to determine the actual recreational experiences in which the individual will participate. When all aspects of an activity (cognitive affective, social, physical) are understood through careful activity analysis, it can be determined if indeed that activity will accomplish the goals set or if it can be modified to do so.[20]

According to Hutchison and Lord, objectives of community-based recreation programs may be both general, in the case of an entire program or service, and specific, when an individual's skills need upgrading. They offer the following examples to illustrate how these two types of objectives may be developed.

I. Program objective for an individual: to be able to reach five places of interest in the community independently using the transit system.
   Enabling objectives:
   1. To obtain information regarding how to get to destination "A" by bus
   2. To go to destination by bus with an advocate
   3. To go to destination by bus without an advocate
   4. To repeat enabling objectives 1–3 in terms of four other places of interest in the community
II. Program objective for a group of children: to develop social play skills.
   Enabling objectives for an individual child:
   1. To play beside one other child at the sand table at least twice in a one-hour play period
   2. To play with one other child at the sand table at least twice (sharing toys or building together)[21]

Environmental Goal Determination

As indicated in the previous assessment section, determining external factors that may pose barriers to the client is an extremely important undertaking. Once these factors

have been initially determined, it is important to specify the objectives that must be met in overcoming these obstacles. A systematic plan may then be developed for the removal of these impediments to leisure participation. Carter, Frost, and Hoffman have developed a decision-making process for the elimination of five common external problems inhibiting the provision of therapeutic recreation service in the community.[22] These problems are: (1) the identification of appropriate clientele, (2) attitudinal and architectural accessibility, (3) transportation, (4) appropriate program provision, and (5) financial resources. To facilitate the resolution of these barriers, a decision-making model is used. Figure 11.3 shows the decision-making process for identification of appropriate clientele (issue 1).

After the completion of this problem-clarification stage, a management checklist may be employed to operationalize the decision-making process as related to each of the critical issues. (Figure 11.4). In using this

FIGURE 11.3. Decision-Making Model

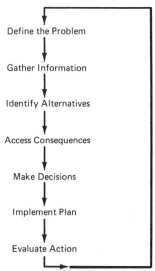

SOURCE: Based on Marcia Jean Carter, Bob Frost, and Judy Hoffman, "Closing the Gap: Community Programs for Special Populations," *Expanding Horizons in Therapeutic Recreation* VI (1978), p. 199.

FIGURE 11.4. Management Checklist for Community Special Recreation Programs

DECISION PRIORITY	CRITICAL ISSUES	ASSESSMENT		IMPLEMENTATION PLAN
		Positive	Negative	
I. Clientele				
	Identification			
2	Demographic survey	Information accurate	Time consuming	Secure list
1	Resource lists	List available	Confidentiality	Develop survey
3	Word of mouth	Personal touch	Lacks reliability	Distribute
	Involvement			
___	Advisory			
___	Media contact			
___	Personal contact			
___	Assume established programs			
	Maintenance			
___	Program variety			
___	Consumer input			
___	Record keeping/evaluating			
II. Accessibility				
	Attitudinal			
___	Advocate group			
___	Exposure			
___	Education			
	Architectural			
___	Legislation			
___	Consultation			
	Equipment/supplies			
___	Self-made			
___	Purchase adapted			
___	Modify			
III. Transportation				
	Usability			
___	Legislation			
___	Volunteer			
___	Profit making			
___	Private			
___	Agency sponsored			
	Cost			
___	Budget allocation			
___	Fund raising			
___	Fees/charges			
___	Cost sharing			
___	Private solicitation			

(*continued*)

IV. Programming

Staff
___ In-service programs
___ Salary incentive
___ Recognition procedures
___ Feedback channels
___ Recruitment/evaluation
___ Innovative services
___ High-risk activities
___ Leisure education
___ Homebound programs
___ Cooperative programming

V. Financial Resources

Direct Revenue
___ Budget preparation
___ Political channels
___ Program justification

Indirect revenue
___ Grants
___ Community resources
___ Solicitation

SOURCE: Marcia Jean Carter, Bob Frost, and Judy Hoffman, "Closing the Gap: Community Programs for Special Populations," *Expanding Horizons in Therapeutic Recreation VI,* Gerald Hitzhusen, ed. (Columbia, Mo.: Department of Recreation and Park Administration, University of Missouri, 1979), p. 200.

tool, the far-left column is provided for prioritizing decisions, while the far-right column is used to identify a realistic plan of action.[23]

Witt has suggested a similar goal-development process, which assigns responsibilities to specific individuals. The worksheet shown in Figure 11.5 represents a sample plan for achieving goals related to the transportation needs of an orthopedically disabled child. This form was developed for use in each of six areas identified on pp. 293–294.[24]

IMPLEMENTATION

After appropriate individual and environmental goals have been established, the therapeutic recreation specialist initiates programs and implements plans that will directly involve the participant in various community-based leisure opportunities. The following section describes this implementation phase by overviewing the recreation-integration process, discussing new roles that the therapeutic recreation specialist will adopt within this framework, and providing examples of actual programs and services that portray the application of the community-based model.

The Recreation-Integration Process

It would be futile to discuss the practice of therapeutic recreation in the community without an overview of the integration or mainstreaming process. Indeed, there has been so much recent thought, discussion,

FIGURE 11.5. AEBLE Planning Form

Date 8–21–81

Name of Child: Ernie S.   Age 11   Sex M   Disability Spinal Cord Trauma

Name of Interviewer: Michael A.   Position/Title Teacher   Name of Facility Crockett Elem. School

Factor (s) to be corrected: 1. Community Recreation Sources

2. Transportation Systems

Goal	Strategy	Responsibility	Date Begun	Date Completed	Evaluation
1. To increase the availability of recreation programs that Ernie can participate in at the local community recreation center.	(1a) Contact local recreation center.	(1a) Teacher	9–1–81	9–15–81	(a) Talked to director. She's very supportive.
	(1b) Determine what programs are offered.	(1b) Teacher, recreation leader	9–15–81	9–16–81	(b) A large realm of programs are offered.
	(1c) Determine which programs or activities Ernie is interested in.	(1c) Ernie, Teacher	9–16–81	9–16–81	(c) Swimming and chess.
	(1d) Modify activities if necessary.	(1d) Teacher, recreation leader	9–16–81	10–5–81	(d) Join chess club and get qualified instructor.
2. To develop an appropriate and adequate transportation system for Ernie to use to get to and from the recreation center.	(2a) Get bus schedule and fare rates.	(2a) Teacher	9–1–81	9–2–81	(2a)Talked to bus company.
	(2b) Determine where Ernie can get on a bus.	(2b) Teacher, recreation leader	9–1–81	9–2–81	(2b)Talked to bus company.
	(2c) Determine if Ernie is able to get on and off a bus.	(2c) Teacher and Ernie	9–3–81	9–5–81	(2c)Ernie is able to get on and off the bus.

SOURCE: Division of Recreation and Leisure Studies, *Manual for the Utilization of the Assessment of Environmental Barriers to Leisure Experiences* (Denton, Texas: North Texas State University, 1982).

and at times debate concerning the involvement of disabled persons in regular recreation programs that a great deal of the recent therapeutic recreation literature has addressed this subject. The following statements provide a working definition of the recreation integration or mainstreaming process and serve to illustrate its depth and complexity.

> The mutual acceptance and interaction of disabled and nondisabled individuals is a goal of mainstreaming. Yet a broader definition considers mainstreaming to be a developmental, step-by-step process. This process entails careful planning to develop a disabled person's skills and decision making abilities, to initiate interagency cooperation, to train staff, to educate able-bodied consumers and the community.[25]

> In other words, we are mainstreaming not people, but the system.[26]

Differences of opinion exist among therapeutic recreation specialists concerning the number of phases in the recreation-integration process, but there is general agreement that it is *sequential* in nature. Spinak conceptualizes this progression from segregated to integrated programs as one involving institutional programming, recreation programs "for" the disabled in society, recreation programs "with" the disabled in society, and integrated programs in the normalized area of society.[27]

Thompson presents a slightly longer continuum involving institutional participation, specialized program participation, transitional participation, specialized community-based participation, regular community participation, and independent community participation.[28] In a similar vein, Hutchison and Lord view recreation integration as passing from segregated experiences to physical and finally social integration. Their steps include:

1. Upgrading experiences in institutions
2. Segregated experiences in advocate associations
3. Segregated upgrading experiences in community settings
4. Upgrading experiences in the community
5. Integrated experiences in the community with advocacy and support
6. Integrated experiences in the community with little or no advocacy
7. Ongoing community involvement[29]

Stensrud has suggested that recreation-integration might follow this model (Figure 11.6.)

Before concluding our discussion of the nature of the recreation-integration process, it may be helpful to review some general guidelines relative to this procedure.

1. The involvement of disabled persons in various recreation programs is both a process and an ultimate goal. Therefore, one individual could conceivably be involved in several activities simultaneously.
2. Separate programs should be seen as stepping stones to participation in regular activities, as outlined in the previous models.
3. The integration process is applicable to a wide variety of disabilities including visual and auditory impairments, emotional problems, and physical conditions.
4. Not everyone would benefit from immediate placement in independent, community-based programs. However, as in principle 2, separate programs should be viewed as prerequisites to community involvement.
5. Successful participation in community-based recreation opportunities is best achieved by the formation of small groups of disabled persons.
6. Grouping different disabilities together does not constitute successful recreation integration. Disabled and nondisabled persons should be free to interact.

FIGURE 11.6. Sequential Recreation-Integration Streams

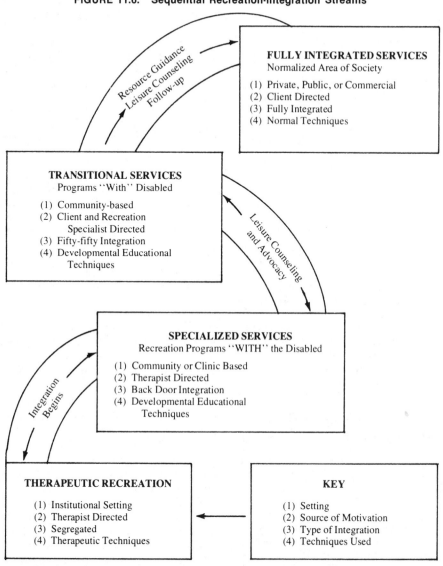

SOURCE: Carol Stensrud, "Sequential Recreation Integration Streams," *Leisurability* 5, no. 2 (1978), 29.

7. Disabled persons should have access to activities that are appropriate to their age.

8. The involvement of disabled persons can best be achieved by a *cooperative* approach involving family members, advocate associations, and institutional and social service personnel.[30]

Role of the Therapeutic Recreation Specialist

It is obvious from the preceding discussion that the community-based therapeutic recreation specialist will have to provide an array of services to a variety of clients along the previously described integration continuum. Providing these services will necessitate the adoption of several new roles on the part of community-based therapeutic recreation personnel. Thompson has succinctly outlined many of these functions in his discussion of role changes for the therapeutic and community recreator in the 1980s. He states:

> The therapeutic recreationist has generally become an influential catalyst in the community mainstreaming movement, very similar to the role of the special educator in the public school system. It appears that those professionals have been at the forefront of mainstreaming efforts in both public schools and community services. Many of these people have assumed a very assertive advocacy role as an advocate, catalyst, trainer, consultant, facilitator, coordinator, educator, enabler, and basically a more versatile role in assisting other individuals, groups and organizations showing interest in mainstreaming programs. It is imperative that the interested and committed therapeutic recreator become more interested, aware, involved and knowledgeable of community programs, political processes, organizational structures, funding resources in the community, interagency cooperation relationships and advocacy organizations. In addition, "a courtship, if not a marriage" with community recreation specialists is critical in fully developing the community's potential for meeting the needs of its handicapped citizens. The therapeutic recreation specialist can play a valuable role in terms of being a resource person or trainer to those program leaders representing community park and recreation departments, youth serving agencies, allied disciplines and rehabilitation centers.[31]

Other authors have also underscored the necessity of expanding roles beyond that of direct service provision in community-based settings. Howe-Murphy states:

> As the change from the traditional separateness of therapeutic-general services to a step-by-step, non-stigmatizing continuum of services emerges, and as the ecological approach to services becomes pronounced, the roles of recreators will change as well. Contingent upon specific community needs, therapeutic recreators, particularly will be called upon and, indeed, should take the lead in providing general staff in-service training programs, consultation, public awareness programs and advocacy in conjunction with community residents. Where direct service provision remains important, awareness of those determinants that promote independence, skill development and social integration must be developed and maintained. New concepts in programming to provide transitional programs certainly will provide new challenges requiring creative problem solving.[32]

Both of the preceding position statements strongly emphasize that community-based therapeutic recreation specialists must work closely with other persons having direct client contact in varied settings. Lindley recognizes some unique challenges that may occur when community therapeutic recreation specialists work with clients who are wholly or in part subject to the supervision of an institution.[33] In cases where the institution is totally responsible for the care of the individual, he suggests that adequate institutional administrative support be given to budget allocation for transportation, insurance, staff, equipment, supplies, and time to visit community recreation agencies. In situations where clients are not totally involved in residential programs, community-based therapeutic recreation personnel could conduct clinics in leisure-skill development and involve the clients directly in community recreation resources. When discharge takes place, referral to community activities should be implemented.

Based upon the preceding discussion, it is apparent that the activities of the therapeutic recreation specialist in the community model must center upon (1) the provision of pre- and postdischarge institutional leisure education, (2) in-service training of general recreation staff personnel, and (3) advocacy measures in the community. Much information is beginning to appear in the literature relative to these three types of services. The following represents brief examples of how to provide each of these types of service in the community model of therapeutic recreation.

Leisure Education. Ross has developed a comprehensive framework for post-discharge preparation and training for clients who have had little experience with active community-based leisure participation. He suggests nine areas that should be addressed by the community-based therapeutic recreation specialist (in co-operation with residential facility staff).

1. Awareness of Leisure
   What it is
   How it *feels*
   Work/leisure distinction
2. Time Budgeting
   Daily and weekly time expenditure
3. Resources
   a) Personal
      Transportation, money, time, leisure skills, life skills
   b) Community
      Programs, facilities, leisure options, support services (counseling, volunteer services, leisure companion)
4. Leisure Interests/Experiences
   Past participation
   Current participation
   Projected participation
5. Setting Goals and Incremental Objectives
   Specific to leisure interests/experiences (step 4) and resources (step 3)
6. Planning
   Development of a leisure plan
   Goals and objectives (step 5) operation-

ally defined with standards for measurement and evaluation
7. Implementation of Leisure Plan
8. Evaluation
   Ongoing and final evaluation
9. Assessment of Progress and Modification/Establishment of New Goals and Objectives[34]

An excellent example of one such cooperative approach to leisure education is the joint partnership developed by the Northwest Special Recreation Association of Chicago and the Northwest Suburban Special Education Organization. In this arrangement special recreation personnel organize and lead community-based activities for mentally retarded, hearing and visually impaired, multiply handicapped, learning disabled, and emotionally disturbed children. They also assume responsibility for support services such as reservation of facilities, development of flyers, and surveys of parents as to the needs of their children. In turn, school staff members jointly lead activities, provide supervision, and discipline and evaluate programs.[35]

Staff Training. Stanley provides an extremely useful plan for training general recreation staff and creating community acceptance of disabled participants. She makes the following concrete suggestions/recommendations for achieving these two goals.

Survey staff as to what they feel is necessary for them to be comfortable with disabled participants.

Begin training with attitude awareness and sensitization experiences.

Arrange for staff observation of, or participation with, disabled persons involved in recreational activities.

Review characteristics of various disabilities and emergency health care procedures.

Meet individually with the activity leader to review functional assessments of the participants.

Sensitize non-disabled participants through simulation exercises.

Demonstrate aids and modified recreation devices. Invite disabled guest speakers into programs.

Arrange for the disabled participant and/or family member to meet with the activity leader beforehand.[36]

Advocacy. A common theme in the literature related to community therapeutic recreation service is that therapeutic recreation specialists must serve as *advocates* for their clients. Advocacy may be defined as:

> A process directed toward improving the quality of goods and services rendered to consumers and an advocate as a person who generates and sustains the advocacy process. Functions include analysis, critique, planning, organizing, informing, etc.[37]

There are several distinct roles that may be played within this advocacy framework by therapeutic recreation specialists. According to Edginton and Compton, these include:

The *initiator, strategist or organizer* who assists a disabled person or group of disabled persons in making concrete plans to be involved in existing community recreational opportunities

The *ombudsman* who gathers information concerning disabled persons' legal rights to leisure services

The *mediator or arbitrator* who negotiates if no response is obtained from existing providers of leisure services

The *lobbyist* who seeks to persuade those making decisions to consider the leisure rights of disabled persons

The *counselor* who informs groups or individuals about existing leisure resources

The *educator* who seeks to make the public aware of the recreational needs of the disabled

The *analyst or evaluator* who monitors whether or not an agency has met its objectives in serving the leisure needs of disabled persons.[38]

Program Tracks

Although this section is addressed from the standpoint of a therapeutic recreation specialist employed by a municipal recreation department, the principles outlined here are applicable to those who work in other community settings, such as advocate associations and schools.

Once the community-based therapeutic recreation specialist has a thorough knowledge of the integration process and the potential roles he or she might perform in its implementation, an important decision must be made. This decision revolves around which clusters of activities will be organized into programmatic units and what the specific points of contact will be between the community therapeutic recreation specialist and the participant. Since client needs in such programs tend to be extremely diverse, program offerings that can meet a broad range of individual goals are necessary. A popular approach to programming, which capitalizes on the notion of sequential tracks as previously described, is the *continuum* model. An example of this paradigm is the mainstreaming progression developed by the Division of Therapeutic Recreation of the Cincinnati Recreation Commission. Table 11.1 illustrates this model.

This continuum can accommodate large numbers of persons with divergent needs and move them progressively toward self-sustained leisure participation. To illustrate, severely mentally retarded children may participate in the Level I program for an extended period of time, while physically handicapped children may rapidly acquire the requisite skills in this program to acceler-

TABLE 11.1. **Division of Therapeutic Recreation Continuum for Mainstreaming**

Level I	Level II	Level III	Level IV
Program for persons still exhibiting basic needs who need a 1:1 or 1:2 ratio, not possessing basic sensory-motor and/or self-help skills	Program for persons possessing sensory-motor skills, able to begin functioning in a group situation and begin learning basic fine and gross motor skills for high-level recreation activities	Programs for persons possessing skills necessary to learn high-level recreation activities	Integration
	EVALUATION REQUIREMENTS		
Sensory-motor skill assessment	Individualized fine and gross motor skill assessment	Individualized evaluation of sport and leisure skills achieved	
Optional: Self-help skill assessment as needed Body awareness skill assessment	Individual socialization skill assessment Basic activity skill assessment	Group socialization skill assessments	

SOURCE: Catherine Burdett and Mary E. Miller, "Mainstreaming in a Municipal Recreation Department Utilizing a Continuum Method," *Therapeutic Recreation Journal* 13, no. 4 (1979), 46.

ate their advancement through Levels II–IV. It is also important to note that some participants will be involved in several activities at different levels simultaneously.

In designing such programmatic offerings in the community-based model, the therapeutic recreation specialist has a plethora of activities from which to choose. An important consideration in the selection of activities should be the concept of *transfer*. Specifically, activities should be selected that will enable the participants to achieve their goals in a variety of settings under a wide range of conditions. Hutchison suggests the following ways to maximize the potential transfer benefits of community-based therapeutic recreation programs.

1. Ensure that special programs are meaningful and relevant. Techniques include: involving participants in the choice of activities and making certain that offerings are skill and age appropriate.
2. Design "special" programs which resemble integrated settings as closely as possible. Characteristics to consider include: client ratio, complexity, novelty, and structure of tasks.
3. Teach meaningful generalizations rather than specific skills or concepts. For example, if an objective of a program is to improve physical fitness, participants should learn that fitness transcends specific exercises and involves such things as cardiovascular strength and endurance, proper nutrition, and positive mental health.
4. Include opportunities for free play and creativity in programs which have large amounts of training, direction and structure. Techniques such as problem solving and guided discovery facilitate transfer and generalization.[39]

Depending upon the size of the community and the resources of the therapeutic recreation specialist, it may be desirable to organize program services that extend beyond the traditional boundaries of the municipal department. The following organizational framework utilizes five key program tracks in its community-based model of service. These may be classified as:

1. Institutional services
2. Advocate association services
3. Community-based skill-upgrading programs
4. Homebound individualized services
5. Community-based programs[40]

Before discussing each of these avenues of programming, it is important to outline three important assumptions that influenced the selection of these possible tracks. First, these divisions are not based upon such factors as age, type of disability, or activity. Rather, they were developed in response to the needs of individuals requiring a specific type of recreational service. As such, this system emphasizes an outreach orientation rather than the provision of "packaged" programs. Second, these categories of service were not conceived to be exclusive or static; instead, it was felt that individuals could receive several types of services simultaneously and move freely through the tracks as described in the previous sequential system. Third, this plan allows therapeutic recreation specialists to assume the major responsibility for one or more of these areas of service.

The following section presents a brief discussion of some of the services a community-based therapeutic recreation specialist might provide within each of these program tracks.

Track 1: Institutional Services. There are many ways in which community therapeutic recreation specialists can assist local residential facilities. One method is working with agency staff to develop leisure-counseling/education programs to improve patients' values and attitudes toward leisure, increase their repertoire of postdischarge leisure skills, and improve their knowledge of recreation resources in the community.

One intervention designed to link a psychiatric hospital to a community recreation program has been described by Laudick, McGovern, and Cosgrove.[41] After substantial planning involving the recreation staff of the hospital and the therapeutic recreation staff of a municipal department, four points of contact were made: (1) providing access to community recreation centers, park facilities and schools for the psychiatric patients; (2) having patients participate in community recreation programs under the supervision of staff from both agencies; (3) involving patients nearing discharge as volunteer recreation aides in municipal programs; and (4) having the community-based therapeutic recreation staff provide postdischarge information concerning clients to hospital staff.

Community therapeutic recreation personnel can also provide a valuable referral service to institutions. The recreational opportunities monitored by the therapeutic recreation specialist should include not only the activities offered by his or her department but the range of leisure opportunities available in the entire community. The following three hypothetical examples illustrate the breadth of the referral process.

An amputee recently discharged from a Veterans' Administration hospital is guided to a municipally operated adapted aquatics program.

A paraplegic who has recently moved to a new city is provided with a list of accessible restaurants.

An elderly woman who has suffered a cerebral vascular accident is made aware of a local stroke club.

Track 2: Advocate Associations. Today most major disability groups are represented by volunteer advocate associations. Indeed, in communities of even moderate size it is common to find local agencies and organizations designed to meet the needs of blind, mentally retarded, emotionally disturbed, and orthopedically handicapped persons, substance-abuse clients, and others. There are several responsibilities the community-based therapeutic recreator may assume when working with advocate associations. These activities would vary depending upon whether or not the advocate association employs full- or part-time recreation personnel. A partial list of duties within the advocate association track might include:

Providing consultative services in the area of leisure-skill development to special education classes, day-care and training centers, sheltered workshops, and other facilities operated by local associations

Furnishing information and assistance to families of the disabled person relative to local recreational programs and facilities

Providing community education programs designed to make the public aware of the leisure abilities of a particular disability group

Assisting agency personnel in the development of grant proposals to obtain financial support for in-service training and/or demonstration projects

Developing a referral system with appropriate recording and reporting techniques to place advocate association clients in community-based recreational opportunities

Track 3: Community-Based Skill-Upgrading Programs. As mentioned in the previous recreation-integration section, this track consists of special programs and classes conducted by the community therapeutic recreation specialist exclusively for small groups of disabled persons. When appropriate, trained general recreation staff or volunteers could assist in these efforts. These programs would allow clients progressing from the institutional and advocate association tracks to acquire the physical and social skills necessary to proceed to track 5 (community-based programming). In

addition to assuming the direct referral role described in tracks 1 and 2, the therapeutic recreation specialist coordinating this track would have the following responsibilities:

Developing specific assessment procedures and instruments containing appropriate demographic, leisure interest, and leisure-skill information as outlined in the first section of this chapter

Coordinating regular meetings involving institutional, advocate association, and municipal recreation personnel

Preparing individualized program plans for persons referred from institutions, advocate associations, and other agencies

Developing and maintaining a resource file containing information on other skill-development programs in the community

Identifying external sources of funding for staff development and demonstration projects

Conducting in-service training for regular recreation personnel

Periodically evaluating program offerings and individual treatment plans

Track 4: Homebound Services. In any community there may be hundreds or thousands of individuals who, for physical or financial reasons, have difficulty participating in organized social service or recreational programs. Examples of these persons are:

A man with a high-level spinal cord injury who needs a large amount of supervision and assistance by his family

A senior citizen with very brittle bones who does not want to negotiate icy sidewalks in winter

A recently discharged mental patient who is not a threat to society but nevertheless feels threatened by it

The needs of these and similar individuals can be met on several levels. First, after an initial evaluation by the community therapeutic recreation specialist, the client could be referred to a volunteer who could make weekly visits to the individual, act as a friend, arrange transportation, or physically assist the individual in performing activities. In many cases the volunteer and therapeutic recreation specialist could act as advocates for the disabled person by encouraging agencies to improve their accessibility and to waive or reduce fees when appropriate. The therapeutic recreation specialist, whenever feasible, would encourage the homebound individual to become involved in activities in his or her immediate neighborhood.

Specific tasks and duties that would be performed by the track 4 therapeutic recreation specialist include:

Conducting a survey (possibly using the media and/or social service agencies) to determine the location and needs of the homebound

Developing a monthly newsletter to be mailed to disabled persons that would announce recreational opportunities and contain games, puzzles, and other sedentary activities

Creating a regularly aired show for public television which would reach disabled persons in their homes. Such a program could feature adapted activities, health hints, referral services, etc.

Developing a cadre of volunteers from churches, civic, and service organizations who could phone or make weekly visits to the homebound

Serving as a liaison with other track and community recreation personnel to facilitate the involvement of the client in activities outside the home

Developing inexpensive "homebound recreation kits" with literature (audiotape, braille, or raised letter), crafts supplies, games, horiticultural materials etc. that could be distributed and used in the home

Creating a resource/referral file of activities for the homebound

Developing a lending library of talking books and tapes on recreational activities which could be mailed to disabled individuals upon request.

Track 5: Community-Based Programs.

This track is designed for individuals who are able to participate in regular recreation programs and classes but will need some type of support or minimal assistance. People could enter this track directly or through referral from other tracks. Examples of individuals involved in this level of program include:

A physically disabled child with good swimming skills who needs help changing and moving through the locker room

A partially sighted senior adult who, while able to paint, needs help mixing and distinguishing colors

A deaf adolescent who is physically fit, yet needs help interpreting the instructions in an aerobic exercise class

The major function of the therapeutic recreation specialist in charge of this track is to facilitate the involvement of persons with adequate skills into activities that are offered to the general population. There are many ways in which this goal can be achieved. For example, the specialist in charge of track 5 might explain some of the relevant limitations of the individual to the regular class instructor and suggest some ways to modify the activity. He or she might arrange for a volunteer to accompany the disabled person to the program on the first session. In special cases adapted equipment might be ordered or designed. After a trial period, the client, the volunteer (if needed), the therapeutic recreation specialist, and the regular instructor should meet to determine if the disabled person should continue in this track or possibly be moved to track 3.

Some of the duties that might be performed by the track 5 specialist are:

Conducting preactivity assessments of all clients entering the program

Acting as a liaison between the disabled individual and the regular activity instructor

Recruiting, screening, and training volunteers to work with disabled individuals

Serving as a liaison between other tracks, hospitals, and agencies in seeking new clients for the program

Acting as a resource person and troubleshooter for the regular recreation instructor

Developing and maintaining a resource file of adapted equipment

Conducting periodic assessments of the client's performance in regular recreation programs.

As mentioned, in a given situation the number of tracks that can be served by a municipal department will depend upon the number of trained therapeutic recreation specialists in the department, the size of the community, and factors such as the availability of leisure opportunities and level of support from other community organizations.

PROGRAM EXAMPLES

This section presents examples of some of the programs offered by a progressive municipal therapeutic recreation division. The broad range of its goals and activities for all ages and disabilities should be noted.[42]

YOUTH PROGRAMS

After-School Action. Program Goal: To provide a variety of recreational activities from sports to arts and crafts appropriate for disabled youths six to twenty years of age. All activities will be structured to meet the participant's needs as well as facilitate skill development in an enjoyable atmosphere. Participants may attend any time during the program hours.

Advanced Bowling. Program Goal: To provide advanced instruction to youths nine to seventeen years of age in bowling techniques, including ball-handling skills, scoring, and terminology, to facilitate the future use of bowling as a recreational pastime. Individuals must have successfully mastered the introductory bowling class.

Let's Move. Program Goal: To develop gross motor skills, body awareness, spatial

relationships, and balance and coordination of visually impaired children four to eight years of age.

New Beginnings. Program Goal: To provide mentally retarded youths eleven to fifteen years of age with exposure to a variety of recreational activities using community resources.

Perceptual-Motor Training. Program Goal: To improve perceptual-motor functioning in learning-disabled youths five to fourteen years of age through skill assessment, prescriptive programming, and skill evaluation.

Saturday Play Day. Program Goal: To provide youths five to ten years of age the opportunity to participate in, and develop skills for, a variety of recreational activities including sports, games, crafts, music, and special events.

Swimming Lessons. Program Goal: To provide aquatic instruction to emotionally disturbed youth five to eighteen years of age. Instruction is based on Red Cross standards.

ADOLESCENT/ADULT PROGRAMS

Activity Club. Program Goal: To introduce community leisure resources and promote independence among mentally retarded adolescents and young adults by coordinating group outings.

Adult Recreation. Program Goal: To provide mentally retarded adults fifteen and older with minimum assistance and supervision in the selection of and participation in ongoing activities.

Cooking. Program Goal: To teach the basic skills of food preparation, service, clean up, and menu planning for disabled individuals aged thirteen and older.

Field Practice. Program Goal: To provide physically disabled individuals aged thirteen and older with supervised practice and coaching in all field events of the National Wheelchair Athletic Association, to improve fitness and/or prepare for competition.

Phoenix Club. Program Goal: To provide the opportunity for disabled adults to adjust to acquired handicaps, receive support and assistance, and improve self-image through recreation and leisure activities in the least restrictive environment.

Skeet and Trap-Shooting Clinic. Program Goal: A clinic to be held for wheelchair-bound adults aged eighteen and older designed to teach gun safety, shooting fundamentals, and range work.

Leisure Adult Club. Program Goal: To provide a variety of recreational opportunities to adults aged eighteen and older; to encourage decision making and establish resources for utilizing personal leisure time. The program is operated in conjunction with Comprehensive Mental Health Services.

ALL-AGE PROGRAMS

Swimming. Program Goal: To provide skill instruction, teach aquatic games, and promote awareness of appropriate and safe water conduct. All skills taught according to Red Cross standards.

Tennis. Program Goal: To teach and/or increase tennis skills of participants aged nine and older with an emphasis on individual skill development and a goal of future leisure participation. Special events will be held at the end of each session.

Slimnastics. Program Goal: To provide a structured program of exercise and physical fitness for disabled individuals aged sixteen and older.

Sun Wheelers Swim Team. Program Goal: To provide instruction and coaching to disabled athletes aged thirteen and older who are interested in competitive swimming.

Table Tennis. Program Goal: To provide physically disabled individuals aged thirteen and older supervised practice and coaching in table tennis in preparation for competition or just for fun.

Fitness and Conditioning. Program Goal: To provide physically disabled individuals aged twelve and older the opportunity to maintain and/or improve fitness. The program includes a personalized prescription of exercise, weight training, and aerobic conditioning.

Horticulture. Program Goal: To provide the opportunity to plant, maintain, and harvest a garden under the supervision of qualified staff and volunteers. Participants include clients of MR/DD programs and any others interested.

Outdoor Recreation. Program Goal: To expose youths twelve years of age and older to a variety of outdoor activities including camping, nature hikes, ropes, and initiative activities and water sports.

Slalom. Program Goal: To provide physically disabled adults thirteen and older supervised practice and coaching in the wheelchair slalom, to prepare for competition under the auspices of the National Wheelchair Athletic Association.

Track Practice. Program Goal: To provide physically disabled individuals aged thirteen and older supervised practice and coaching in all track events of the National Wheelchair Athletic Association, to improve fitness and/or prepare for competition.

Wheelchair Basketball. Program Goal: To provide a competitive sports program for physically disabled adults aged sixteen and older. Program includes two scheduled practices, uniforms, transportation, conference dues, and more.

EVALUATION

Once participants have become involved in community-based therapeutic recreation programs, periodic evaluation of their progress must take place. Because this model of service is so new, few standardized evaluation procedures or instruments exist. Nevertheless, this process may be readily undertaken by reviewing the objectives that were developed in the individual- and environmental-assessment and goal-determination phases. For example, changes in the client's functional ability may be measured by using the information obtained through the participant observation form (p. 299) as a baseline. In this fashion social, learning, physical, and self-help skills can be readily evaluated. Likewise, changes in leisure skills and interests can be detected and noted. Environmental factors in the areas of community resources, architectural barriers, family, community, and care-giver support and transportation can be assessed by periodically reviewing the AEBLE worksheet found on p. 293. Answering the questions concerning the availability and quality of service found on p. 295 will also provide an overview of the status of community-based therapeutic recreation services. Finally, a most valid indicator of success is the progression of the individual through the sequential programs and tracks outlined in the implementation phase.

SUMMARY

This chapter has provided an overview of the recent interest in community-based therapeutic recreation programming, examined current trends that have emerged in this area of service, and illustrated the application of the community model through the assessment, planning, implementation, and evaluation phases. Discussion sections were devoted to the recreation-integration process and the role of the therapeutic recreation specialist in this setting. The chapter concluded with several contemporary examples of programs that exemplify this approach to therapeutic recreation service.

NOTES

1. Catherine Andres, "The Status of Municipal Recreation for the Mentally Retarded," *Therapeutic Recreation Journal* 4, no. 1 (1970), I.F.C., 30.

2. *The Whitehouse Conference on Handicapped Individuals,* May 1977 (Washington, D.C.: National Planning and Advisory Council).

3. Christopher R. Edginton and others, "The Status of Services for Special Populations in Park and Recreation Departments in the State of Iowa," *Therapeutic Recreation Journal* 9, no. 1 (1975), 109–16; Gene A. Hayes and Dick Smith, "Municipal Recreation Services for Special Populations in Texas," *Therapeutic Recreation Journal* 7, no. 1 (1973), 23–31; Barbara J. Williams, "The Status of Recreation for Individuals with Handicaps in Oregon Park and Recreation Agencies," *Therapeutic Recreation Journal* 13, no. 2 (1979), 44–47; David R. Austin, James A. Peterson, and Linda M. Peccarelli, "The Status of Services for Special Populations in Park and Recreation Departments in the State of Indiana," *Therapeutic Recreation Journal* 12, no. 1 (1978), 50–58; and Joanne Ardolf Decker, "Who Is Providing Recreation for Mentally Retarded Persons in Rural Communities?" *Leisurability* 10, no. 1 (1983), 36–39.

4. Peter A. Witt, "The Status of Recreation Services for the Handicapped in Canada," *Leisurability* 1, no. 2 (1974), 37–44; Renee Lyons, "A Profile of Municipal Services for Special Populations in Canada," *Leisurability* 8, no. 4 (1981), 14–24; Christopher R. Edginton, Roberta M. McDonald, and Debby A. Smith, "Are Municipal Recreation Services for Special Populations a Priority?" *Leisurability* 5, no. 3 (1978), 4–8; Doris Haist, "Municipal Recreation Services for Special Groups," *Leisurability* 2, no. 4 (1975), 32–37, and Karen J. Haist, Peggy J. Hanly, and Christopher R. Edginton, "A Study of Recreation Services for Special Populations Provided by Service Clubs," *Leisurability* 5, no. 1 (1978), 33–38.

5. W. R. Parkinson, "Community-Based Recreation Provision in the United Kingdom Disabled Users: Participation, Problems, Potential," in *Expanding Horizons in Therapeutic Recreation VII*, ed. Gerald Hitzhusen (Columbia: Department of Recreation and Park Administration, University of Missouri, 1979), pp. 18–27.

6. Helen Jo Mitchell, "A Community Recreation Program for the Mentally Retarded," *Therapeutic Recreation Journal* 5, no. 1 (1971), 3–8; Joseph Abrahams, "1970 Report to the Members of the NTRS-APRS Community Liaison Committee," *Therapeutic Recreation Journal* 5, no. 1 (1971), 9–10; Thomas A. Stein, "Environmental Barriers to Persons with Physical Disabilities," *Therapeutic Recreation Journal* 5, no. 1 (1971), 11–12; and Ardis Stevens, "Recreation in Community Mental Health," *Therapeutic Recreation Journal* 5, no. 1 (1971), 13–18.

7. Karen E. Sugiyama, "Integration: The Recreation Director and the Parents," *Leisurability* 5, no. 3 (1978), 16–18.

8. Doris L. Berryman, Annette Logan, and Bernard Braginsky, *Recreation for Disabled Children: Guidelines for Parents and Friends* (New York: New York University, School for Education, 1971).

9. Dee Dee Hill, *A Therapeutic Recreation Program for the Handicapped* (Richmond, Va.: Division of State Planning and Community Affairs, 1975).

10. John A. Nesbitt, *New Concepts and New Processes in Special Education,* Report on the National Conference and National Institute on New Models of Community Based Recreation and Leisure Programs and Services for Handicapped Children and Youth, Institute Report I (Iowa City: Recreation Education Program, University of Iowa, 1978), pp. 40–44; and David J. Szymanski and Tom Hoffman, "National Institute on New Models for Community Recreation and Leisure for Handicapped Children and Youth," in *Expanding Horizons in Therapeutic Recreation V,* ed. Gerald Hitzhusen (Columbia: Department of Recreation and Park Administration, University of Missouri, 1978), pp. 47–54.

11. Peggy Hutchison, "The Status of Recreation Integration Research," *Leisurability* 10, no. 4 (1983), 26–35.

12. Dan W. Kennedy, David R. Austin, and Ralph W. Smith, *Special Recreation: Opportunities for Persons with Disabilities* (Philadelphia: CBS College Publishing, 1987), pp. 17–18.

13. Kathleen Nolan, "A Comparison of Two Surveys Concerning the Relationship Between the Therapeutic Recreator and the Community Recreator," *Therapeutic Recreation Journal* 12, no. 1 (1978), 48.

14. Jacquelyn Stanley, "A Systematic Approach to Mainstreaming in a Public Recreation Department," *Therapeutic Recreation Journal* 13, no. 4 (1979), 21.

15. Ibid., 22

16. David M. Congdon, Sheila C. Conley, and James A. Duecker, *A Part, Not Apart: A Systematic Approach to Integrated Recreation and Leisure for Developmentally Disabled Adults* (Marion, Ind.: Grant-Blackford Developmental Center, 1981).

17. Division of Recreation and Leisure Studies *Manual for Utilization of the Assessment of Environmental Barriers to Leisure Experiences* (Denton, Texas: North Texas State University, 1982).

18. Peter A. Witt, *Community Leisure Services and Disabled Individuals* (Washington, D.C.: Hawkins and Associates, 1977), 32–33.

19. Renee F. Lyons and Ronald P. Reynolds, *How to Improve Community Leisure Opportunities for Disabled People* (Halifax: Recreation Council for the Disabled in Nova Scotia, 1978), 18–19.

20. Stanley, "Systematic Approach," p. 22.

21. Peggy Hutchison and John Lord, *Recreation Integration: Issues and Alternatives in Leisure Services and Community Involvement* (Ottawa, Ontario: Leisurability Publications, 1979), p. 57.

22. Marcia Jean Carter, Bob Frost, and Judy Hoffman, "Closing the Gap: Community Programs for Special Populations," *Expanding Horizons in Therapeutic Recreation VI,* (1979), p. 199.

23. Ibid., 200–202.

24. Division of Recreation and Leisure Studies, North Texas State University, *Manual for Utilization,* p. 14.

25. Kathleen Collard and Ethel Charboneau-Klein, "A Catalyst to Change," *Therapeutic Recreation Journal* 13, no. 4 (1979), 27.

26. James L. Paul, Ann P. Turnbull, and William M. Cruickshank, *Mainstreaming: A Practical Approach* (Syracuse, N.Y.: Syracuse University Press, 1977), p. 11.

27. Jerry Spinak, "Normalization and Recreation for the Disabled," *Leisurability,* 2, no. 2 (1975), 31–35.

28. Gary Thompson, "Role Changes of the Therapeutic Recreator and the Community Recreator in the Mainstreaming Process," *Expanding Horizons in Therapeutic Recreation VII,* ed. Gerald Hitzhusen et al. (Columbia: Department of Recreation and Park Administration, University of Missouri, 1980), p. 4.

29. Hutchison and Lord, *Recreation Integration,* p. 111.

30. Ronald P. Reynolds, "What Is Normalization and How Can You Do It?" *Parks and Recreation* 14, no. 8 (1979), 33–34, 50.

31. Thompson, "Role Changes," pp. 4–5.

32. Roxanne Howe-Murphy, "A Conceptual Basis for Mainstreaming Recreation and Leisure Services: Focus on Humanism," *Therapeutic Recreation Journal* 13, no. 4 (1979), 17–18.

33. Donald L. Lindley, "Problems of Integrating Therapeutic Recreation Programs into the Community," *Therapeutic Recreation Journal* 6, no. 1 (1972), 8–10.

34. Colin David Ross, "Leisure in the Deinstitutionalization Process: A Vehicle for Change," *Leisurability* 10, no. 1 (1983), 15.

35. Darla Kay and Keven Kendrigan, "Education for Leisure—A Critical Step to Normalization," *Parks and Recreation* 15, no. 4 (1980), 55–59.

36. Stanley, "Systematic Approach," pp. 24–25.

37. Christopher R. Edginton and David M. Compton, "Consumerism and Advocacy: A Conceptual Frame-

work for the Therapeutic Recreator," *Therapeutic Recreation Journal* 9, no. 1 (1975), p. 27.

38. Ibid., pp. 28–29.

39. Margaret L. Hutchison, "Maximizing Transfer Benefits of Special Programs," *Leisurability* 2, no. 4 (1975), 2–8.

40. Ronald P. Reynolds et al., *Therapeutic Recreation Service Delivery Model for the Richmond Department of Recreation and Parks* (Richmond, Va.: Division of Parks and Recreation, Outdoor Recreation Service Section, 1983).

41. Bonnie Laudick, John McGovern, and Susan Cosgrove, "Linking the Hospital and the Local Recreation Agency," *Parks and Recreation* 17, no. 4 (1982), 44–45.

42. Courtesy of the City of Virginia Beach Department of Parks and Recreation, Therapeutic Recreation Unit. Guidelines for community-based therapeutic recreation programs can be obtained from the National Therapeutic Recreation Society.

SUGGESTED READINGS

BARKELY, ALLEN L., and PAMELA ROBINSON. "Ticket to Re-Integration," *Leisurability* 2, no. 3 (1975), 3–10.

BOYD, WALTER, and FRANCES HARTNETT. "Normalization and Its Implication for Recreation Services." *Leisurability* 2, no. 1 (1975), 22–27.

BURDETT, CATHERINE, and MARY MILLER. "Mainstreaming in a Municipal Recreation Department Utilizing a Continuum Method." *Therapeutic Recreation Journal* 13, no. 4 (1979), 41–47.

CARTER, MARCIA JEAN, BOB FROST, and JUDY HOFFMAN. "Closing the Gap: Community Programs for Special Populations." In *Expanding Horizons in Therapeutic Recreation VI*, ed. D. J. Szymanski and G. L. Hitzhusen, pp. 195–203. Columbia: Technical Education Services, University of Missouri, 1979.

EDGINTON, CHRISTOPHER R., and DAVID M. COMPTON. "Consumerism and Advocacy: A Conceptual Framework for the Therapeutic Recreator." *Therapeutic Recreation Journal* 9, no. 1 (1975), 26–31.

FLYNN, ROBERT J., and KATHLEEN E. NITSCH, eds. *Normalization, Social Integration and Community Services*. Baltimore: University Park Press, 1980.

HOWE-MURPHY, ROXANNE. "A Conceptual Basis for Mainstreaming Recreation and Leisure Services: Focus on Humanism." *Therapeutic Recreation Journal* 13, no. 4 (1979) 11–18.

HUTCHISON, PEGGY. "The Status of Recreation Integration Research." *Leisurability* 10, no. 4 (1983), 26–35.

——and JOHN LORD. *Recreation Integration: Issues and Alternatives in Leisure Services and Community Involvement*. Ottawa, Ontario: Leisurability Publications, 1979.

KAY, DARLA, and KEVEN KENDRIGAN. "Education for Leisure—A Critical Step to Normalization." *Parks and Recreation* 15, no. 4 (1980), 55–59.

KENNEDY, DAN W., DAVID R. AUSTIN, and RALPH W. SMITH. *Special Recreation: Opportunities for Persons with Disabilities*. Philadelphia: Saunders College Publishing, 1987.

LAUDICK, BONNIE, JOHN MCGOVERN, and SUSAN COSGROVE. "Linking the Hospital and the Local Recreation Agency." *Parks and Recreation* 17, no. 4 (1982), 44–45.

LYONS, RENEE. "A Profile of Municipal Services for Special Populations in Canada." *Leisurability* 8, no. 4 (1981), 14–24.

PARKINSON, W. R. "Community-Based Recreation Provision in the United Kingdom Disabled Users: Participation, Problems, Potential." In *Expanding Horizons in Therapeutic Recreation VII*, ed. G. Hitzhusen, J. Elliott, D. J. Szymanski, and M. G. Thompson. Columbia: Curators, University of Missouri, 1980. Pp. 18–27.

REYNOLDS, RONALD P. "Normalization: A Guideline to Leisure Skills Programming for Handicapped Individuals." In *Leisure and Handicapped Individuals: Adaptation, Techniques and Curriculum*, ed. Paul Wehman and Stuart Schleien. Baltimore: University Park Press, 1981.

ROSS, COLIN DAVID. "Leisure in the Deinstitutionalization Process: A Vehicle for Change." *Leisurability* 10, no. 1 (1983), 13–19.

"Special Recreation: Programming for Everyone." *Leisure Today*, May–June 1985.

STANLEY, JACQUELYN. "A Systematic Approach to Mainstreaming in a Public Recreation Department." *Therapeutic Recreation Journal* 13, no. 4 (1979), 19–26.

STENSRUD, CAROL. "Sequential Recreation Integration Streams." *Leisurability* 5, no. 2 (1978), 28–33.

SZYMANSKI, DAVID J., and TOM HOFFMAN. "National Institute on New Models for Community Recreation and Leisure for Handicapped Children and Youth."

In *Expanding Horizons in Therapeutic Recreation* V, ed. Gerald L. Hitzhusen, pp. 47–54. Columbia: Department of Recreation and Park Administration, University of Missouri, 1978.

THOMPSON, GARY. "Role Changes of the Therapeutic Recreator and the Community Recreator in the Mainstreaming Process." In *Expanding Horizons in Therapeutic Recreation VII*, ed. G. Hitzhusen, J. Elliott, D. J. Szymanski, and M. G. Thompson. Columbia: Curators, University of Missouri, 1980. Pp. 1–8.

WITT, PETER A. *Community Leisure Services and Disabled Individuals*. Washington, D.C.: Hawkins and Associates, 1977.

WOLFENSBERGER, WOLF. *The Principle of Normalization in Human Services*. Toronto: National Institute on Mental Retardation, 1972.

12

Trends
in Therapeutic Recreation

Throughout this text we have discussed the needs of individuals with varying disabilities, prevalent notions of health and rehabilitation, the spectrum of health-related facilities, and the models and processes that form the basis for therapeutic recreation service. Therapeutic recreation, however, is not a static process. It will continue to grow and develop against an ever-changing backdrop of political, social, and economic change. It is therefore most appropriate to reflect now upon potential courses of action that may be taken as the field refines its mission, attempts to enhance its status within the allied health-care disciplines, develops new standards of professional preparation and practice, and examines its approaches to service delivery.[1]

Before proceeding, three brief caveats are in order. First, the material that follows contains the authors' opinions concerning possible directions that future developments in the field *may* take. Readers are encouraged to form their own alternative opinions and interpretations of these trends. Second, although this material has been organized around major topical areas, a natural overlap exists among many of the major concepts. For example, professional efforts at defining

the field of service would no doubt directly affect the processes of credentialling, educational preparation, developing standards, and ultimately, service delivery. Third, owing to the newness of the field, many key issues have not yet been resolved. Rather than experiencing frustration at this situation, it is hoped that readers will share the authors' excitement in being part of such a vibrant and rapidly emerging human-service profession. Indeed, readers are encouraged to take every opportunity to exert their influence on the development of the field.

Trend 1: Efforts to Define the Philosophical Basis for the Field Will Intensify

Debate about the development of a well-defined occupational philosophy has been prevalent in the field during its emergence as a profession. There are indications that this debate will continue and expand over the next few years. Before examining some of the contemporary factors fueling this controversy, it will be helpful to review briefly the evolution of this issue.

From the late 1930s until the mid 1960s three diverse orientations existed concerning the fundamental nature or purpose of the provision of recreational services to disabled persons.[2] The *hospital recreation* position held that recreation in a medical setting served the same purpose as community recreation—enjoyment and diversion. In contrast, the *recreational therapy* orientation viewed recreation as a treatment tool in the rehabilitation of individuals with disabling conditions. Finally, the term *recreation for ill and handicapped* connoted a community-based orientation to service.

The merger of the National Association of Recreation Therapists, the Hospital Recreation Section of the American Recreation Society, and the Recreation Therapy Section of the American Alliance for Health, Physical Education, and Recreation and Dance into the Council for the Advancement of Hospital Recreation in 1953 and into the National Therapeutic Recreation Society (NTRS) in 1966 had little effect in quieting this debate. In fact, early issues of the National Therapeutic Recreation Society's journal devoted large sections to the opinions of various authors on the nature of therapeutic recreation. The "Is recreation therapy . . . ?" debate stimulated the development of a definition of therapeutic recreation at the Ninth Southern Regional Institute on Therapeutic Recreation in 1969. Central to this definition was the notion of therapeutic recreation as:

> a process which utilizes recreation services for purposive intervention in some physical, emotional, and/or social behavior to bring about a desired change in that behavior and to promote the growth and development of the individual.[3]

Reaction to this statement was swift. The mid-1970s produced many and varied models of service, some utilizing continuum and matrix approaches that conceptualized the process of therapeutic recreation. In 1978 Gunn and Peterson proposed that therapeutic recreation was in fact a *service* that utilized many *processes*.[4]

Position Statements

In an attempt to reach a consensus regarding an occupational philosophy, the NTRS asked Dr. Lee Meyer in 1980 to develop a document entitled "Philosophical Alternatives and the Professionalization of Therapeutic Recreation." This paper outlined the following four possible orientations or positions:

> *Position A (Recreation):* This notion, the earlier viewpoint of hospital recreation, states that therapeutic recreation is simply the provision of recreation services and opportunities to persons with disabling conditions.

> *Position B (Treatment):* This position holds that the primary purpose of therapeutic recreation is to utilize recreation experiences and opportunities to help treat or ameliorate effects of illness or disability.

> *Position C (Treatment/Education/Recreation):* This view states that therapeutic recreation services are designed to assist individuals to establish and express independent leisure lifestyles. The three types of services offered within this model are therapy, leisure education, and recreation participation.

> *Position D (Treatment and Recreation):* This position states that therapeutic recreation is both the provision of recreation services and opportunities for treatment and the provision of recreation services to persons with disabling conditions.[5]

Position C (Treatment/Education/Recreation) was formally adopted by the membership of the NTRS in 1982, but response to a poll on the subject was marginal, and the acceptance of the position far from unanimous. With this in mind, it may not be surprising that the debate concerning the fundamental nature of therapeutic recreation continues as this book is being written.

Divergent Opinions

Three articles in the 1985 issue of the *Therapeutic Recreation Journal* are testimony to this current controversy. In the first, Sylvester challenges the treatment component of the model adopted by the NTRS by pointing out that a therapeutic recreation specialist who conducts therapy with a client may, in fact, be interfering with that individual's freedom and ability to enjoy leisure:

> In brief, benefits associated with leisure . . . often materialize only when the activity is freely engaged in for its own sake. Yet, when the same activity is professionally prescribed and controlled for treatment purposes, when it becomes a professional means aimed at functional ends, the results are seemingly decreased.[6]

In a similar vein, Mobily strongly advocates an expanded view of the meaning of the term *therapeutic* to include growth and prevention as well as remedy or cure. Stressing the notion of recreation as a "means rather than an end," he too feels that therapeutic recreation practitioners must continually "seek to induce in their clients perceptions of control, responsibility and freedom."[7]

In an article titled appropriately "The Dilemma of an Unresolved Philosophy in Therapeutic Recreation," Halberg and Howe-Murphy view therapeutic recreation as being at a crossroads in terms of its professional identity. They point out that philosophical beliefs will eventually determine if therapeutic recreation aligns itself with the allied health professions or the larger recreation and leisure profession or be independent of both fields. In their opinion, the field to date has been successful in defining its parameters of service (what the field does and how) but has not yet resolved internal issues such as the recreation-therapy dichotomy or reached consensus regarding our view of the nature of human beings, orientations to leisure, or approaches to intervention.[8]

While some of the preceding material may appear abstract to the reader, no individual activity could be more important than the development of an acceptable occupational philosophy. The adoption of such a philosophical base is, in fact, necessary if we are to define our relationship to other disciplines, choose among credentialling options (licensure, certification, registration), develop standards of practice and professional preparation, decide what types of research studies to conduct, and choose among possible treatment techniques to use with our clients.

Philosophical Exercises

To assist readers in monitoring trends in the development of a philosophical basis for therapeutic recreation and help them clarify their own views of the nature of therapeutic recreation, the following exercises are suggested.

> Examine each of the four philosophical alternatives described on p. 316. What are the strengths and weaknesses of each?
>
> Which area(s) of service—therapy, leisure education, or recreation—would be most prevalent in the custodial, medical-clinical, therapeutic milieu, education and training, and community models of therapeutic recreation? Defend your answer.
>
> Are there current societal trends that may cause the existing philosophical position statement to be altered? If so, list and briefly describe these trends.

Trend 2: The Credentialling Movement Will Expand and Accelerate

Over the past several years the field of therapeutic recreation has intensified its efforts to increase its status and maintain high standards of service to clients through various forms of credentialling. In general, it has sought to set and meet standards of accredition, registration, certification, and licensure. A brief review of these terms and the field's response follows.

Accreditation

This term, as noted in an earlier chapter, refers to "the process by which an agency or organization evaluates and recognizes an institution as meeting predetermined qualifications or standards."[9] Programs of professional preparation in therapeutic recreation at the baccalaureate level must meet both the general standards set by the National Recreation and Park Association's Council on Accreditation *and* the following list of competencies established by the council on accreditation of the National Recreation and Park Association in cooperation with the American Association for Leisure and Recreation.

Knowledge of human anatomy and physiology

Understanding of the nature and etiology of illness and disability

Understanding of and ability to use basic medical and psychiatric terminology

Understanding of the attitudes and self-concepts of disabled persons toward themselves and toward their illness or disability

Understanding of the societal attitudes toward illness and disability

Understanding of the bio-psycho-social limitation imposed by illness and disability as related to leisure involvement

Knowledge of various assistive techniques related to specific illnesses or disabilities including, but not limited to, transfer techniques, ambulation, self-help skills, signing, orientation, and mobility

Knowledge of the health-care delivery systems

Understanding of the role of therapeutic recreation as a component of health-care systems

Knowledge of the legal issues in delivering services for special populations

Knowledge of local, state, and federal (national) laws, regulations, and standards regarding recreation services for special populations

Knowledge of appropriate interagency and intraagency referral procedures to meet individual client needs

Understanding of a variety of treatment approaches and their implications for therapeutic recreation programming

Understanding of the concept of habilitation, rehabilitation, maintenance, and prevention as related to therapeutic programs

Understanding of the concept of a continuum of therapeutic recreation service

Ability to conceptualize and plan appropriate therapeutic recreation programs for diverse special need populations

Ability to conduct client-assessment procedures and analyze and interpret results for programming

Ability to design individual treatment and program plans

Knowledge of the theory and technique of therapeutic intervention including, but not limited to, reflective listening, reality therapy, nondirective therapy, transactional analysis, and behavior modification

Knowledge of various adaptive devices and equipment

Ability to demonstrate and translate medical-record charting techniques

Knowledge of the credentialling process related to therapeutic recreation

Understanding of ethical and professional behavior related to therapeutic recreation

Understanding of the role of the therapeutic recreation professional as an advocate for services for special populations[10]

The accreditation process is sometimes criticized for promoting minimal standards, discouraging innovation in curriculum design, and failing to ensure successful performance by professionals; nevertheless, there are several arguments in favor of accreditation that the authors find convincing.

1. Accreditation improves the quality of professional preparation.
2. Accreditation assists in the successful building of a public image of therapeutic recreation as a profession.
3. Accreditation provides reliable information to NCTRC and licensure boards for certification and licensure purposes.
4. Accreditation assists in neutralizing political and group pressures from internal and external sources.
5. Accreditation helps to overcome diversity in therapeutic recreation courses and curricula in some programs of study in relation to other health professions.
6. Accreditation reflects the scope of therapeutic recreation.
7. Accreditation facilitates communication with other professional accrediting agencies.
8. Accreditation discourages governmental involvement in control of curricula.[11]

By the end of the 1980s forty-seven programs of study in therapeutic recreation had been accredited nationally. Many professionals were considering applying for accreditation, and others were going through the accreditation process. The authors feel that as employers and the general public gain an increased knowledge of the accreditation process and specify graduation from an accredited university as a requirement for employment, the accreditation movement will gain momentum. Consequently, accredited programs of professional preparation in therapeutic recreation will prove to be the rule and not the exception in the future.

Certification, Registration, and Licensure

Certification is a voluntary and national process "by which a governmental or nongovernmental agency grants recognition to an individual who has met certain predetermined qualifications set by a credentialling agency or association."[12] Registration is "the process by which qualified individuals are listed on an official roster maintained by a governmental or nongovernmental agency."[13] Licensure is "the process by which an agency of government grants permission to persons meeting predetermined qualifications to engage in a given occupation and use a particular title."[14]

Currently the only certification plan for therapeutic recreation personnel is administered by the National Council for Therapeutic Recreation Certification. Its two-tiered standards designate individuals as meeting either the professional or paraprofessional qualifications based on the criteria of professional preparation and experience. (See Appendix D.) Similarly, many states administer their own registration programs through professional societies. Only two states, Utah and Georgia, have licensing laws.

In debating which form of credentialling would best serve the profession, several questions must be addressed.

How would the geographic and career mobility of therapeutic recreation personnel be affected by various credentialling plans?

What effect would the variation among states relative to the organization and operation of state boards and agencies have on plans for licensure?

Who is ultimately responsible for administering therapeutic recreation credentialling—the profession or the government?

Can the field currently define "quality therapeutic recreation service"?

Can therapeutic recreation document financial accountability?

Can we adequately delineate the functions performed by entry-level therapeutic recreators?[15]

Will written examinations improve the quality of therapeutic recreation education and the practice of therapeutic recreation service?

The authors feel that the following statement by Dr. Marcia Jean Carter represents an insightful response to these and other questions concerning current credentialling efforts.

Increased public demands for the assurance of practitioner competence as well as practitioners' interest in professional recognition have contributed to the growth and concern for an appropriate credentialling program for therapeutic recreators. A credentialling trend exists. Licensure for therapeutic recreators is a premature priority. Therapeutic recreators lack the solid theoretical and practical base and the political astuteness to develop and maintain or justify the existence of state licensure. A more appropriate posture for the present is to coordinate licensure and certification efforts of the National Council on Therapeutic Recreation Certification and state licensure boards.[16]

Trend 3: The Development of Professional Standards and the Practice of Accountability Will Become Essential Features of Therapeutic Recreation Service

While widespread interest in health and human service standards is largely a post-World War II phenomenon, there is ample evidence that concern about such laws and regulations has reached epic proportions. Much of the impetus for this concern has been from consumers and the government, who have raised serious questions regarding the availability of care, the quality of services when rendered, and the cost of these services. A sampling of recent events illustrates today's movement toward *accountability, quality assurance,* and *cost containment:*

Consumers are becoming increasingly involved in outreach services and in shaping health policies and procedures at many levels.

Governmental influence is being exerted through Professional Standards Review Organizations, which monitor the services received by recipients of Medicare, Medicaid, and maternal and child health care. Specifically, these organizations determine whether hospitalization (1) is medically necessary, (2) is of appropriate duration, and (3) meets recognized professional standards of quality.

Congress has approved a prospective-pricing plan, termed Diagnostic Related Groupings (DRGs), for most Medicare inpatient services. This concept bases reimbursement to the medical facility upon patient cost data as determined by diagnosis, treatment, and age of the patient. Many individuals feel that private insurance carriers will follow suit.

Current Action

The field of therapeutic recreation's response to this trend has been swift and mounted on two fronts. First, it has moved to develop its own sets of standards. For example, since 1979 the National Therapeutic Recreation Society has published *Guidelines for Community-Based Recreation Programs for Special Populations, Standards of Practice for Therapeutic Recreation Service,* and *Guidelines for Administration of Therapeutic Recreation Service in Clinical and Residential Facilities.* Second, it has lobbied to have therapeutic recreation service included in the standards of various regulatory bodies that monitor health-care service.

Notable examples of activities and accomplishments of the NTRS include:

Initiated dialogue with Medicare policy officials to determine their understanding of therapeutic recreation service and developed appropriate methods to influence Medicare operations so that decisions about coverage of therapeutic recreation service were consistent throughout the Medicare system.

Developed guidelines and determined resources to be used by therapeutic recreation professionals when seeking reimbursement for services.

Created a committee charged with the task of developing a standard-of-practice document including assessment procedures, treatment goals/objectives, treatment methodologies and evaluation procedures for various settings, hospital service areas, and disabilities.

Reviewed the Accreditation Manual for Hospitals and Consolidated Standards of the Joint Commission on Accreditation of Hospitals.

The newly formed American Therapeutic Recreation Association has also been vitally concerned with issues of accountability. Its efforts to date include the formation of the following standing committees concerned with standards and accountability:

Joint Commission on Accreditation of Hospitals/Commission on Accreditation of Rehabilitation Facilities Standards Committee Purpose: To maintain relationships with JCAH and CARF, monitor standards, provide input to these bodies, and inform membership regarding their standards.

Quality-Assurance Committee Purpose: To recommend procedures, publications, and ways of informing members about appropriate quality-assurance activities.

Reimbursement Committee Purpose: To recommend procedures, publications, and other methods of informing members about third-party reimbursement.

Legislation Committee Purpose: To monitor legislation and develop and present testimony to represent ATRA's position on legislation, regulation, and other legislative activities.

Future Action

In seeking to develop standards and have these standards accepted by administrators and accrediting bodies, the field of therapeutic recreation must first meet the challenge of determining what specific standards ensure quality. Specifically, it must develop concrete measures of such concepts as improvement in health status and enhancement of patient satisfaction. Secondly, efforts must be made to reduce the confusion that has arisen from attempts to make the multiple standards of therapeutic recreation practice compatible with diverse agency and organization standards. We must also make certain that our standards are sufficiently high to ensure a level of service that demands approval and acceptance from other health-care professionals. Clearly, more research is needed to validate the standards in existence today. Empirical studies of the therapeutic recreation process and continuum discussed in earlier chapters would enable us to identify important elements of practice that should be included in our standards. Investigations must focus on *outcome* (the ultimate effects upon the consumer), *process* (whether adequate service has been provided), and *structure* (the adequacy of facilities, personnel, supplies and equipment, etc.).[17]

Similarly, *fiscal accountability* will also be of particular concern to the profession. If recent publications are a predictor of future trends, therapeutic recreation specialists will be concerned not only with third-party reimbursement and DRG prospective pricing but with effective risk management, productivity analysis, marketing, and fund raising from private foundations. Indeed, our professional-preparation curriculums may well include supplementary courses in health administration, business, marketing, and mass communications.

West and Thorn outline strategies they feel must be undertaken by therapeutic recreation specialists in the future with respect to fiscal accountability:

1. We should increase the knowledge and understanding we have of the organization and financing of the service systems and agencies which provide therapeutic recreation services.

2. We should demonstrate a commitment to providing a reasonable quality of service to those most in need of services instead of attempting to be all things for all people.

3. We should increase revenue generations to cover the cost of our services in inpatient, outpatient, home health, and community settings by third-party reimbursement, donations, grants, and fund-raising projects.

4. We should produce research which demonstrates the therapeutic value and cost effectiveness of therapeutic recreation service for individuals with certain illnesses or disabilities.

5. We should determine what business we are in, what our unique product is, and accordingly market therapeutic recreation services to consumers, physicians, third-party payers, administrators, and allied disciplines.

6. We should improve the efficiency and effectiveness of service delivery by the use of management techniques such as cost efficiency/effectiveness analysis, and productivity measurement.

7. We should continue to develop innovative programs such as community reintegration, preventive care/wellness, and others which demonstrate the unique contribution of therapeutic recreation services to becoming and staying healthy.

8. We should improve our management of personnel, supplies, equipment, and facilities to improve services delivered and reduce costs.

9. We should organize and unite our professionals through networks and professional organizations to be more proactive in anticipating and responding to change

and to strategically advance our profession in service to our clients.[18]

In short, the new and rapidly emerging profession of therapeutic recreation faces the challenge of responding to changing public, private, and governmental demands for accountability. To meet this challenge it must continue its efforts to develop reliable, valid, and externally acceptable standards of practice.

Trend 4: Our Efforts at Professional Preparation Will be Analyzed and Refined

The field of therapeutic recreation is only beginning to develop its knowledge base and determine the most effective means to impart needed skills and abilities to students. There is general agreement that the competencies mentioned in the earlier discussion of accreditation form the basis for therapeutic recreation practice. However, the profession appears to be struggling with some very basic problems concerning the preparation of its practitioners. As a relatively new field, therapeutic recreation has not yet developed the large body of knowledge that other occupations possess. Therefore, the books, journals, and other instructional materials available to our students may be limited by comparison with other professions. Other problems arise when we borrow information from related disciplines and attempt to apply it to our field. The recent controversy over leisure counseling is one such example of a problematic area. Although more programs of professional preparation are being developed, there is a lack of uniformity in therapeutic recreation curricula. Recent studies, in fact, have found a range of from one to nine course offerings in undergraduate programs of professional preparation.[19]

Recent concern has also been focused on the degree to which our educational programs have (or have not) emphasized the values and ethics that form the basis for professional practice. Other issues have evolved around the appropriateness of faculty credentials and faculty-student instructional ratios. Debate has also continued relative to the degree of specialization of coursework at the graduate and undergraduate level. Likewise, programs have varied greatly in their emphasis on therapeutic recreation theory and practice. Some educators have emphasized a specialist or clinical approach to professional preparation in contrast to the generalist orientation maintained by others.

Earlier we outlined some of the trends in professional preparation that we hope will continue. These trends are reflected in the following list of characteristics and goals for academic education for therapeutic recreation.

1. Emphasis should be placed on developing behaviors which cannot readily be acquired on the job.
2. Broad problem-solving approaches, rather than specific procedures, should be emphasized.
3. Knowledge based upon scientific theory should be constantly integrated into our curriculums.
4. Classroom and field-learning experiences should be stressed.
5. Objectives should be carefully chosen, operationalized, and grouped into learning modules.
6. Students should be alerted to constantly changing societal trends and client needs.[20]

Trend 5: The Roles and Functions of Therapeutic Recreation Specialists Will Expand

Earlier chapters of this text revealed emerging societal trends and shifting practices in the delivery of health-care services that will greatly affect the profession of therapeutic recreation. The following section explores the effects these changes may have upon the daily activities of therapeutic recreation personnel and reveals some of the challenges our field faces in the future.

The Social and Political Arena

It is apparent from the trends described in earlier chapters that today's therapeutic recreation specialists must understand the total health-care delivery system, not just their specialty. Furthermore, therapeutic recreation personnel must be able and willing to change society's attitudes toward disability and treatment while monitoring and influencing legislation. In this latter capacity members of the field will have to assume the roles of *advocates* and *change agents* to ensure that therapeutic recreation service is included in the regulations of the federal government and private insurance carriers. To achieve this end, we must understand and participate in the legislative process described in Chapter 3 of this text.

Public awareness of our field will be a primary goal, particularly in light of the imminent changes in hospital boards also described in Chapter 3. Therapeutic recreation personnel, in fact, will have to be prepared to occupy positions of influence on governmental boards and committees and voluntary philanthropic and professional organizations. The very existence of our field could well depend upon these activities.

Health, Wellness, and Prevention

The therapeutic recreation specialist of the 1980s and 1990s must adhere to the concept of health as complete well-being rather than a mere lack of illness. Therefore, the physical, mental, social, and emotional well-being of the client should be our chief goal. Therapeutic recreation personnel must focus on leisure goals, values, and lifestyles. Prevention of disability will become a central goal of the profession. Destructive patterns of behavior, such as overeating, lack of exercise, emotional stress, and job tension leading to coronary thrombosis, as described in Chapter 2, will be the basis for intervention by trained therapeutic recreation personnel. Many therapeutic recreation specialists will find employment beyond hospital walls in clinics and community-based programs of health maintenance in the next decade.

Interactions with Consumers and Other Professionals

Changes are currently taking place concerning the manner in which we approach and interact with the recipients of our service. Specifically, therapeutic recreation specialists are relying less on physician-centered orientations where the orders or prescriptions of an M.D. dictate the type of intervention. Rather, therapeutic recreation personnel are assuming an active role in developing their own strategies with appropriate guidance from medical practitioners. Similarly, a more comprehensive picture is being obtained of the client's vocational, educational, sexual, social, and leisure functioning before treatment. Consequently, today's therapeutic recreation specialist will have to develop more comprehensive and sophisticated assessment and program-evaluation instruments. These instruments must be sensitive enough to detect each client's personal reaction to disease or illness, as described in the introductory chapter. Likewise, therapeutic recreation professionals must continually examine their own reaction to individual clients. Indeed, we must realize that the therapeutic use of self is a powerful tool that transcends the activities we employ. Trends in human service, such as the normalization/integration movement, must be foremost in our minds. The implications of this orientation are clear. Parents' groups will play a central role in monitoring our services to mentally retarded children. Groups of disabled consumers will also provide guidance to our efforts in clinical and community settings.

Therapeutic recreation specialists must understand the nature and implications of disabilities yet avoid the damaging process of labeling. Programs must be based on residual interests and abilities rather than disabilities. New activity programs must be developed and stereotyped activities, age inappropriate pursuits, and overly competitive sports avoided. In the future therapeutic recreation specialists will rely heavily upon the previously described technique of activity analysis to meet specific treatment objectives. Follow-up, aftercare, and outpatient services will occupy central positions in the health-care delivery of the next several years.

Therapeutic recreation has a vital role and interest in these services. As we move toward the 1990s, practitioners in the field will also have to interact with an increasing number of highly specialized members of the allied health field, including dance, music, and art therapists, in addition to "multimedia" disciplines such as occupational therapy. In these interactions we must be prepared to articulate our mission and interpret the nature of our services. Potential boundary disputes and occasional instances of overlap will have to be resolved. As our field expands, more and more therapeutic recreation specialists will find themselves in managerial positions requiring advanced skills and training. As one-person departments decrease, tomorrow's specialists will need to possess budgeting, supervision, accounting, and other administrative abilities.

Service Settings

There is every indication that the right-to-treatment concept and the move toward deinstitutionalization will cause a shift from custodial approaches to human service in favor of the therapeutic community, milieu therapy, and education and training models. The implications of this trend for the field of therapeutic recreation are profound. One obvious consequence will be a sharp increase in the provision of therapeutic recreation service in facilities such as halfway houses, detention centers, training schools, and workshops. Neighborhood health centers, clinics, and outpatient treatment centers will also employ a significant number of our personnel. Owing to the short-term nature of these facilities, programming will be particularly challenging. Briefer, less frequent contact will necessitate the development of new assessment techniques, planning strategies, and methods of implementation and evaluation. New duties of the therapeutic recreation specialist will center on family education, early diagnosis and prevention of illness, home visitation, and aftercare and training. In addition to our traditional role as activity provider, we will increasingly serve as public relations specialists, advocates, community planners, educators/teachers, and referral-service coordinators. In short, therapeutic recreation specialists will be "catalyst innovators" and "resource leaders."

A particularly promising area for practicing therapeutic recreation specialists appears to be the provision of consultation services. Indeed, it appears that all three types of consulting (special population, colleague, and agency centered), as described in Chapter 5, will increase. In the future it may be commonplace for therapeutic recreation specialists to be employed on a part-time consultancy basis by several agencies. Such individuals will need to be well versed in techniques of entrepreneurship and business practices.

Several developments in medical care and treatment will create promising new areas of service for today's (and tomorrow's) practitioners. Hospice programs for terminally ill persons represent a most challenging point of contact. Detoxification and substance-abuse treatment will no doubt increase over the next several years. New interventions in treating persons with brain injuries will also necessitate the provision of therapeutic recreation service. Respite and day care for children and adults with disabilities also promises to be a fruitful area of employment. While opportunities for service in public school settings are currently limited, developments such as the *Education for All Handicapped Children Act* may serve to stimulate employment in this area. A major

challenge to the field of therapeutic recreation is to facilitate a shift in correctional recreation from a diversional to a rehabilitative emphasis. As this transition comes about, more and more personnel will be necessary to provide recreational services in correctional facilities and in pre- and postrelease centers.

Community-based voluntary advocate associations, such as organizations for visually impaired, mentally retarded, and mentally ill persons, are also beginning to realize the benefits of employing therapeutic recreation specialists. In the coming years professionals will serve these organizations at the local, state, and national level. Over the past ten years there has been a proliferation of small, private, for-profit hospitals providing mental health treatment. These facilities have been and will continue to be employers of therapeutic recreation specialists. Not only will those specialists have to be well versed in the theory and practice of therapeutic recreation but they will also have to possess a strong business sense in providing fee-based services.

Possibly the fastest growing area for therapeutic recreation service may be the municipal recreation department. Whether the title of their program is therapeutic recreation, adapted recreation, special populations programs, or another term, more and more local recreation and parks departments are seeking the service of qualified therapeutic recreation specialists. Indeed, as the number of aged individuals residing in the community increases and persons with varied disabilities return home due to better care, the opportunities for community-based therapeutic recreation will grow dramatically.

Research and Demonstration

Research efforts generate the information that constitutes the body of knowledge of the therapeutic recreation field. Systematic investigations also solve problems that confront the field, such as which path of credentialling is most desirable, what competencies practitioners should possess, and which definition of therapeutic recreation is most appropriate. Research, in fact, is the responsibility of all professionals in the field of therapeutic recreation. There is every indication that this responsibility will increase in the future.

One fruitful area of research may well be demonstration projects funded by governmental bodies or private foundations. While support for these endeavors has been uneven in the past, funding should increase as the field grows in stature and credibility. It is the authors' prediction that joint endeavors involving university personnel, practitioners, and community agencies will predominate. Popular topics for research and demonstration could well include the following:

The integration of persons with disabilities into various community-based recreation programs

Determining the basic leisure needs of special population members.

Developing techniques to increase consumer involvement in recreation planning, decision making, and operation

Investigating the relationship between leisure education and vocational success

Determining the factors that influence the employment choices of therapeutic recreation specialists

While these and many other questions are important avenues of investigation, therapeutic recreation specialists cannot ignore research in the broader recreation and parks field. They will certainly, for example, increase their contributions to publications such as the *Journal of Leisure Research,* which studies the leisure-participation patterns of various groups of disabled and nondisabled individuals.

Computer literacy promises to be a central theme of pre- and in-service training in therapeutic recreation. Although the application of computer technology to the field has just begun, several exciting areas are already beginning to emerge. Examples include the use of computer software to facilitate activity analysis, client charting and record keeping, and leisure assessments such as interest finders and attitude scales.

As we move toward the next decade, research efforts will increase in three main topical areas. First, considerable time will be devoted to developing reliable and valid assessment and evaluation instruments. Second, numerous studies will be aimed at determining what actually constitutes "good and acceptable" practice in the field of therapeutic recreation. Third, as the internal and external accountability pressures in the field increase, substantial effort will have to be made to demonstrate the overall effectiveness of therapeutic recreation service.

One result of this heightened activity will most likely be an increase in the number of journals and other publications that contain therapeutic recreation research. At present there are currently scarcely a half dozen periodicals that regularly publish studies pertaining to therapeutic recreation, but this number will rapidly grow as our body of knowledge expands. Furthermore, as computer technology increases and therapeutic recreation literature proliferates, the need for centralized information retrieval and referral centers will become acute. The authors would not at all be surprised to see such centers appear at regional, national, and international points over the next several years. In short, the therapeutic recreation specialist of tomorrow will be an active producer and consumer of research.

Trend 6: The Contrast Between Clinical and Community Therapeutic Recreation Service Will Diminish

Over the past several years there has been a tendency to define the roles therapeutic recreation specialists perform on the basis of the settings in which they practice. This trend has been particularly noticeable in referring to the functions of clinical and community-based therapeutic recreation specialists. Those in hospitals, physical rehabilitation centers, and training facilities have been labeled clinical practitioners; those in municipal recreation departments, advocate association centers, and other community-based facilities have been designated community therapeutic recreation personnel. In the opinion of the authors, the use of these terms to *contrast* modes of therapeutic recreation service has led to a misinterpretation of the roles and functions of specialists in these two settings. Furthermore, this dichotomy has caused discussion of such topics as professional preparation and standards to center on community *versus* clinical service.

Problems: Roles and Settings

At this time there appear to be several problems associated with identifying the roles of therapeutic recreation specialists around the *settings* in which they are employed. A brief outline and discussion of these potential drawbacks follow.

One major problem involves defining the boundaries of clinical and community settings. Specifically, where do the parameters of the clinic end and those of the community begin? To illustrate: Is a therapeutic recreation specialist directing an infant-stimulation program in a local association for mentally retarded persons providing a clinical or a community therapeutic recreation service? Similarly, is a therapeutic recreation specialist in a community mental health outpatient clinic automatically providing clinical services? While substantial debate continues concerning the philosophical orientation of the field, a majority of professionals surveyed in 1982 agreed that therapeutic recreation service included recreation therapy and leisure education with appropriate overlap between areas. No distinction appeared on the basis of setting. Rather, it was felt that therapeutic recreation practitioners should be educated and otherwise prepared to provide *any* of these

services, in *any* setting, to *any* group of clients.

A second problem appears to have emerged from the misconception that community programs are chiefly diversional in nature, while programs in medical or rehabilitation settings are wholly prescriptive, intervention oriented, and individualized. Although personnel in medical settings are striving, most justifiably, to respond to issues of accountability, many community-based therapeutic recreation programs serve an identical developmental purpose. Many of today's municipally employed therapeutic recreation personnel conduct individual client assessments, develop specialized program goals, and work closely with other specialized disciplines to meet the specific leisure needs of their participants. The Individualized Educational Plans (IEP) utilized by therapeutic recreation specialists in public school settings are one such example of systematic, goal-oriented programming.

A third problematic area concerns professional training. Specifically, does the field wish to establish separate tracks of professional preparation within its university degree programs? Should universities offer a clinical or community degree option? As employment opportunities and career goals of therapeutic recreation practitioners change, the authors feel that the answer to these questions is no.

A final, subtle misconception is that clinical therapeutic recreation personnel are somehow more responsible for knowing the *whys* of programming, but community personnel need only to concern themselves with the *hows*. In certain instances this misconception has led students aspiring to employment in community settings to question the relevance of course work in subjects such as anatomy and kinesiology. There appear to be two shortcomings to this line of thinking. First, it is difficult or impossible to predict where a professional will provide therapeutic recreation service over the span of an entire career. Second, and of more importance, community-based specialists must be as aware of the physical and psychological functioning of human beings as their counterparts employed in clinical settings are.

Resolution

As members of the profession become increasingly cognizant of these and other potential drawbacks of the community/clinical dichotomy, the field will likely deemphasize distinctions that are currently being made. To be sure, differences in emphasis among the recreation, leisure-education, and therapy areas will continue. The distinction, however, will be largely one of degree rather than orientation to service.

This discussion of trends concludes our introduction to the helping profession of therapeutic recreation. The authors hope that the reader shares their excitement in being part of this young and rapidly developing profession. As a therapeutic recreation specialist, you will be providing an extremely valuable service. We trust that this effort will bring with it the very deepest of personal satisfaction.

SUMMARY

This chapter has identified several contemporary issues and trends in the field of therapeutic recreation and reflected upon potential courses of action the profession might take in meeting these challenges. Once again, the reader is cautioned that much of the preceding material represents the authors' opinion concerning future directions. Readers are again invited to form their own opinions and interpretations of these trends and to actively participate in the field's growth and development.

NOTES

1. For a complete discussion of these and other contemporary issues, see Ronald P. Reynolds and Gerald S. O'Morrow, *Problems, Issues, and Concepts in Therapeutic Recreation* (Englewood Cliffs, N.J.: Prentice-Hall, Inc., 1985).

2. Lee E. Meyer, "Philosophical Alternatives and the Professionalization of Therapeutic Recreation" (Paper submitted as part of the Philosophical Statement Task Force of the National Therapeutic Recreation Society, May 1980), p. 2.

3. "Therapeutic Recreation Position Paper" (Developed at the Ninth Southern Regional Institute on Therapeutic Recreation, University of North Carolina, 1969).

4. Scout Lee Gunn and Carol Ann Peterson, *Therapeutic Recreation Program Design: Principles and Procedures* (Englewood Cliffs, N.J.: Prentice-Hall, 1978), p. 11.

5. These positions are extracted from a survey conducted by the NTRS in the summer of 1981.

6. Charles D. Sylvester, "Freedom, Leisure and Therapeutic Recreation: A Philosophical View," *Therapeutic Recreation Journal* 18, no. 1 (1985), 11–12.

7. Kenneth E. Mobily, "A Philosophical Analysis of Therapeutic Recreation: What Does It Mean to Say

"We Can be Therapeutic"? part 2, *Therapeutic Recreation Journal* 18, no. 2 (1985), 2.

8. Kathleen J. Halberg and Roxanne Howe-Murphy, "The Dilemma of an Unresolved Philosophy in Therapeutic Recreation," *Therapeutic Recreation Journal* 19, no. 4 (1985), 7–16.

9. U.S. Department of Health, Education and Welfare, *Health Resource Statistics 1976–1977*, DHEW publication no. (PHS) 79-1509 (Washington, D.C.: U.S. Government Printing Office, 1977), p. 6.

10. Council on Accreditation, *Standards and Evaluative Criteria for Recreation, Parks Resources and Leisure Services Baccalaureate Curricula* (Alexandria, Va: National Recreation and Park Association, 1981), pp. 9–10.

11. Ronald P. Reynolds and Gerald S. O'Morrow, *Problems, Issues, and Concepts in Therapeutic Recreation* (Englewood Cliffs, N.J.: Prentice-Hall, 1985), pp. 74–75.

12. U.S. Department of Health, Education and Welfare, *Credentialling Health Manpower*, DHEW publication no. (05) 77-50057 (Washington, D.C.: U.S. Government Printing office, 1977), p. 4.

13. DHEW, *Health Resource Statistics*, p. 6.

14. Ibid., p. 7.

15. Marcia J. Carter, "State Licensure: Trend or Fad?"

(Paper presented at the National Therapeutic Recreation Institute, Congress of Parks and Recreation, Louisville, October 24, 1982).

16. Ibid.

17. Jack Zusman, "Mental Health Service Quality Control," *Archives of General Psychiatry* 13, no. 11 (1972), 497–506.

18. Ray E. West and Bernie Thorn, "Guest Editorial," *Therapeutic Recreation Journal* 18, no. 4 (1984), 11–12.

19. Peterson, *Accreditation Report,* App. B; and Peterson and Connolly, "Professional Preparation," pp. 40–41.

20. Reynolds and O'Morrow, *Problems, Issues, and Concepts,* pp. 144–45.

SUGGESTED READINGS

ANTHONY, PATRICIA. "The Recreation Practitioner as Change Agent and Advocate for Special Populations." *Leisurability* 12, no. 1 (1985), 19–23.

BULLOCK, CHARLES C., and MARCIA JEAN CARTER. "Status Report: Continuing Professional Development Program for Therapeutic Recreators." *Therapeutic Recreation Journal* 15, no. 2 (1981), 46–49.

CARTER, MARCIA JEAN. "Issues in Continuing Professional Competence of Therapeutic Recreators." *Therapeutic Recreation Journal* 18, no. 3 (1984), 7–10.

———. "Registration of Therapeutic Recreators: Standards from 1956 to Present." *Therapeutic Recreation Journal* 15, no. 2 (1981), 4–10.

COMPTON, DAVID M. "Research Priorities in Recreation for Special Populations." *Therapeutic Recreation Journal* 18, no. 1 (1984), 9–17.

HALBERG, KATHLEEN J., and ROXANNE HOWE-MURPHY. "The Dilemma of an Unresolved Philosophy in Therapeutic Recreation." *Therapeutic Recreation Journal* 19, no. 3 (1985), 7–16.

JAMES, ANN. "Historical Perspective: The Therapy Debate." *Therapeutic Recreation Journal* 14, no. 1 (1980), 13–16.

LYNCH, BONNIE L. "Team Building: Will It Work in Health Care?" *Journal of Allied Health* 10, no. 4 (1981), 240–47.

McDOWELL, C. FORREST. "Wellness and Therapeutic Recreation: Challenges for Service." *Therapeutic Recreation Journal* 20, no. 2 (1986), 27–38.

NAVAR, NANCY, and JULIE DUNN, eds. *Quality Assurance Concerns for Therapeutic Recreation.* Urbana-Champaign: University of Illinois, Department of Leisure Studies, 1981.

O'MORROW, GERALD S. "Therapeutic Recreation Accreditation: Its Problems and Future." *Therapeutic Recreation Journal* 15, no. 2 (1981), 31–38.

PETERSON, CAROL A. "Pride and Progress in Professionalism." In *Expanding Horizons in Therapeutic Recreation VIII,* ed. G. L. Hitzhusen. Columbia: Technical Education Services, University of Missouri, 1981. Pp. 1–9.

———. "Therapeutic Recreation in the Eighties: Excellence, Existence or Extinction." *National Therapeutic Recreation Society Newsletter* 6, no. 1 (1981), 3–5.

———, and PEG CONNOLLY. "Professional Preparation in Therapeutic Recreation." *Therapeutic Recreation Journal* 15, no. 2 (1981), 39–45.

REITTER, MARY S. "Third Party Reimbursement: Is Therapeutic Recreation Too Late?" *Therapeutic Recreation Journal* 18, no. 4 (1984), 13–19.

REYNOLDS, RONALD P., and GERALD S. O'MORROW. *Problems, Issues, and Concepts in Therapeutic Recreation.* Englewood Cliffs, N.J.: Prentice-Hall, 1985.

SESSOMS, H. DOUGLAS. "Therapeutic Recreation Service: The Past and Challenging Present." In *Extra Perspectives: Concepts in Therapeutic Recreation,* ed. L. L. Neal and C. R. Edginton. Eugene: Center of Leisure Studies, University of Oregon, 1982. Pp. 1–14.

THORSTENSON, WILLIAM. "Beyond Professionalism." In *Recreation and Leisure: Issues in an Era of Change,* ed. Thomas L. Goodale and Peter A. Witt. State College, Pa.: Venture Publishing, 1980. Pp. 269–79.

VAN ANDEL, GLEN E. "Professional Standards: Improving the Quality of Services." *Therapeutic Recreation Journal* 15, no. 2 (1981), 25–30.

WEISS, CAROL, JUDITH BIEBER, CAROLYN PETERSON, and LINDA WOLD. "Danger: Therapeutic Recreation at Work." *Therapeutic Recreation Journal* 17, no. 1 (1983), 12–17.

WEST, RAY E., ed. *Issues and Guidelines for Establishing Third-Party Reimbursement for Therapeutic Recreation.* Alexandria, Va.: National Recreation and Park Association, 1981.

Appendix A
Introduction to Charting

Charting presents a written picture of occurrences and situations pertaining to a patient. All records are strictly confidential and are not to be read or discussed by anyone except the physician or persons directly caring for the patient in a health-care facility.

Charting is required for each medication, treatment, or nursing procedure. Accounts of the patient's condition and activities must be charted accurately and in clear, meaningful terms. Terse statements are essential. The chart is a legal document and is the property of the health facility. The law requires that a record be kept of patient care. Charting must be done so that it is comprehensible days, months, or years later if it must be used in court. That is why standardized charting terms are used. Each health-care worker knows and recognizes the meaning of these terms, and they are not likely to be misconstrued in court. Viewed from a legal standpoint, charting is one of the most significant duties that health workers and you will perform.

Accounts of the patient's condition and response to care and treatment are hand printed or written and signed with the hand-written signature of the person doing the charting. Only standard medical abbreviations and terms are used. If you are in doubt about abbreviations, consult a medical dictionary or books of terms and abbreviations.

It is possible to make an error when charting. Since the chart is a legal document, an erasure is not permitted. If a word is wrong or misspelled or something is written on the wrong chart, you may correct it by drawing one line through the incorrect word or sentence and writing the word *error* above it; then proceed with the charting. After completing the account, sign the chart with one initial and last name and your title (C.T.R.S.).

From a therapeutic recreation specialist's perspective the following offers some general rules for charting:

1. Entries on the patient's chart should be printed or handwritten. After completing the account, sign the notation with one initial and last name including title.

2. Ditto marks may *not* be used.

3. Do not erase. If a mistake is made, a single line is drawn through the mistake and the word *error* is printed above it. Charting is then continued in a normal manner.

4. Be exact in charting time, effect, and results of all care and treatment procedures.

5. Describe clearly and concisely patient behavior and concerns.

6. Leave no blank lines in the charting. Draw a line, if necessary, through the center of an empty line or part of a line.

7. Check with the health facility to learn the color of ink used for charting because of microfilming.

8. Use standard abbreviations.

9. Use present tense. Never future tense such as "patient to be ambulated." It is not always necessary to use the term *patient* on the chart; the chart belongs to the patient, and all notations are about the patient.

10. Do not falsify a patient's chart; legal action can be taken against anyone who does or anyone who helps another to do so.

11. Spell correctly. If you are not sure about the spelling of a word, use the dictionary.

More and more hospitals are converting to the computer system for charting. It is wise for the specialist to become familiar with basic computer usage.

ABBREVIATIONS

There are many commonly used abbreviations. Below are a list of a few abbreviations with meanings. Others can be found in a dictionary or books of medical terminology.

$\overline{aa}$ of each

a.c. before meals

ad. lib. as needed

A.M. morning

amb. ambulatory, walking

amt. amount

approx. approximately (about)

b.i.d. twice per day

B.M.R. basal metabolic rate

B.P. blood pressure

C. centigrade

$\overline{c}$ with

ca cancer

C.D. communicable disease

cmpd. compound

c/o complains of pain

DC discontinue

dr. dram (measurement)

ECG (EKG) electrocardiogram (tracing of heart function)

EEG electroencephalogram (brain wave tracing)

exam examination

ext. extract

fld. fluid

G.I. gastrointestinal (stomach and intestines)

gm. gram (measurement)

gr. grain (measurement)

h. hour

hi-cal high calorie

hi-vit high vitamin

hgb hemoglobin

H_2O water

h.s. bedtime

involv. involuntary (without knowledge of)

I & O intake and output

IV intravenous (within vein)

kg. kilogram (weight)

lab. laboratory

lb. pound

liq. liquid

L.L.Q. left lower quadrant (left lower section of abdomen)

L.U.Q. left upper quadrant

med. medical (or medication)

mid. middle

min. minute

no. number

noc. night

O_2 oxygen

O.B. obstetrics

O.R. operating room

o.d. right eye

o.u. each eye

oz. ounce

o.s. left eye

p. pulse

Ped. or Peds or Pedi pediatrics

per by or through

p.o. per or by mouth

post-op post-operative (after surgery)

p.r.n. when necessary

pre-op pre-operative (before surgery)

psych psychology

pt. patient

q.d. everyday

q.h. every hour

q.i.d. four times a day

q.o.d. every other day

R or resp. respirations

R.L.Q. right lower quadrant (right lower quarter of abdomen)

R.U.Q. right upper quadrant of abdomen

ss one-half

stat at once

tab tablet

TL team leader

TPR temperature, pulse, respiration

via by way of

wt weight

NUMBERS AND SYMBOLS

There are in addition to abbreviations, numbers and symbols commonly used in charting. Some of the more frequently used ones are as follows:

ī	one	v̄ı̄ı̄	seven
īı̄	two	v̄ı̄ı̄ı̄	eight
īı̄ı̄	three	īx̄	nine
īv̄	four	x̄	ten
v̄	five	x̄ı̄	eleven
v̄ı̄	six	x̄ı̄ı̄	twelve, etc.
+ , &	and	īss	one and one-half
>	greater than	℥ īı̄ı̄	three ounces
<	less than	ʒ īı̄	two drams
ʒ	**dram**	number	#, no.
℥	ounce	c̄	with
gr	grain	s̄	without

TERMINOLOGY

To assist the student in the development of behavior terminology, a guide of words or phrases used to describe behavior is provided. It is not all-inclusive, but it is a start and should be considered only as an introduction.

APPEARANCE
Unkempt
Neat and clean
Takes pride in appearance

BEHAVIOR

IN RELATION TO THERAPEUTIC
RECREATION ACTIVITIES
Shows interest in activities
Sits, unless directed into activities
Initiates activities
Remembers rules and directions
Shows initial ability to comprehend directions
Moves slowly or sluggishly
Rigid
Hyperactive

Responds inadequately to a situation
Participates easily in activities
Maintains attention span
Conflicts with or defies authority
Reacts to competition
Becomes involved (enjoys the activity, desires to win, and so on)
Reacts to winning or losing

IN RELATION TO OTHER PATIENTS
AND/OR PERSONNEL
Tries to be friendly with others
Attempts to manipulate others
Is withdrawn
Seeks attention
Forms specific friendships
Forms relationships with the rest of the group

IN RELATION TO EMOTIONAL BEHAVIOR
AND ITS APPROPRIATENESS

Is impatient

Loses temper frequently

Is easily upset

Laughs or smiles at funny comments or events

Giggles or smiles to himself or herself for no apparent reason

Irritable or grouchy

Depressed

Tearful

Shy or aloof

Suspicious

Immature

Hostile

Aggressive

Helpless

Dependent

Overconscientious

Selfish

Autistic

Anxious

Hostile

IN RELATION TO INDIVIDUAL BEHAVIOR
CHARACTERISTICS

Hallucinatory

Delusional

Memory and retention

Orientation

Intellectual functioning

Quality of judgment

Affect

Sexual identification

Physical complaints

Quality of associations

Ambivalence

Characteristics of self-image

Frequently tries doors and exits

CONVERSATION

Hypertalkative

Initiates conversation

Quiet, but responds to verbal approach

Refuses to speak

Is able to express himself or herself adequately and appropriately

Talks of death

Exhibits pattern to subject matter

Mentions future plans

INTENSITY SCALING OF TERMS USED TO DESCRIBE PERSONALITY*

VERBAL HOSTILITY		even-tempered	irritable
venomous	soft-spoken	peaceable	grouchy
abusive	complimentary	harmless	petulant
threatening	praising	inhibited	grudging
derisive	flattering	placating	civil
derogatory	mealy-mouthed	cringing	inoffensive
scornful	apple-polishing		unresentful
sarcastic	eulogistic	HOSTILE ATTITUDES	agreeable
argumentative		malicious	gentle
overcritical	PHYSICAL HOSTILITY	embittered	gracious
nagging	murderous	quarrelsome	conciliatory
outspoken	assaultive	surly	ingratiating
frank	destructive	provocative	oily
tactful	combative	resentful	fawning
	hot-blooded		

*Arnold H. Buss, "The Scaling of Terms Used to Describe Personality," *Journal of Consulting Psychology* 21, no. 5 (1957), 361–69.

ANXIETY

terrified
panicky
agitated
tremulous
apprehensive
tense
fretful
uneasy
composed
calm
nonchalant
unconcerned
cool
bland
stolid
imperturbable
phlegmatic

MOOD

euphoric
elated
frivolous
buoyant
gay
jovial
light-hearted
cheerful
placid
sober
serious
solemn
mirthless
grave
gloomy
brooding
dejected
disconsolate
despondent
hopeless

GUILT

self-condemning
self-reproachful
remorseful
ashamed
chagrined
regretful
concerned
indifferent
unfeeling
unreformed
cynical

unrepentant
hardened
shameless
conscienceless
unscrupulous
incorrigible

SELF-ESTEEM

self-exalting
pompous
conceited
boastful
vain
cocky
confident
self-respecting
modest
unassuming
humble
self-doubting
self-effacing
self-deprecatory
forlorn
self-abasing

IDEATION

delusional
ruminative
day-dreaming
fanciful
musing
contemplative
thoughtful
matter-of-fact
literal
unreflective
unimaginative
stolid
vacuous

IMPULSIVENESS

incontinent
reckless
rash
impetuous
excitable
hasty
abrupt
restless
mobile
spontaneous
self-possessed
cool-headed

amenable
adaptable
conventional
persistent
habit-bound
stubborn
persevering
unbending
mulish

EMOTIONAL WARMTH

overindulgent
doting
affectionate
sentimental
tender
sympathetic
kindly
considerate
cool
unresponsive
detached
unfeeling
hardened
rejecting
frigid

SOCIABILITY

intrusive
meddlesome
gregarious
convivial
intimate
comradely
companionable
agreeable
accessible
hesitant
reserved
bashful
reticent
retiring
shrinking
seclusive
withdrawn
solitary
isolated

DOMINANCE

dictatorial
autocratic
high-handed
masterful

deliberate
controlled
restrained
staid
overcautious
retarded
sluggish

FLEXIBILITY

spineless
yielding
changeable
forceful
assertive
decisive
cooperative
assenting
conforming
compliant
acquiescent
imitative
deferent
timid
meek
servile

AMBITION

grandiose
pretentious
aspiring
enterprising
persistent
eager
self-satisfied
complacent
lackadaisical
indifferent
listless
indolent
apathetic
lethargic

Appendix B
Drug Therapy

Drugs occupy a prominent place in the care and treatment of individuals. Their use as a therapeutic agent has been known throughout the ages. The science of pharmacology is a highly developed medical field. The number of different drugs manufactured commercially for distribution has increased enormously in recent years. As each new drug is added, its composition, physiological action, uses, and dosage are recorded in the *Materia Medica, Pharmacopea,* and *Physicians' Desk Reference* (drug reference publications). Furthermore, any one drug can have as many as four names: its trademark, its official name, its chemical name, and its generic name.

When a newly developed drug is prepared for clinical testing, it's given an official name or so-called generic name. Once the drug has passed its tests and is ready for the medical marketplace the company assigns it a new trade or proprietary name. This is what is called a brand name. Usually brand names are catchy, easy to pronounce and easy to remember. Generic names are often tongue twisters. For example, Valium is a household word, but few people would recognize its generic name, diazepam. How about Tylenol vs. acetaminophen or Darvon vs. propoxyphene? You can see why doctors and others would opt for the easy-to-spell, pronounce-and-remember brand-name version.

Drugs are put up as tablets, capsules, powders, or fluids. They are given usually by mouth, occasionally by rectum. Drugs may be inhaled or rubbed into the skin (inunction). They may be injected (parenteral) into the skin (intradermal), under the skin (subcutaneous), or into the muscle (intramuscular). Lastly, drugs may be introduced into a vein (intravenous therapy) or into the peritoneum (intraperitoneal therapy). The method of administration is partially determined by the age of the individual, his or her orientation, and degree of consciousness and the disease. The role of administering the drug affects the optimal dosage of the drug. And the effect (or action) of the drug on the body may be *systemic* (affecting the whole body) or *local* (affecting a specific area).

The quickest and most profound results are obtained by hypodermic injection and are given (1) when an immediate effect from the drug is desired, (2) when for any reason it is inadvisable or impossible to administer the drug by mouth, and (3) when the chemical nature of the drug is such that it is rendered ineffective by the action of the digestive juices. The slowest results are obtained from inunction.

Listed below are some of the more commonly used drugs that therapeutic recreation specialists may encounter in working with special populations in various settings. The student will note that each drug is listed under the body system it influences; thereafter, in the first column the brand name is given, followed by the generic name in parentheses and the drug's class or pharmacologic action. However, a few drugs are not classed. The second column indicates the principal therapeutic use of the drugs, and the third column reflects the drug's commonly observed side effects. Although many side effects may be associated with the drug other than those listed, the ones listed are for the attention of the therapeutic recreation specialist.

Drug	Use	Side Effect
Cardiovascular System		
Aldomet (methyldopa) antihypertensive	Treats mild to severe hypertension	Hemolytic anemia; sedation; decreased mental acuity; dry mouth; nasal stuffiness
Dilantin (phenytoin) antiarrhythmic	Treats atrial and ventricular arrhythmias of various causes	Ataxia; lethargy; severe hypotension; rash diplopia; nystagmus; nausea; vomiting
Inderal* (propranolol hydrochloride) antiarrhythmic and anti-hypertensive	Treats supraventricular, ventricular, and atrial arrhythmias	Fatigue; lethargy; increased airway resistance; congestive heart failure
Isordil (isosorbide dinitrate) antianginal	Treats acute angina, prophylaxis in situations likely to cause angina attack, chronic ischemic heart disease	Headaches; dizziness; ankle edema; palpitations; flushing
Lanoxin* (digoxin) cardiacglycoside	Increases cardiac output in acute and chronic congestive heart failure; controls rate of ventricular contraction in atrial fibrillation and flutter	Fatigue; general muscle weakness; agitation; hallucinations; blurred vision; nausea
Lopressor (metoprolol tartrate) antihypertensive	Treats mild to severe hypertension	Fatigue; lethargy; nausea
Minipress (prazosin hydrochloride) antihypertensive	Treats mild to moderate hypertension; severe chronic congestive heart failure	Dizziness; palpitations; nausea
Nitroglycerin (nitroglycerin) antianginals	Treats chronic angina	Headaches; dizziness; flushing; palpitations
Procardia (nifedipine) antianginal	Management of variant angina and chronic angina pectoris	Dizziness; light-headedness; flushing; headaches; nausea; heartburn
Pronestyl (procainamide hydrochloride) antiarrhythmic	Management of atrial and ventricular arrhythmias	Severe hypotension; nausea; vomiting;
		Diarrhea; bitter taste in mouth; anorexia; maculopapular rash; fever; myalgia
Autonomic Nervous System		
Artane (trihexyphenidyl hydrochloride) cholinergic blocker	Treats Parkinsonism and extrapyramidal reactions associated with neuroleptic drugs	Dry mouth; nausea; nervousness; blurred vision; dizziness
Cogentin (benztropine mesylate) cholinergic blocker	Treats acute dystonic reaction (reaction to neuroleptic drugs)	Dry mouth; nausea

*Drugs most frequently taken by the elderly.

Drug	Use	Side Effect
Central Nervous System		
Aspirin (acetylsacicylic acid) nonnarcotic analgesic	Treats mild to moderate pain; alleviates inflammation of rheumatoid arthritis, osteoarthritis, gout, and other conditions	Tinnitus and hearing loss; nausea; skin rash; vomiting; hypersensitivity manifested by anaphylaxis and/or asthma
Dalmane* (flurazepam hydrochloride) sedative	Induces sleep and provides sedation and relief of anxiety	Daytime sedation; dizziness; drowsiness; disturbed coordination; headaches
Dilantin (phenytoin) anticonvulsant	Treats generalized grand mal seizures and nonepileptic seizures	Initial nausea; weight loss; nervousness; skin rash
Dilantin with phenobarbital anticonvulsant†	Controls convulsions	
Elavil (amitriplyline hydrochloride) antidepressant	Treats depression, anxiety, tension, fear, psychomotor retardation	Drowsiness; dizziness; blurred vision; dry mouth; constipation; urinary retention; sweating; headaches
Haldol (haloperidol) antipsychotic	Treats psychotic disorders, modifies thought disorders, blunts affect, and behavior associated with psychomotor and lessens symptoms of paranoia agitation, hallucinations, delusions, and autistic behavior	Severe extrapyramidal reactions (high incidence); blurred vision; dry mouth
Indocin (indomethacin) nonsteroidal antiinflammatory	Treats moderate to severe arthritis	Headaches; dizziness; vertigo; blurred vision; nausea; vomiting; diarrhea
Librium (chlorizepoxide hydrochloride) antianxiety	Treats mild to moderate anxiety and tension; relaxes skeletal muscles; and treats and prevents alcohol-withdrawal symptoms	Drowsiness; lethargy; hangover; skin rash; constipation
Marplan (isocarboxazid) antidepressant	Treats depression	Dizziness; anorexia; headaches; overactivity; skin rash
Motrin (ibuprofen) nonsteroidal antiinflammatory	Treats arthritis and gout	Nausea; headaches; dizziness
Mellaril* (thioridazine hydrochloride) antipsychotic	Same as Haldol; in addition, controls anxiety, agitation, and confusion	Sedation (high); ocular changes; blurred vision; dry mouth; constipation; urinary retention; cholestatic jaundice; mild photosensitivity; exfoliative dermatitis
Mysoline (primidone) anticonvulsant	Treats generalized grand mal seizures and psychomotor seizures	Drowsiness; ataxia; diplopia; nausea; vomiting

†Anticonvulsant drugs prevent or reduce the frequency or severity of seizures of idiopathic epilepsy or seizures secondary to drugs. There are a wide range of anticonvulsant drugs designed for specific seizure disorders.

(continued)

Drug	Use	Side Effects
Central Nervous System (*Continued*)		
Norpramin (desipramine hydrochloride) antidepressant	Treats depression	Drowsiness; dizziness; blurred vision; dry mouth; constipation; sweating
Phenobarbital (luminal) anticonvulsant	Treats all forms of epilepsy	Drowsiness; lethargy; hangover
Stelazine (trifluoperazine hydro-chloride) antipsychotic	Treats anxiety state, agitation, confusion	Extrapyramidal reactions (high incidence); ocular changes; blurred vision; dry mouth; constipation; mild photosensitivity; cholestatic jaundice; exfoliative dermatitis; skin rash
Thorazine (chlorpromazine hydrochloride) antipsychotic	Same as Haldol and Mellaril	Extrapyramidal reactions (moderate incidence); sedation (high incidence); ocular changes; blurred vision; dry mouth; constipation; urinary retention; cholestatic jaundice; mild photosensitivity; exfoliative dermatitis
Tofranil (imipramine hydrochloride) antidepressant	Treats depression	Drowsiness; dizziness; blurred vision; dry mouth; constipation; sweating; urinary retention
Tylenol and Tylenol with codeine #1, 2, 3, and 4 (acetaminophen) narcotic and opioid analgesics	Relieves moderate to severe pain	Tylenol alone: rash and urticaria; Tylenol with codeine: dizziness; sedation; nausea; constipation; and dry mouth
Valium (diazepam) anticonvulsant/antianxiety	Treats epilepsy and controls anxiety	Drowsiness; ataxia; fatigue; mild nausea; dizziness
Xanax (alprazolam) antianxiety	Reduces anxiety and tension; relaxes skeletal muscles; prevents and treats alcohol-withdrawal symptoms	Drowsiness; light-headedness
Hormonal Agents		
Insulin* antidiabetic	Treats diabetes mellitus, especially juvenile onset (insulin dependent), and maturity onset (noninsulin dependent)	Hypoglycemia; hyperglycemia (rebound effect); lipoatrophy; lipohypertrophy; anaphylaxis
Hydrochuril (hydrochlorothiazide) diuretics (concern with body's water and salt volume)	Treats edema and hypertension	Dehydration; hypokalemia; asymptomatic hyperuricemia; hyperglycemia
Lasix* (furosemide) diuretic	Treats heart failure and hypertension	Dehydration; hypokalemia; asymptomatic hyperuricemia; hyperglycemia

Drug	Use	Side Effects
Others		
Levopa and Larodopa (levodopa) uncategorized	Treats idiopathic Parkinsonism and Parkinsonian syndrome and cerebral arteriosclerosis	Dyskinetic movements; involuntary grimacing; head movements; ataxia; tremors; muscle twitching; psychiatric disturbances; memory loss; anxiety; fatigue; depression; delirium, hallucinations; nausea; vomiting; anorexia
Sinemet (levodopa-carbidopa) uncategorized	Treats idiopathic Parkinsonism and Parkinsonian syndrome	Dystonic; dyskinetic movements; involuntary grimacing; head movement, myoclonia body jerks; ataxia
Tagamet (cimetidine) gastrointestinal	Treats duodenal ulcer	Mental confusion; dizziness; mild and transient diarrhea; exfoliative dermatitis

SOURCE: Based on data from *Drugs,* 2nd ed. (Springhouse, Pa.: Springhouse Corporation, 1986).

SUGGESTED REFERENCES

ALBANESE, JOSEPH A. *Nurses' Drug Reference* (2nd ed.). New York: McGraw-Hill Book Co., 1982.

HAKN, ANNE B., et al. *Pharmacology in Nursing* (15th ed.). St. Louis: C. V. Mosby Co., 1982.

LOEBL, SUZANNE, et al. *The Nurses Drug Handbook* (3rd ed.). New York: John Wiley & Sons, 1983.

Physicians' Desk Reference (37th ed.). Oradell, N.J.: Medical Economics Co., 1983.

Appendix C
Organizational Leadership and Awards

ORGANIZATIONAL LEADERSHIP

Those who have been responsible for the leadership of their respective organizations by serving as chairman or president are as follows:

Chairman, Hospital Recreation Section—American Recreation Society

Malcoln Randall (1949–50)
Carolyn N. Lyle (1950–51)
Thomas H. Rickman, Jr.(1951–52)
C. C. Bream, Jr. (1952–53)
Dorothy Taaffe (1953–54)
Fred M. Chapman (1954–55)
Edith L. Ball (1955–56)
James F. Pratt (1956–57)
Lillian Summers (1957–58)
Lillian Summers (1958–59)
Albert J. Meuli (1959–60)
Sidney H. Acuff (1960–61)
John J. Gehan (1961–62)
Frances Cleary (1962–63)
Gerald S. O'Morrow (1963–64)
Francis W. Heinlen (1964–65)
Fred Humphrey (1965–66)

SOURCE: *The Hospital Recreation Section: Its History 1948–64.* Washington, D.C.: American Recreation Society, n.d., and personal knowledge.

Chairman, Recreation Therapy Section—American Association For Health Physical Education and Recreation (now American Alliance for Health, Physical Education, Recreation and Dance)

B. J. Rudquist (1952–53)
B. J. Rudquist (1953–54)
Martin W. Meyer (1954–55)
Martin W. Meyer (1955–56)
Cecil W. Morgan (1956–57)
Cecil W. Morgan (1957–58)
Robert C. Boyd (1958–59)
Thomas J. Clark (1959–60)
Wayne Nichols (1960–61)
Jeannette C. McGranaham (1961–62)
Morton Thompson (1962–63)
John Roan (1963–64)
Martin W. Meyer (1964–65)

SOURCE: *Journal of Health, Physical Education and Recreation* from 1951 to 1964 and personal communication with Martin W. Meyer, January 17, 1986.

President, National Association of Recreational Therapists, Inc.

Floyd E. McDowell (1953–54)
Frank Longo
William T. Lawler
Philip Walsh
Steve Chiovaro
Edward Karpowicz
Hayden Walker
Charlotte L. Cox
Samuel Seabolt
William L. Smith
Anne K. Bushart

SOURCE: Charlotte L. Cox and Virginia Dobbins, "Before the Merger: The National Association of Recreational Therapists (1953–1967)," *Therapeutic Recreation Journal* 4, no. 1 (1970), 3–8, and personal communication with Samuel Seabolt, May 5, 1987. The years of presidency, other than as shown above for Mr. McDowell, have been purposely left out since some individuals served more than one term but the exact years are unknown. However, their order of presidency as indicated above is correct.

President, National Therapeutic Recreation Society

Ira Hutchison (1966*)
John Logue (1966–67)
Fred Humphrey (1967–68)
William L. Smith (1968–69)
Gerald S. O'Morrow (1969–70)
John A. Nesbitt (1970–71)
Sidney H. Acuff (1971–72)
Jerry D. Kelly (1972–73)
William A. Hillman, Jr. (1973–74)
Jean R. Tague (1974–75)

Richard L. Stracke (1975–76)
Lee E. Meyer (1976–77)
Gary M. Robb (1977–78)
Gerald S. Fain (1978–79)
David C. Park (1979–80)
Carol A. Peterson (1980–81)
Jacquelyn Vaughan (1981–82)
Viki S. Annand (1982–83)
Ann James (1983–84)
Jerry Dickason (1984–85)
David M. Compton (1985–86)
Michal A. Lord (1986–87)
Sandra Mayfield (1987–88)
Fred Humphrey (1988–89)
*Served only a partial term as a result of accepting the position of executive secretary, NTRS/NRPA. Other executive secretaries have been David C. Park (1968–75) and Yvonne Washington (1975–present).

SOURCE: Files of the National Therapeutic Recreation Society, National Recreation and Park Association, and National Therapeutic Recreation Society; *NTRS Newsletter* 12, no. 2 (Winter 1987), 1,2.

President, American Therapeutic Recreation Association, Inc.

Peg Connolly (1984–85)
Ray E. West (1985–86)
Bernard E. Thorn (1986–87)
Ann Huston (1987–88)

SOURCE: Personal communication with Peg Connolly, May 7, 1987.

AWARDS

Since its inception, NTRS has recognized the desirability of honoring certain of its members, citizens, organizations, and institutions that have rendered outstanding service to the society and the fields of endeavors it represents. (Information regarding the qualifications for any specific award may be obtained by writing the National Therapeutic Recreation Society.) The following individuals and organizations have been recipients of the various awards.

Distinguished Service Award

Sidney H. Acuff (1970)
David R. Austin (1985)
Edith L. Ball (1974)

Doris L. Berryman (1973)
Anne K. Bushart (1970)
Marcia Jean Carter (1987)
Fred M. Chapman (1971)
Rose Hanzlicek (1982)
Francis Heinlen (1969)
Helen Jo Hillman (1982)
William A. Hillman (1977)
Gerald Hitzhusen (1981)
Fred Humphrey (1971)
Ira Hutchison (1971)
Jerry D. Kelley (1978)
Lee E. Meyer (1979)
John A. Nesbitt (1972)
Gerald S. O'Morrow (1977)
David C. Park (1981)

Martha Peters (1984)
Carol Ann Peterson (1982)
Gary M. Robb (1979)
Samuel Seabolt (1976)
Jay Shivers (1983)
Ed Supina (1986)
Jean R. Tague (1977)
Jacquelyn Vaughan (1978)

SOURCE: National Therapeutic Recreation Society, *NTRS Newsletter*, 12, no. 2 (Winter 1987), 5; and personal communication with Yvonne Washington, November 17, 1987. (No DSA was given in 1975 or 1980.)

Member of the Year Award

Marcia Jean Carter (1981)
Nancy Edwards (1984)
Patrick Griffen (1980)
Nancy Navar (1982)
Robert Parker (1983)
John W. Shank (1986)
Ray E. West (1985)
Joe Wilson (1987)

SOURCE: National Therapeutic Recreation Society, *NTRS Newsletter*, 12, no. 2 (Winter 1987), 7; and personal communication with Yvonne Washington, Novermber 17, 1987.

Individual Citation (Nonmember of NTRS)

Cliff Bream (1974)
Alto Brenner (1980)
Myrtice Cook (1971)
William deGraveller (1977)
Beatrice Hill (1987)
Wayne Hollenbaugh (1985)
Albert Incani (1969)
Rafer Johnson (1972)
Tim Nugent (1972)
Janet Pomeroy (1970)
Dr. Howard Rusk (1973)
Lois Timmins (1976)
Marion Wurster (1979)

SOURCE: National Therapeutic Recreation Society, *NTRS Newsletter*, 12, no. 2 (Winter 1987), 6; and personal communication with Yvonne Washington, November 17, 1987. (No award given in 1978 or from 1981 to 1984.)

Certificate of Recognition (Member, NTRS)

M. Jean Keller (1987)
Sharon McIntyre (1987)
Barbara Sirvis (1985)
Lisa Turpel (1987)

SOURCE: National Therapeutic Recreation Society, *NTRS Newsletter*, 12, no. 2 (Winter 1987), 7; and personal communication with Yvonne Washington, November 17, 1987.

Institutions or Organizations Receiving Citations

Bing Crosby Youth Fund, Carmel, Calif. (1972)

Board of Governors, American Red Cross, Washington, D.C. (1974)

Camp Allen, New Hampshire (1979)

Courage Center, Golden Valley, Minn. (1984)

DARE (Diversified Activity and Recreation Enterprises), Tacoma, Wash. (1986)

Hayward Area Recreation and Park District, Hayward, Calif. (1978)

Joseph P. Kennedy Foundation, Washington, D.C. (1973)

National Easter Seal Society, Chicago, Ill. (1980)

New Jersey Office of Community Recreation for Handicapped Persons, Department of Community Affairs (1985)

North Suburban Special Recreation Association, Highland Park, Ill. (1975)

North American Riding for the Handicapped Association, Cheff Center for the Handicapped, Augusta, Maine (1976)

Paralyzed Veterans of America, Washington, D.C. (1987)

Project Chips, Parks and Recreation Department, Buffalo, N.Y. (1983)

Programs for Mentally Retarded and Physically Handicapped, Department of Recreation, Washington, D.C. (1971)

U.S. Bureau of Education for the Handicapped, Department of Education, Washington, D.C. (1975)

Recreation Center for the Handicapped, San Francisco, Calif. (1982)

Sigma Sigma Sigma National Sorority (1984)

Teaching Center for Casa Colina Hospital, Pomona, Calif. (1977)

Therapeutic Recreation Association of Milwaukee County, Milwaukee, Wis. (1983)

Timberlawn Psychiatric Center, Dallas, Texas (1986)

Topeka Resource Center for the Handicapped, Topeka, Kansas (1987)

Very Special Arts, Washington, D.C. (1987)

Veterans Administration Hospital, Bedside Network, Radio/Television Guild, New York, N.Y. (1972)

Veterans Administration Hospital, Central Office, Washington, D.C. (1981)

SOURCE: National Therapeutic Recreation Society, *NTRS Newsletter,* 12, no. 2 (Winter 1987), 6; and personal communication with Yvonne Washington, May 18 and November 17, 1987.

Appendix D
National Council
for Therapeutic Recreation
Certification

STANDARDS

The purpose of the National Council for Therapeutic Recreation Certification is to (1) establish national evaluation standards for the certification and recertification of individuals who possess the competencies of the therapeutic recreation profession; (2) grant recognition to individuals who voluntarily apply and meet the established standards; and (3) monitor adherence to the standards by certified therapeutic recreation personnel.

A *major in therapeutic recreation or major in recreation with an option in therapeutic recreation* refers to the completion of a degree that includes the following courses:

1. Nine (9) semester units or twelve (12) quarter units of therapeutic recreation content courses, *and*

2. Nine (9) semester units or twelve (12) quarter units of general recreation content courses, *and*
(There must be at least three (3) content courses in therapeutic recreation and three (3) content courses in recreation.)

3. Completion of supportive courses to include a minimum of eighteen (18) semester hours or twenty-seven (27) quarter hours from four (4) of the six (6) areas—adaptive physical education, biological/physical sciences, human services, psychology, sociology, or special education *and*

4. Completion of a minimum 360-hour field-placement experience in a clinical, residential, or community-based therapeutic recreation program under an *agency* field-placement supervisor who is certified by NCTRC at the therapeutic recreation specialist professional level.

A *major in recreation* refers to the completion of a degree that includes the following courses:

1. Nine (9) semester units or twelve (12) quarter units of general recreation courses, *and*
(There must be at least three (3) content courses in recreation.)

2. Completion of supportive courses to include a minimum of eighteen (18) semester hours or twenty-seven (27) quarter hours from four (4) of these six (6) areas—adaptive physical education, biological/physical sciences, human services, psychology, sociology, or special education.

DEGREE PROGRAMS

Therapeutic Recreation Specialist— Professional (minimum requirements)

Baccalaureate degree or higher from an accredited college or university with a major in therapeutic recreation or a major in recreation with an option in therapeutic recreation (Degree must be verified by an official transcript.)

Therapeutic Recreation Specialist— Professional Provisional (minimum requirements) (nonrenewable certification)

This professional provisional is for applicants whose transcripts indicate a *degree* with a major in therapeutic recreation or a major in recreation with an option in therapeutic recreation, but the completed courses do not meet the standards for a major or option in therapeutic recreation.

Baccalaureate degree or higher from an accredited college or university with a major in therapeutic recreation, a major in recreation with an option in therapeutic recreation, or major in recreation. The academic preparation *must* include *one* of the following:

1. Nine (9) semester units or twelve (12) quarter units of therapeutic recreation content courses *or*
2. Nine (9) semester units or twelve (12) quarter units of general recreation content courses *or*
3. A combination of nine (9) semester units or twelve (12) quarter units of therapeutic recreation and recreation content courses.

This alternative permits temporary certification for a two- (2) year provisional period. In order to maintain certification a person must acquire the necessary academic preparation as defined by the therapeutic recreation specialist professional standards within this two-year period.

Baccalaureate degree or higher from an accredited college or university with a major in recreation. (Degree must be verified by an official transcript.) This alternative permits temporary certification while a person acquires the two years of full-time paid experience in a clinical, residential, or community-based therapeutic recreation program. In order to maintain certifica-

tion a person must complete the work experience within this two- (2) year period.

Therapeutic Recreation Specialist— Professional Equivalency (minimum requirements)

Baccalaureate degree or higher from an accredited college or university. (Degree must be verified by an official transcript.)

1. A degree in one of the following areas: art education, dance, drama, early childhood education, music education, physical education, psychology, rehabilitation, sociology or special education *and*
2. Five (5) years of full-time paid experience in a clinical, residential, or community-based therapeutic recreation program *and*
3. Eighteen (18) semester hours or twenty-seven (27) quarter hours of upper-division or graduate credits in therapeutic recreation/recreation courses. (All courses must be verified by an official transcript.)

Therapeutic Recreation Assistant— Paraprofessional (minimum requirements)

A. Associate degree from an accredited educational institution with a major in therapeutic recreation or a major in recreation with an option in therapeutic recreation. (Degree must be verified by an official transcript.)
B. Associate degree from an accredited educational institution with a major in recreation *plus* one (1) year of full-time paid experience in a clinical, residential, or community-based therapeutic recreation program. (Degree must be verified by an official transcript.)

Therapeutic Recreation Assistant— Paraprofessional Equivalency (minimum requirements)

A. Associate degree or higher from an accredited educational institution with:

1. Major in one of the following areas: allied health, art education, dance, drama, gerontology, human services, mental health, music education, or physical education *and*

2. One year of full-time paid experience in a clinical, residential, or community-based therapeutic recreation program *or*

B. Completion of the NTRS 750-hour training program for therapeutic recreation personnel with verification by an official certificate of completion *or*

C. Four (4) years of full-time paid experience in a clinical, residential, or community-based therapeutic recreation program.

Additional information regarding the requirements associated with the therapeutic recreation assistant and other terms used within the requirement can be obtained by writing:

National Council for Therapeutic Recreation Certification
P.O. Box 16126
Alexandria, Va. 22302
PHONE: (703) 820-3993

Appendix E
Therapeutic Recreation Resources

ASSOCIATIONS AND ORGANIZATIONS SERVING SPECIAL POPULATIONS*

GOVERNMENT

Administration on Aging
330 C St., SW
Washington, D.C. 20201

Architectural and Transportation Barriers
Compliance Board
330 C. St., SW, Room 1010
Washington, D.C. 20201

Children's Bureau, Office of Child Development
300 Independence Av., SW
Washington, D.C. 20201

National Clearinghouse on Post-Secondary Education
for Disabled People
1 DuPont Circle
Washington, D.C. 20036

*For a publication which furnishes details on over twenty thousand national and international nonprofit trade and professional associations, social welfare and public affairs organizations, religious, sports and hobby groups, see Katherine Gruber, ed. *The Encyclopedia of Associations*, Vol. 1, 21st ed. (Detroit: Gale Research Company, 1987). Other volumes include the associations and organizations found in volume 1 by city and state, a supplement to volume 1 concerned with associations and organizations in the process of being formed, and a volume concerned solely with international organizations.

National Council on the Aging, Inc.
600 Maryland Av., SW, West Wing 100
Washington, D.C. 20024

National Institutes of Health
9000 Rockville Pike
Bethesda, Maryland 20010

National Institute of Mental Health
11A-20 Parklawn Bldg.
5600 Fishers Lane
Rockville, Maryland 20857

National Institute of Neurological and
Communicative Disorders and Stroke
National Institute of Health
Bldg. 31, Room 8A-06
Bethesda, Maryland 20205

National Park Service
Department of Interior
18th and C St., N.W.
Washington, D.C. 20240

President's Committee on Mental Retardation
Washington, D.C. 20201

President's Committee on Employment of the
Handicapped
1111 20th St., N.W., Room 606
Washington, D.C. 20036

Veterans Administration
810 Vermont Av., N.W.
Washington, D.C. 20420

PROFESSIONAL

Academy of Dentistry for the Handicapped
211 East Chicago, Suite 2133
Chicago, Illinois 60611

American Academy of Physical Medicine and
Rehabilitation
1425 W. Fairview Av.
Dayton, Ohio 45406

American Alliance of Health, Physical Education,
Recreation, and Dance
1900 Association Drive
Reston, Virginia 22091

American Art Therapy Association
1980 Isaac Newton Square, South
Reston, Virginia 22090

American Association for Music Therapy
PO Box 359
66 Morris St.
Springfield, New Jersey 07081

American Association for Rehabilitation Therapy
Box 93
North Little Rock, Arkansas 72216

American Association of University Affiliated
Programs for the Developmentally Disabled
1234 Massachusetts Av., NW
Suite 813
Washington, D.C. 20005

American Camping Association
Bradford Woods
5040 State Rd., 67 North
Martinsville, Indiana 46151

American Congress of Rehabilitation Medicine
30 N. Michigan Av.
Chicago, Illinois 60602

American Correctional Association
4321 Hartwick Rd.
College Park, Maryland 20740

American Corrective Therapy Association
259-08, 148th Rd.
Rosedale, New York 11422

American Dance Therapy Association
2000 Century Plaza, Suite 108
Columbia, Maryland 21044

American Health Care Association
1200 15th St., NW
Washington, D.C. 20005

American Hospital Association
840 North Shore Dr.
Chicago, Illinois 60611

American Nurses' Association
2420 Pershing Rd.
Kansas City, Missouri 64108

American Occupational Therapy Association
1383 Piccard Dr., Suite 301
Rockville, Maryland 20850

American Orthotic & Prosthetic Association
1440 N. St., NW
Washington, D.C. 20005

American Physical Therapy Association
1111 North Fairfax St.
Alexandria, Virginia 22314

American Psychiatric Association
1400 K St., NW
Washington, D.C. 20005

American Psychological Association
1200 17th St., NW
Washington, D.C. 20036

American Public Health Association
1015 8th St., NW
Washington, D.C. 20036

American Speech-Language Association
10801 Rockville Pike
Rockville, Maryland 20852

American Therapeutic Recreation Association
2021 L St., NW, Suite 250
Washington, D.C. 20036

Council on Accreditation of Rehabilitation Facilities
2500 North Pontano Rd.
Tucson, Arizona 87515

Council for Exceptional Children
1920 Association Dr.
Reston, Virginia 22031

Gerontological Society of America
1411 K St., NW
Washington, D.C. 20005

Joint Commission on Accreditation of Hospitals
875 North Michigan Av.
Chicago, Illinois 60611

National Association of Activity Professionals
PO Box 274
Park Ridge, Illinois 60068

National Association of Activity Therapy and
Rehabilitation Program Directors
Box 111
Independence, Iowa 50644

National Association of Drama Therapy
19 Edwards St.
New Haven, Connecticut 06511

National Association for Music Therapy
910 Kentucky Av.
Lawrence, Kansas 66044

National Association for Poetry Therapy
1029 Henhawk Rd.
Baldwin, New York 11510

National Association of Physical Therapists, Inc.
PO Box 367
West Covina, California 91793

National Association of Vocational Education for
Special Needs Personnel
University of Nebraska
300 West Nebraska Hall
Lincoln, Nebraska 65888

National Correctional Recreation Association
Blackburn Correctional Complex
311 Spurr Rd.
Lexington, Kentucky 40511

National Council for Therapy and Rehabilitation
through Horticulture
9220 Wightman Rd., Suite 300
Gaithersburg, Maryland 20877

National Recreation and Park Association
3101 Park Center Dr.
Alexandria, Virginia 22302

National Rehabilitation Association
633 South Washington St.
Alexandria, Virginia 22314

National Therapeutic Recreation Society
3101 Park Center Dr.
Alexandria, Virginia 22302

Section for Rehabilitation Hospitals and Programs
c/o American Hospital Association
875 North Michigan Av.
Chicago, Illinois 60611

SERVICE

Alcoholics Anonymous
PO Box 459
Grand Central Station
New York, New York 10017

American Allergy Association
PO Box 7273
Menlo Park, California 94026

American Association for the Deaf
PO Box 105
Talladega, Alabama 35160

American Association of Retired Persons
215 Long Beach Boulevard
Long Beach, California 90801

American Association on Mental Deficiency
(AAMD)
5101 Wisconsin Av., NW
Washington, D.C. 20016

American Cancer Society, Inc.
90 Park Av.
New York, New York 10016

American Coalition of Citizens with Disabilities
1346 Connecticut Av., NW
Room 817
Washington, D.C. 20036

American Council on Alcoholism
8501 Lasalle Rd., Suite 301
Towson, Maryland 21204

American Diabetes Association
PO Box 25757
1660 Duke St.
Arlington, Virginia 22313

American Federation of the Physically
Handicapped, Inc.
1376 National Press Building
Washington, D.C. 20004

American Foundation for the Blind
15 East 16th St.
New York, New York 10011

American Geriatrics Society
10 Columbus Circle, Suite 1470
New York, New York 10019

American Heart Association
7320 Greenville Av.
Dallas, Texas 75231

American Lung Association
1740 Broadway
New York, New York 10019

American National Red Cross
17th and D Sts., NW
Washington, D.C. 20006

American Paralysis Association
PO Box 187
Short Hills, New Jersey 07078

American Rheumatism Association
1314 Spring St., NW
Atlanta, Georgia 30309

American Spinal Injury Association
250 East Superior St., Room 619
Chicago, Illinois 60611

Arthritis and Rheumatism Foundation
10 Columbus Circle
New York, New York 10019

Association for the Aid of Crippled Children
345 East 46th St.
New York, New York 10017

Association for Children with Learning
Disabilities
4156 Library Rd.
Pittsburgh, Pennsylvania 15234

Association for Retarded Citizens
PO Box 6109
Arlington, Texas 76006

Association for the Severely Retarded
7010 Roosevelt Way, NE
Seattle, Washington 98115

Braille Institution
741 North Vermont Av.
Los Angeles, California 90029

The Candlelighters Foundation
2025 Eye St., NW, Suite 1011
Washington, D.C. 20006

Council for Learning Disabilities
PO Box 40303
Overland Park, Kansas 66204

Council of Organizations Serving the Deaf
PO Box 894
Columbia, Maryland 21044

Down's Syndrome Congress
1640 W. Roosevelt Rd., Room 156E
Chicago, Illinois 60608

Epilepsy Foundation of America
4351 Garden City Dr.
Landover, Maryland 20785

Federation of the Handicapped, Inc.
211 W. 14th St.
New York, New York 10011

Foundation for Children with Learning
Disabilities
PO Box LD 2929
Grand Central Station
New York, New York 10016

Information Center for Individuals with
Disabilities
20 Park Plaza, Room 330
Boston, Massachusetts 02116

Joseph P. Kennedy, Jr. Foundation
1701 K St., NW, Suite 205
Washington, D.C. 20006

Muscular Dystrophy Associations of America, Inc.
810 7th Av.
New York, New York 10019

Myasthenia Gravis Foundation, Inc.
230 Park Av.
New York, New York 10017

National Amputation Foundation
12-45 150th St.
Whitestone, New York 11357

National Association of the Deaf
814 Thayer Av.
Silver Spring, Maryland 20910

National Association of Developmental
Disabilities Council
1234 Massachusetts Av., NW
Suite 203
Washington, D.C. 20005

National Association for Retarded Citizens
2709 Avenue E, East
Arlington, Texas 76011

National Association for the Deaf
814 Thayer Av.
Silver Spring, Maryland 20910

National Association of the Physically
Handicapped, Inc.
6473 Grandville Av.
Detroit, Michigan 48228

National Congress of Organizations for the
Physically Handicapped, Inc.
1627 Deborah Av.
Rockford, Illinois 61103

National Council on Rehabilitation
1790 Broadway
New York, New York 10019

National Council on Senior Citizens
925 15th St., SW
Washington, D.C. 20005

National Easter Seal Society for Crippled
Children and Adults
2023 West Ogden Av.
Chicago, Illinois 60612

National Federation of the Blind
218 Randolph Hotel Building
Des Moines, Iowa 50309

National Foundation For the Blind
800 2nd Av.
New York, New York 10017

National Foundation for Neuromuscular Diseases
250 West 57th St.
New York, New York 10019

National Genetics Foundation, Inc.
250 W. 5th St.
New York, New York 10019

National Head Injury Foundation
280 Singletary Lane
Framingham, Massachusetts 01701

National Hemophilia Foundation
110 Green St., Room 406
New York, New York 10012

National Hospice Organization
1901 North Fort Myer Dr., Suite 902
Arlington, Virginia 22209

National Information Center on Deafness
Gallaudet College
Kendall Green
Washington, D.C. 20002

National Institute for Advanced Study in
Teaching Disadvantaged Youths.
Room 112, 1126 16th St., NW
Washington, D.C. 20036

National Institute of Senior Centers
c/o National Council on the Aging
600 Maryland Av., SW
Washington, D.C. 20024

National Kidney Foundation
2 Park Av.
New York, New York 10016

National Mental Health Association
1021 Prince St.
Arlington, Virginia 22314

National Multiple Sclerosis Society
205 E. 42nd St.
New York, New York 10017

National Paraplegia Foundation
333 North Michigan Av.
Chicago, Illinois 60601

National Rehabilitation Information Center
(NARIC)
Catholic University of America
4407 8th St., NE
Washington, D.C. 20064

National Society for the Prevention of
Blindness, Inc.
79 Madison Av.
New York, New York 10016

Orton Dyslexia Society
724 York Rd.
Baltimore, Maryland 21204

Self Help for Hard of Hearing People, Inc.
PO Box 34889
Washington, D.C. 20034

Society for the Rehabilitation of the Facially
Disfigured, Inc.
550 1st Av.
New York, New York 10016

United Cerebral Palsy Association
66 E. 34th St.
New York, New York 10016

*RECREATION AND COMPETITIVE SPORTS**

INFORMATION CENTERS AND CLEARINGHOUSES

Accent on Information
PO Box 700
Gillum Rd. and High Dr.
Bloomington, Illinois 61701

American Athletic Association of the Deaf
3916 Lantern Dr.
Silver Spring, Maryland 20902

American Camping Association
Bradford Woods
Martinsville, Indiana 46151

International Committee of the Silent Sports
Gallaudet College
Florida Avenue and 7th St., NE
Washington, D.C. 20002

Indoor Sports Club
1145 Highland St.
Napoleon, Ohio 43545

National Arts and the Handicapped
Information Service
Arts and Special Constituencies Project
National Endowment for the Arts
2401 E St., NW
Washington, D.C. 20506

National Association of Sports for Cerebral Palsy
United Cerebral Palsy Association, Inc.
66 E 34th St.
New York, New York 10016

National Committee/Arts for the Handicapped
1701 K St., NW, Ste. 801
Washington, D.C. 20006

National Handicapped Sports and Recreation
Association
4105 E. Florida Av., 3rd Floor
Denver, Colorado 80222

National Inconvenienced Sportsmen's Association
3738 Walnut Av.
Carmichael, California 95608

National Park Service
Division of Federal and State Liaison
Department of the Interior
Washington, D.C. 20240

National Wheelchair Athletic Association
40-24 62nd St.
Woodside, New York 11377

Outdoor Recreation Technical Assistance
Clearinghouse
Heritage Conservation and Recreation Service
Department of the Interior
Washington, D.C. 20240

President's Council on Physical Fitness and Sports
400 6th St., SW
Washington, D.C. 20201

Special Olympics, Inc.
1701 K St., NW
Washington, D.C. 20006

*For a publication which considers a variety of topics
from career information for the handicapped, to
sources of legal information for the handicapped, to rehabilitation facilities, to sports and game organizations
for the handicapped, see Judith Norback, ed. *Source-
book of Aid for the Mentally and Physically Handicapped*
(New York: Van Nostrand Reinhold Co., 1983).

ACTIVITIES

Baseball

National Beep Ball Association
730 Hennepin Av., Ste. 301
Minneapolis, Minnesota 55403

Basketball

National Wheelchair Basketball Association
c/o Stan Labanowich
110 Seaton Bldg.
University of Kentucky
Lexington, Kentucky 40506

Biking

Western Electric Co., Hawthorne Works
Medical Engineering Division
Cicero and Cermak Rd.
Chicago, Illinois 60650
(Manufactures a "cricket" mechanism [battery powered], which emits a series of sounds enabling a blind person to follow a sighted companion on a bike. Designed for long-distance rides.)

The Funway Co.
15940 Warwick Rd.
Detroit, Michigan 48223

Bowling

National Association of Sports for Cerebral Palsy
United Cerebral Palsy Association of Connecticut
c/o Craig Huber
1 State St.
New Haven, Connecticut 06511

American Wheelchair Bowling Association
c/o Don Pinault
2424 N. Federal Hwy., Ste. 109
Boynton Beach, Florida 33435

American Blind Bowling Association
150 N. Bellaire Av.
Louisville, Kentucky 40206
(Publishes an instruction brochure for sighted instructors, a bowling lesson manual in braille, and a quarterly periodical, *The Blind Bowler*, in print, braille, and cassette.)

Cycling

Wheelchair Motorcycle Association
101 Torrey St.
Brockton, Massachusetts 02401

Flying

American Wheelchair Pilots Association
c/o John Green
3953 W. Evans Dr.
Phoenix, Arizona 85023

Handicapped Flyers International
1117 Rising Hill
Escondido, California 92025

Golf

National Amputee Golf Association
St. Joseph's Hospital
11705 Mercy Blvd.
Savannah, Georgia 31406

U.S. Blind Golfer's Association
c/o Patrick Browne
225 Varonne St., 28th Floor
New Orleans, Louisiana 70112

Riding

Cheff Center for the Handicapped
c/o Lida L. McCowan
Augusta, Michigan 49012

National Foundation for Happy Horsemanship for the Handicapped
Box 462
Malvern, Pennsylvania 19355

North American Riding for the Handicapped Association
c/o Diana Seacord
Thistlecroft, Park St.
Mendon, Massachusetts 01756

Skiing

BOLD, Inc.
Blind Outdoor Leisure Development
533 E. Main St.
Aspen, Colorado 81611
(Teaches blind children and adults to ski at centers throughout the United States.)

National Amputee Skiing Association
3738 Walnut Avenue
Carmichael, California 95608

National Handicapped Sports and Recreation Association
4105 E. Florida Av., 3rd Floor
Denver, Colorado 80222

Winter Park Handicapped Skier Program
Winter Park Recreational Association
PO Box 36
Winter Park, Colorado 80482

New England Handicapped Sportsmen's Association
PO Box 2150
Boston, Massachusetts 02106

Ski for Light, Inc.
1455 W. Lake St.
Minneapolis, Minnesota 55408

Softball

National Wheelchair Softball Association
c/o Dave Van Buskirk
PO Box 737
Sioux Falls, South Dakota 57101

Track

National Track and Field Committee for the Visually
Impaired
4244 Heather Rd.
Long Beach, California 90808

Other

Handicapped Artists of America, Inc.
8 Sany Lane
Salisbury, Massachusetts 01950

PUBLICATIONS

DIRECTORIES

American Annals of the Deaf
814 Thayer Av.
Silver Spring, Maryland 20910
Published: Monthly; April issue includes Directory
        Programs and services for the deaf

*Directory of Agencies Serving the Visually
Handicapped*
American Foundation for the Blind
15 W. 16th St.
New York, New York 10011
Published: Biannually

*Guide to Federal Benefits and Programs for
Handicapped Citizens and Their Families*
Association for Retarded Citizens
National Governmental Affairs Office
1522 K St., Ste. 516
Washington, D.C. 20005

JOURNALS, MAGAZINES, AND NEWSLETTERS

The following list of publications was assembled
to give the instructor and the student an idea of
the extensive body of literature that concerns
itself with rehabilitation. This list does not pre-
tend to be exhaustive. Further, a majority of these
periodicals have published articles on recreation
and therapeutic recreation in the rehabilitation
process.

Adapted Physical Activity Quarterly
Aging
American Archives of Rehabilitation Therapy
American Corrective Therapy Journal
American Journal of Art Therapy
American Journal of Corrections

American Journal of Mental Deficiency
American Journal of Nursing
American Journal of Occupational Therapy
American Journal of Orthopsychiatry
American Journal of Psychiatry
American Journal of Psychology
American Journal of Public Health
American Journal of Sociology
Behavior Research and Therapy
Camping Magazine
Children Today
Community Mental Health Journal
Exceptional Children
Federal Probation
Geriatrics
Hospital and Community Psychiatry
Hospitals
International Rehabilitation Review
Journal of Applied Rehabilitation Counseling
Journal of Counseling Psychology
*Journal of Criminal Law, Criminology and Police
Science*
Journal of Gerontology
Journal of Health and Social Behavior
*Journal of Physical Education, Recreation, and
Dance*
Journal of Learning Disabilities
Journal of Leisure Research
Journal of Rehabilitation
Leisurability
Leisure Today
Mental Hygiene
Mental Retardation Abstracts
Mental Retardation News
MR/Mental Retardation
NAPH Newsletter (National Association of

Physically Handicapped)
NAPT Journal
New Outlook for the Blind
Nursing Outlook
Palaestre
Parks and Recreation
Pathfinder, The (National Rehabilitation Information Center)
Performance
Physical Therapy
Programs for the Handicapped
Prison Journal

Psychological Abstracts
Rehabilitation Literature
Rehabilitation Record
Scene (Braille Institute of America, Inc.)
Social Work
Sports 'N Spokes
Talking Book Topics
Therapeutic Recreation Journal
Today's Health
Update (National Library Services for the Blind and Physically Handicapped)

FOUNDATIONS

The following foundations are involved with the handicapped in some manner. More specific information can be obtained by writing each individual foundation. This is not an exhaustive list.

Alexander Graham Bell Association for the Deaf
3417 Volta Pl., NW
Washington, D.C. 20007

This association awards a variety of scholarships through various internal award committees as follows: The Lucile A. Abt Meritorious Award, The Lucile A. Abt Scholarship Award, The Monticello College Foundation Scholarship Award, The Oral Deaf Adults Section Scholarship Award, The Volta Meritorious Award, and The Volta Scholarship Award.

Edyth Bush Charitable Foundation, Inc.
650 Barnett Bank Bldg.
PO Box 1967
Winter Park, Florida 32790

George Harrington Trust
c/o Boston Safe Deposit and Trust Co.
1 Boston Pl.
Boston, Massachusetts 02106

Gross (Stella B.) Charitable Trust
c/o Bank of the West
PO Box 1121
San Jose, California 95108

The Jacob and Annita France Foundation, Inc.
6301 N. Charles St.
Baltimore, Maryland 21212

John W. Anderson Foundation
2402 Cumberland Dr.
Valparaiso, Indiana 46383

Lowe Foundation
c/o Luis D. Rovira
State Judicial Bldg.
2 East 14th Av.
Denver, Colorado 80203

McGraw Foundation
PO Box 578
Palatine, Illinois 60067

UOP Foundation
Ten UOP Plaza
Des Plaines, Illinois 60016

Wahlstrom Foundation, Inc.
2429 Post Rd.
Southport, Connecticut 06490

Index

Name Index

Menninger, W. C., 3, 90
Meuli, A. J., 340
Meyer, L. E., 316, 341
Meyer, M. W., 340
Meyerson, L., 12
Mobily, K. E., 113, 317
Moore, W. E., 116
Morgan, C. W., 340
Morgan, J., 87
Mosey, A. C., 244
Mosher, R., 274
Moss, S. L., 140
Musgrove, D. G., 144

Navar, N., 342
Nesbitt, J., 157, 341
Nichols, W., 340
Nugent, T., 342

O'Morrow, G. S., 119, 340, 341
Ortom, D. J., 103
Ovans, P. M., 273

Paré, A., 86
Park, D. C., 94, 341
Parker, R., 342
Pavlov, I. P., 90
Peters, M., 119, 131, 132, 143
Peterson, C. A., 119, 131, 132, 316, 341, 342
Phillips, B. E., 111, 119
Pinel, P., 87
Pomeroy, J., 342
Porch, B. E., 181
Pratt, J. F., 340
Priest, E. L., 275

Randall, M., 340
Rathbone, F., 15
Rathbone, J. L., 119
Rawson, H. E., 276
Reagan, R., 227
Reynolds, R. P., 103, 202, 288
Rickman, T. H., Jr., 340
Ridgway, R. F. L., 90
Roan, J., 340
Robb, G. M., 112, 113, 119, 184, 341, 342
Ross, C. D., 303
Rousseau, A., 87
Rubin, R., 176
Rudquist, B. J., 340
Rusalem, 114
Rush, B., 88, 97
Rusk, H. A., 180, 342

Salk, S. K., 15
Schlotter, B. E., 90, 123
Schnorr, J. M., 272
Seabolt, S., 341, 342
Semmons, O. G., 231
Sessoms, H. D., 119
Shank, J. W., 342
Sheley, J. F., 42, 69
Shivers, J. S., 119, 342
Sirvis, B., 342
Smith, D. A., 262
Smith, R. W., 113, 119, 285
Smith, W. L., 341
Soulek, M., 13
Spinak, J., 300
Stanley, J., 286, 295, 303
Stein, T. A., 119
Stensrud, C., 279, 300
Stewart, M. W., 119
Stoudenmire, J., 276

Stracke, R. L., 341
Summers, L., 340
Supina, E., 342
Svendsen, M., 90, 123
Sylvester, C. D., 113, 317

Taaffee, D., 340
Tague, J. R., 341, 342
Taulbee, L., 199
Teaff, J. D., 154
Teeters, N. K., 101
Thompson, G., 300
Thompson, G., 302
Thompson, M., 340
Thorn, B., 321, 341
Tillick, P., 15
Timmins, L., 342
Tissot, C., 89
Touchstone, W. A., 186
Tubbs, H. R., 140
Turpel, L., 342

Van Andel, G. E., 113, 119, 184
Vaughan, J., 341, 342

Walker, H., 341
Walsh, P., 341
Washington, Y., 341
Watson, J. B., 90
West, R. E., 152, 321, 341, 342
Wickenden, W., 115, 116
Williams, L. R., 103
Wilson, J., 342
Wilson, W., 22
Winston, C., 22
Witman, J., 276
Witt, P. A., 288, 298
Wolfensberger, W., 114
Wurster, M., 342

Zilboorg, H., 88

Subject Index